Brain Asymmetry and Neural Systems: Clinical Neuroscience

Brain Asymmetry and Neural Systems: Clinical Neuroscience

Editor: Margaret Ramon

AMERICAN
MEDICAL PUBLISHERS
www.americanmedicalpublishers.com

AMERICAN
MEDICAL PUBLISHERS
www.americanmedicalpublishers.com

Cataloging-in-Publication Data

Brain asymmetry and neural systems : clinical neuroscience / edited by Margaret Ramon.
p. cm.
Includes bibliographical references and index.
ISBN 978-1-63927-605-9
1. Cerebral dominance. 2. Neural circuitry. 3. Nervous system. 4. Neurosciences.
5. Clinical neuropsychology. 6. Neurophysiology. I. Ramon, Margaret.
QP385.5 .B73 2023
612.825--dc23

American Medical Publishers,
41 Flatbush Avenue,
1st Floor, New York,
NY 11217, USA

ISBN 978-1-63927-605-9 (Hardback)

Contents

Preface

Clinical neuroscience refers to a subfield of neuroscience which focuses on the scientific study of fundamental mechanisms that underly disorders and diseases of the central nervous system and brain. It aims to develop new methods of conceptualizing and diagnosing such disorders and developing new therapies. The human nervous system is divided into two symmetric halves, but a closer examination of the brain reveals functional and anatomical lateralization. Brain asymmetry is detected in terms of behavior, structure and function. Experiential, evolutionary, genetic, developmental and pathological factors are hypothesized to have a role in this lateralization. Defects in brain asymmetry are linked to a variety of neurological disorders, and certain disorders exacerbate the brain asymmetries. Various disorders related with brain asymmetries include schizophrenia and dyslexia. This book explores all the important aspects of brain aging in the present day scenario. Those with an interest in this field would find it helpful.

This book has been the outcome of endless efforts put in by authors and researchers on various issues and topics within the field. The book is a comprehensive collection of significant researches that are addressed in a variety of chapters. It will surely enhance the knowledge of the field among readers across the globe.

It gives us an immense pleasure to thank our researchers and authors for their efforts to submit their piece of writing before the deadlines. Finally in the end, I would like to thank my family and colleagues who have been a great source of inspiration and support.

Editor

1

The Brain's Asymmetric Frequency Tuning: Asymmetric Behavior Originates from Asymmetric Perception

Arianna Felisatti [1,*], David Aagten-Murphy [1,2], Jochen Laubrock [1,3], Samuel Shaki [4] and Martin H. Fischer [1]

1 Department of Psychology, University of Potsdam, Karl-Liebknecht-Strasse 24-25 House 14, D-14476 Potsdam OT Golm, Germany; murphy@neuraltrain.de (D.A.-M.); jochen.laubrock@mhb-fontane.de (J.L.); martinf@uni-potsdam.de (M.H.F.)
2 Neuraltrain GmbH, Friedrichstr. 68, 10117 Berlin, Germany
3 Department of Psychology, Brandenburg Medical School Theodor Fontane Fehrbelliner Straße 38, 16816 Neuruppin, Germany
4 Department of Behavioral Sciences and Psychology, Ariel University, Ariel 40700, Israel; samuel_shaki@hotmail.com
* Correspondence: ariannafelisatti@uni-potsdam.de

Abstract: To construct a coherent multi-modal percept, vertebrate brains extract low-level features (such as spatial and temporal frequencies) from incoming sensory signals. However, because frequency processing is lateralized with the right hemisphere favouring low frequencies while the left favours higher frequencies, this introduces asymmetries between the hemispheres. Here, we describe how this lateralization shapes the development of several cognitive domains, ranging from visuo-spatial and numerical cognition to language, social cognition, and even aesthetic appreciation, and leads to the emergence of asymmetries in behaviour. We discuss the neuropsychological and educational implications of these emergent asymmetries and suggest future research approaches.

Keywords: asymmetry; global/local; spatial frequencies; temporal frequencies; embodied cognition

---

1. Introduction

> *"The universe is asymmetric and I am persuaded that life, as it is known to us, is a direct result of the asymmetry of the universe or of its indirect consequences."*
>
> —Louis Pasteur

Decades of research have revealed that our symmetrical anatomical arrangement of body, eyes, and brain obscures many surprising asymmetries in how our bodies sample the external world and later act upon it. In this review, we aim to address how sensory asymmetries interact with and drive functional changes and—in turn—influence and shape our behaviours, preferences, and even our cultural norms. We begin by describing behavioral, neuropsychological, neuroimaging, and comparative evidence for behavioral asymmetries that result from competition between global and local visual processing. Then, we describe models of processing asymmetries that aim to account for these findings. Based upon these reported results, we then introduce a new theoretical model to account for how brain functional lateralization, spatial frequency tuning, and object location in the external world relative to the observer interact to generate asymmetrical actions. This model is subsequently applied to higher-level cognitive asymmetries to illustrate its broader viability and explanatory power. We end our review by listing a few implications and outstanding questions.

2. Global vs. Local Perception

A growing number of studies suggest that perceptual and behavioral asymmetries originate from hemispheric lateralization. The left hemisphere is more efficient in the selection of fine detail, while the right hemisphere is predominant in the selection of coarse elements [1–3]. Due to the cross-over of the optic fibres, each visual hemi-field projects to the contralateral brain hemisphere. Here, we will specifically review studies on visuo-spatial processing to explain how this organization shapes the development of several cognitive domains.

We begin our review by reminding readers of a seminal behavioral study conducted by Navon (1977) [4]. He presented artificially created hierarchical stimuli in the centre of participants' visual field (see Figure 1, central panel). The stimuli were letter-shaped figures made from many smaller letters, and participants had to respond either to the global or the local letter information with assigned button responses. Importantly, global and local letters could be either response-incongruent or response-congruent (without necessarily being identical). Navon (1977) [4] reported an overall processing speed advantage for the global level, and asymmetrical interference, which was stronger from the global to the local level than in the reverse direction. Together, these findings suggested a coarse-to-fine visual processing sequence. An aspect of the stimuli influencing the salience of the global/local level is the low-pass/high-pass filter. The low-pass filtered images (see Figure 1, left panel) retain the unifying big global structure while removing the numerous little details. On the contrary, high-pass filtered images (see Figure 1, right panel) retain the numerous little details while removing the unifying big global structure. Since this seminal work, there have been numerous behavioural, neuropsychological, neuroimaging, and comparative studies of these "global precedence" and "global/local interference" effects. We review this research here selectively to illustrate the current understanding of visual processing asymmetries.

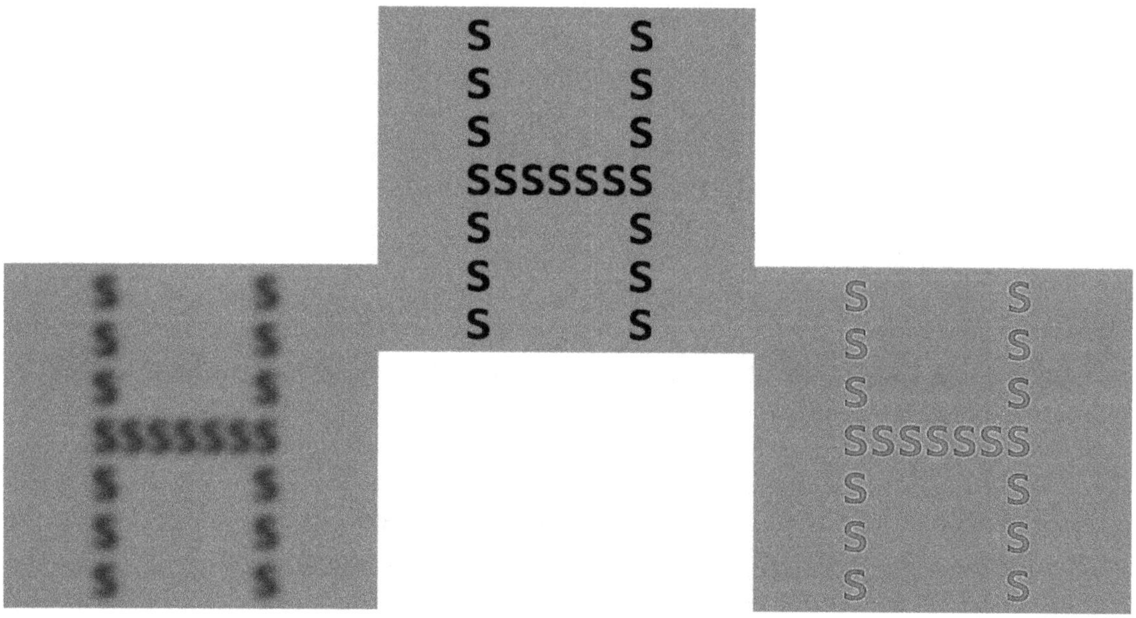

Figure 1. Example of hierarchical stimulus before and after a low-pass/high-pass filter. Central panel: example of hierarchical stimulus with letter "H" at the global level and letter "S" at the local level. Left panel: low-pass filtered stimulus. Right panel: high-pass filtered stimulus.

2.1. Behavioral Evidence

In addition to the Navon task, there are multiple other sources of behavioural evidence for hemispheric lateralization for global/local processing. Neural development is associated with progressive maturation of the *corpus callosum*, which is a bundle of fibres supporting inter-hemispheric communication. Investigation of hemispheric asymmetries in healthy populations relies on the use of lateralized stimulus presentation by means of hemi-field paradigms (consider Reference [5] for meta-analysis and Reference [6] for methodological considerations). Global stimuli are better perceived when briefly shown on the left side of the fixation point. However, local stimuli are better perceived when briefly displayed on the right side of the fixation point [7–11]. In addition, handedness, which is related to hemispheric asymmetry, influences local/global processing. In everyday life, we use our dominant hand to deal with fine-scale and uni-manual tasks [12]. By testing right-handers, Stanković and Nešić (2018) [13] reported how contraction of the right hand, activating the left hemisphere, correlated with enhanced attention for local stimuli.

Hemispheric specialization for holistic and analytic processing has been considered related to functional lateralization for words and faces. While word recognition recruits the visual word form area, usually confined to the left hemisphere, face recognition recruits the visual face form area, typically found in the right hemisphere (consult Reference [14] for a review). Behavioral experiments using visual half-field tasks showed a right visual field advantage during lexical decision and a left visual field advantage in judging similarities of faces [15]. According to the most influential account, known as *input asymmetry principle*, the hemispheric predominance for high-level processes is motivated by the types of information required at lower levels [16]. Recently, Brederoo and colleagues (2020) [17] provided evidence to this account reporting correlation between local features and word processing on the left hemisphere, and between global form and face processing on the right hemisphere. Even within the domain of language, holistic processing results in the right visual field advantage as a consequence of left hemisphere involvement [18]. Even if the pattern of right/left predominance for global/holistic processing seems to be stable at the population level, introduction of factors such as handedness and hemispheric dominance for language are linked to completely mirrored or atypical patterns [19–22]. Whatever the direction of the lateralization, its strength is associated with cognitive performances and, as a consequence, with evolutionary advantages [22].

Another example for behavioral asymmetries is pseudo-neglect in bisection tasks. Healthy adults have a tendency to mark the perceived center of visually presented lines to the left of their true center [23]. While this bias is generally interpreted as evidence for an attentional asymmetry, cognitive and motoric factors may also contribute. Depending on the nature of the visual stimulus, higher-level processes may be assessed with the bisection task [24]. For example, when healthy adults mark the midpoints of visually perceived long words, their marks are too close to the beginning of the letter string. This bias is larger than expected from pseudo-neglect and possibly reflects attentional scaling as part of lexical access processes [25–27]. When the stimulus is a long string of digits, its perceived center depends on digit magnitude with a left bias for smaller numbers and a right bias for larger digits, as well as a tendency to bisect plain horizontal lines toward the larger of two different flanker digits [28]. Moreover, the habitual reading direction [29–31] and recent spatial experience [32] are known to influence visuospatial biases in bisection or exploration tasks. For example, the tendency to start reading on the left side of a page in Western cultures seems to induce an anchoring effect for the subsequent bisection judgments with lines and words but not with geometric figures [29]. Relatedly, McManus, Edmondson, and Rodger (1985) [33] evaluated the perceived balance in compositions of abstract shapes. They found that participants marked the balance point of an artistic image slightly to the left of center but that there was considerable inter-individual variability. We will return to aesthetic asymmetries below.

2.2. Neuropsychological Evidence

Consider the evidence from neuropsychology in support of hemispheric lateralization for global/local processing. People with occipital, temporal, or parietal brain damage but intact primary visual functions report dissociable performance, depending on the lateralization of their damage (Reference [34] for review). In the bisection task described above, neurologically damaged patients mark the perceived midpoints of horizontally extended plain lines ipsilesional [35–37]. Thus, they seem to ignore the spatial extent of the stimulus into their contralesional visual field.

Left-side and right-side brain-damaged patients also show difficulties in detecting detail and coarse elements, respectively [38,39]. The corpus callosum plays a crucial role. It supports inter-hemispheric communication but also enhances inter-hemispheric interference between representations [40,41]. Interference between global and local processing, which is present in healthy subjects, disappears in patients with a cut corpus callosum [42]. A lesion in the posterior part of the corpus callosum results in selective copying of global elements when using the left hand (controlled by the right hemisphere), and in selective copying of local details when employing the right hand (controlled by the left hemisphere, [43]). The higher number of callosal fibres projecting from the right to the left cortex rather than vice versa seems to be the anatomical expression of asymmetric inhibitory control between the two brain hemispheres [44,45]. We will return to this asymmetry below.

There are other domains of lateralized visual processing, which we briefly mention. First, *apperceptive agnosia*, the inability to identify unique exemplars of an object under varying illumination or angles of observation or to copy an object, and *prosopagnosia*, the inability to recognize familiar faces, are usually associated with bilateral or right unilateral occipito-temporal lesions [46,47]. Secondly, *visual associative agnosia*, the ability to see and even copy an object without appreciating its meaning, as well as *pure alexia*, the inability to read printed words in the absence of object and face recognition deficits, and with, otherwise, intact language processing, appear to be associated with bilateral or left unilateral occipito-temporal lesions [48]. The N170 EEG potential that reflects the early categorization of faces, familiar objects, or words is right-lateralized for faces, bilateral for objects, and left-lateralized for word-like stimuli.

2.3. Neuroimaging Evidence

Hemispheric lateralization of global/local processing is further supported by neuroimaging studies. Low-pass filtered images, which retain global structure while removing detail, more strongly engage the right cortical hemisphere, whereas high-pass filtered images, which retain detail while removing global structure, more strongly engage the left cortical hemisphere ([49], see Reference [3] for review). As mentioned in the paragraph on behavioral evidence, even the hemispheric specialization for face and language processing, has been shown to reflect asymmetric processing of low-level properties rather than category-specific knowledge. Left and right occipito-temporal cortical areas are more strongly activated by sine-wave gratings that are frequency-matched to word and face images, respectively [50]. The well-established left hemispheric preference for language, or, more generally, for conspecific communication observed across mammalian species [51,52], and also the right-hemispheric preference for visuo-spatial processing [53], may both build on this early specialization to which we will return in greater detail below.

2.4. Comparative Evidence

Lastly, consider the evidence from comparative psychology in support of lateralized global/local processing. Brain lateralization is not a peculiarity of the human brain. All vertebrates have lateralized brains, birds included [51,54]. In daily routines, not only mammals but also birds, amphibians, and fish show biases in two activities that are essential for survival [55]. Feeding is associated with rightward behavior, driven by the left hemisphere [56–58]. Conversely, avoidance of predators and identification of conspecifics are associated with leftward behavior, controlled by the right hemisphere [59–61]. Sovrano (2004) [62] noticed that fish prefer using the left-eye monocular field with familiar stimuli and the right-eye monocular field with unfamiliar stimuli, suggesting right/left hemisphere superiority in discriminating global/local aspects of the visual input, respectively.

The origin of these many perceptual, cognitive, and motoric biases can be found in the fundamental features of a perceptual system driven by global/local processing mechanisms. A left-hemisphere predominance in discrimination between targets that are similar in local features (grains vs. grit), distinguishable through detailed comparison, and a right-hemisphere superiority in discrimination based on larger changes (e.g., predators vs. conspecifics, [63,64]), which is distinguishable through a coarse comparison. Thus, a wide range of non-human species shows functional asymmetries resembling those present in humans with the right and left hemisphere specialized for holistic and analytic processing, respectively. Hemispheric functional asymmetry is supported by an evolutionary explanation since it is present in all vertebrates and entails important advantages: (1) Increase of neural capacity, (2) avoidance of useless duplication of functions, and (3) possibility to execute more tasks simultaneously without interference [64–67].

3. Global/Local Processing and Spatial Frequencies

Every visual percept consists of a hierarchical structure with local elements embedded within global ones ([4], see Reference [2], for a review and Reference [68], for recent meta-analysis). For instance, a forest is made up of many trees, a flock is made up of many sheep, and a word is made up of many letters. As a result, local and global image components can be conveyed by different ranges of *spatial frequencies* (SFs), [1,69–72]. SF is a measure of how often a sine wave pattern of light intensity repeats per unit of distance across the visual field. Much like complex sounds can be constructed from the superposition of simple periodic waves of *temporal frequencies* (TFs), complex visual stimuli can be thought of as being composed of different spatial frequencies with various orientations and phases. Perceptual systems solve the inverse task known as decomposition. The hierarchical composition of natural stimuli is heavily exploited by convolutional neural networks, which is the currently most successful "artificial intelligence" object detection models [73,74]. These are explicitly motivated by hierarchical processing in human object perception and closely correspond to the feed-forward pass in the human ventral stream [75].

It is well known that complex sounds can be decomposed by Fourier transform into their frequency spectra, which is a task approximated by the cochlea and primary auditory cortex (A1). Similarly, complex visual stimuli can be decomposed into their underlying spatial frequency spectra that contains information about the energy or power of the individual frequencies. Simple cells in early visual cortex seems (V1) can be conceptualized as spatial frequency analyzers. In any visual scene, coarse shapes represent few dark-light oscillations across space (Low SF range, LSFs, see Figure 1, left panel), while fine details correspond to many dark-light cycles per unit of space (High SF range, HSFs, see Figure 1, right panel). Spatial frequencies are some of the lowest-level visual features used in perception, providing the basis for processes such as edge detection or texture discrimination. In visual processing, the identification of a stimulus is made possible by re-integration of different SFs, resulting in a characteristic power spectrum, and other higher-order combinations of simple features.

LSFs are preferentially conveyed by the fast-transmitting *magnocellular* visual channels and activate the anterior half of the calcarine fissures, linked to the peripheral visual field, while HSFs are conveyed by slower-transmitting *parvocellular* visual channels and activate the posterior part of the occipital lobe, linked to foveal vision. The processing speed difference between magnocellular and parvocellular streams amounts to 10 ms in typically developing adults but can be as large as 40 ms ([76], cited in Reference [77]). In line with models of visual recognition [78–80], the well-established coarse-to-fine processing sequence [81] is explained by faster access of the LSFs to higher-order visual areas in the brain's *dorsal* stream. These areas can, in turn, modulate the subsequent processing of the HSFs, which are transmitted more slowly to the brain's *ventral* stream.

It is generally accepted that two broad visual streams process information relatively independently. The dorsal stream is concerned with vision for action and the ventral stream is concerned with vision for perception [82]. The dorsal stream is linked to motion processing and visuo-spatial transformation, which is preferably signaled by magnocellular cells and mainly relies on fast processing of low spatial frequencies across the visual field. The function of the ventral stream is linked to processing of color and form, texture, and general object perception, and preferably draws on parvocellular cells, foveal processing, and high spatial frequencies. The division of the visual field into a high acuity fovea driving ventral stream analysis of object details and a low acuity periphery specialized in signaling scene gist [83] and transients for dorsal stream processing has likely evolved to optimize bandwidth and energy, and is the main reason for overt attention expressed by eye movements [84]. Peripheral vision selects objects of interest as saccade targets for close inspection by foveal vision. Peripheral selection and foveal inspection occur in parallel, but selection is usually faster than inspection [85].

However, only a few studies have linked the two visual streams to hemispheric asymmetries. Notably, Stevens et al. (2012) [86] discuss a general pattern of right/left asymmetry of form-specific versus form-abstract visual processing, and demonstrate that the left para-hippocampal place area is relatively more involved in form-abstract conceptual/semantic processing of complex visual scenes, while the right para-hippocampal place area is involved in relatively more form-specific perceptual processing. With respect to the function of the dorsal stream, Pisella et al. (2011) [87] reported a right-hemispheric dominance for visual remapping–important for saccade programming, and Sheremata et al. (2010) [88] found that only the right posterior parietal cortex codes visual short-term memory load independent of the visual stimulus, which is consistent with the finding that hemi-spatial neglect, a deficit in contra-lesional attentional processing, which typically involves damage to right-hemisphere parieto-temporal lobes. Stephan et al. (2007) [89] provide neurophysiological evidence for asymmetric information transfer and hemispheric recruitment in ventral and dorsal streams, respectively, during induced task-driven lateralization. Despite these findings, clearly plenty remains to be explored. Taken together, there appears to be some evidence that visuo-spatial cognitive processes primarily drawing on LSF information are right-lateralized, whereas processes related to object semantics and language, primarily relying on HSF information, are left-lateralized.

The complementary processes of frequency analysis and re-integration constitute a multi-modal working principle of the brain. The brain is lateralized not only for spatial but also for temporal frequencies [90–92] since birth [93]. The left brain hemisphere is predominant in extrapolating relatively fine signals and from short time windows (high TFs) while the right brain hemisphere is superior in processing relatively coarse signals and from long time windows (low TFs). Consistent insight for this specialization comes from developmental neuropsychology and, in particular, from *Autism Spectrum Disorder*. People with autism tend to report a co-morbidity that consists of atypical perception in the visual and in the auditory domains with enhanced ability to process local features [94–96].

3.1. Hemispheric Lateralization for SF Processing and Previous Models

Given that global and local processing are associated with a preference for LSF and HSF, respectively, and with the perceptual and behavioral asymmetries we discussed in part 1, it follows that there should also be asymmetries for SF processing. Although the data are consistent with functional asymmetries for SF processing (see Reference [3] for review), current models are inconsistent about the mechanism underlying this hemispheric tuning. Before describing these models, it is important to clarify the experimental tasks in which lateralization emerges. The interactions between hemispheric engagement and SF bands were found in activities characterized by high cognitive demand (e.g., identification, recognition, and copying). Instead, when the tasks had almost exclusively perceptual characteristics (e.g., contrast sensitivity tests, detection, sensory summation), the hemispheres showed comparable SF tuning [97]. More involvement of the right hemisphere is registered only under high perceptual uncertainty (e.g., perceptually degraded stimuli, see Reference [98] for a review). This implies that SF channels in V1 are symmetric and that processing differences originate beyond the early perceptual level.

Several important, and inter-related, theories regarding the organization of our perceptual processing have emerged in recent decades that considerably reframed older arguments such as those from classical Gestalt psychology. While these modern accounts heavily intersect, they predominantly focus on different ideas about functional lateralization, SF processing biases between the hemispheres, and the emergence of conscious perception. The models we review include Sergent's model [1], the Dual Filtering by Frequency hypothesis (DFF, [90,99], the reverse hierarchy theory of perceptual learning (RHT, [100–102], and the coarse-to-fine processing hypothesis (CTF, [103]).

3.1.1. Sergent's Model

Sergent (1982) [1] postulated that hemispheric sensitivity to different SF bands is symmetric during early stages of processing, becoming asymmetric during later stages. When performance requires higher cognitive effort, the right hemisphere deals more efficiently with LSF content conveyed through the fast magnocellular stream. On the other side, the left hemisphere becomes predominant in processing HSF content, made available later, through the slow parvocellular pathway.

3.1.2. Dual Filtering by Frequency (DFF)

The observation that hemispheric asymmetries for SF processing depend on the relative and not absolute SF ranges led Robertson and Ivry [90] (see Reference [99]) to advance the DFF hypothesis. In contrast with Sergent's (1982) [1] original theory, DFF states that even high-cognitive tasks are characterized by a first stage in which SFs processing is symmetric in the brain. In the first stage, low-level sensory information is sent to both hemispheres so that attention filters the SF range most relevantly for the current activity. Only in the second stage, the right/left hemispheres act as asymmetric filters to emphasize the lower/higher SFs, but relative to the initially selected SF band. The DFF theory postulates the presence of dynamic mechanisms between low-level processing by SF channels and high-level attentional selection of these channels [104]. This is well supported by evidence on flexible preference of the same SFs by the different hemispheres, depending on the reference SF range involved in the stimulus set [105].

3.1.3. Reverse Hierarchy Theory (RHT)

This theory of perceptual learning originally set out to link the rapid capture of conceptual gist —in the absence of access to its constituent features—with the generalization (or lack thereof) of training effects in perceptual learning tasks [101]. In contrast to the anatomical hierarchy, where vision is assembled from simple cells into increasingly complex and broad receptive fields, the Reverse Hierarchy Theory argues that perception proceeds rapidly and implicitly to high-order summaries before cognitive feedback directs attention to the serial processing of relevant detail in the scene. This framework was later expanded to also encompass auditory perception and broadened to cover conscious perception in general. A key component of this theory is the trade-off between convergent activities (linking several diverse, low-level exemplars to the same high-level category) and divergent activities (assigning highly similar, low-level exemplars to distinct high-level categories). Depending on the specific task driving current perception, the categorization may be accurate enough to enable further higher-level processing and decision-making. Alternatively, serial, attention-driven processing of details in the scene may be desirable. When learning how to optimally solve a new perceptual task (i.e., in perceptual learning), both knowing the correct level of detail to process the stimuli and the depth of this level determine generalizability. The more low-level the details required (needing access to earlier stages of the visual hierarchy), the more difficult the learning, the greater the potential gain, but the less any learning generalizes to other perceptual tasks.

3.1.4. Coarse-To-Fine Processing (CTF)

While highly related, the Coarse-to-Fine Processing hypothesis for perception places less emphasis on learning and on the "gist" or high-level representation belonging to a specific category, and, instead, takes a Bayesian approach of gradually refining a representation from coarse to fine. Bayesian approaches encompass both descriptive accounts, discussing how different levels of hierarchy interact, as well as more concrete computational accounts that attempt to lay out an inverted (high-low) competitor to traditional computational accounts of perception (e.g., signal detection theory). For example, the account by Ding and colleagues (2017) [106] examined joint distributions of two judgements (differing in complexity) and found that the best model to describe behaviour reflected visual perception as the retrospective decoding of high-to-low features from visual working memory.

Like in RHT, low-level details are decoded only when required. However, here, the recall of noisy, less-reliably encoded low-level features is explicitly constrained by memory for higher-level features. Generally, many fluctuations in low-level features will be behaviourally irrelevant, and instead reflect inconsequential events like subtle sway in our posture, changes in lighting conditions, or micro saccades. The higher-level stimulus features (e.g., a person's mouth being in a smile) are more relevant, more categorical, and easier to store in working memory than the precise alignment or the precise shade of their right upper lip. Nevertheless, although differing slightly in interpretation, both the Bayesian CTF hypothesis and the RHT emphasize a global representation being perceived first, which is followed by slower, serial processing of details.

3.2. Brain's Asymmetric Frequency Tuning (BAFT) as Generalized Account of a Perceptual Processing

All theoretical models of cortical visual processing sketched above share the assumption that the functional lateralization for SFs processing emerges beyond the sensory level. In other words, both hemispheres are endowed with an equal ability to process all ranges of SFs during early processing stages, but with different efficiency in emphasizing low or high SF information for the creation of a percept that is suitable for the current task. It is reasonable to assume the presence of asymmetric cortical circuits with common components, rather than strictly unilateral components underlying the visual and auditory hemispheric tuning of our brains, especially when we think about its adaptive function for ensuring symmetrical sensory sensitivity and, at the same time, enhancing our capability to perform parallel and distinct computations (see Reference [54] for a review on encoding asymmetry).

It is important to consider that brains are embodied and encode sensory and motor inputs within a body-centred spatial reference frame. According to the recently popular *embodied cognition perspective*, cognition is supported by modal representations that originate from reciprocal exchanges between the organism and the surrounding environment [107–110]. Embracing and developing this view, the recently proposed *brain's asymmetric frequency tuning* model [111] treats lateralization for SF processing as a congenital aspect of the mind that influences learning and cognition through interaction with sensory and motor constraints imposed by the body. Which implications does the functional asymmetry driven by SFs have on cognition? BAFT addresses this question and derives testable predictions. We briefly describe the components of the model before explaining its specific contributions within different cognitive domains.

BAFT relies on three fundamental facts that were already established above: (1) The vertebrate brain spontaneously analyses SF information to create a coherent percept and to inform the distinction between vision for perception and vision for action, (2) SF processing is lateralized with the left and right brain hemispheres predominantly selecting high and low SFs, respectively, (3) due to the cross-over of the optic fibers at the level of the optic chiasm (partial in humans and total in animals with laterally located eyes), information from each hemi-field projects to the contralateral hemisphere that, in turn, drives attentional orienting toward the contralateral space. Figure 2 graphically represents the three components of the BAFT model.

Previous models on brain asymmetries for SFs processing have focused on the mechanism underlying the second assumption. Instead, BAFT integrates this mechanism with the hemispheric control of spatial attention (assumption 3), thus, linking the SF tuning principle to spatial biases in behavior. In addition, BAFT considers functional brain asymmetry for frequency processing to be a universal constraint that interacts with embodied and contextual factors, thus, shaping all levels of knowledge representation (for details of this theoretical framework, see References [112–114]). The structure of the visual system, the asymmetry in SF selection, and the asymmetry of attentional orienting, naturally lead to an optimal representation of fine detail in the right visual field and coarse features in the left visual field. BAFT, incorporating this implication, explains several behavioral consequences of these perceptual asymmetries driven by SFs lateralization in different cognitive domains.

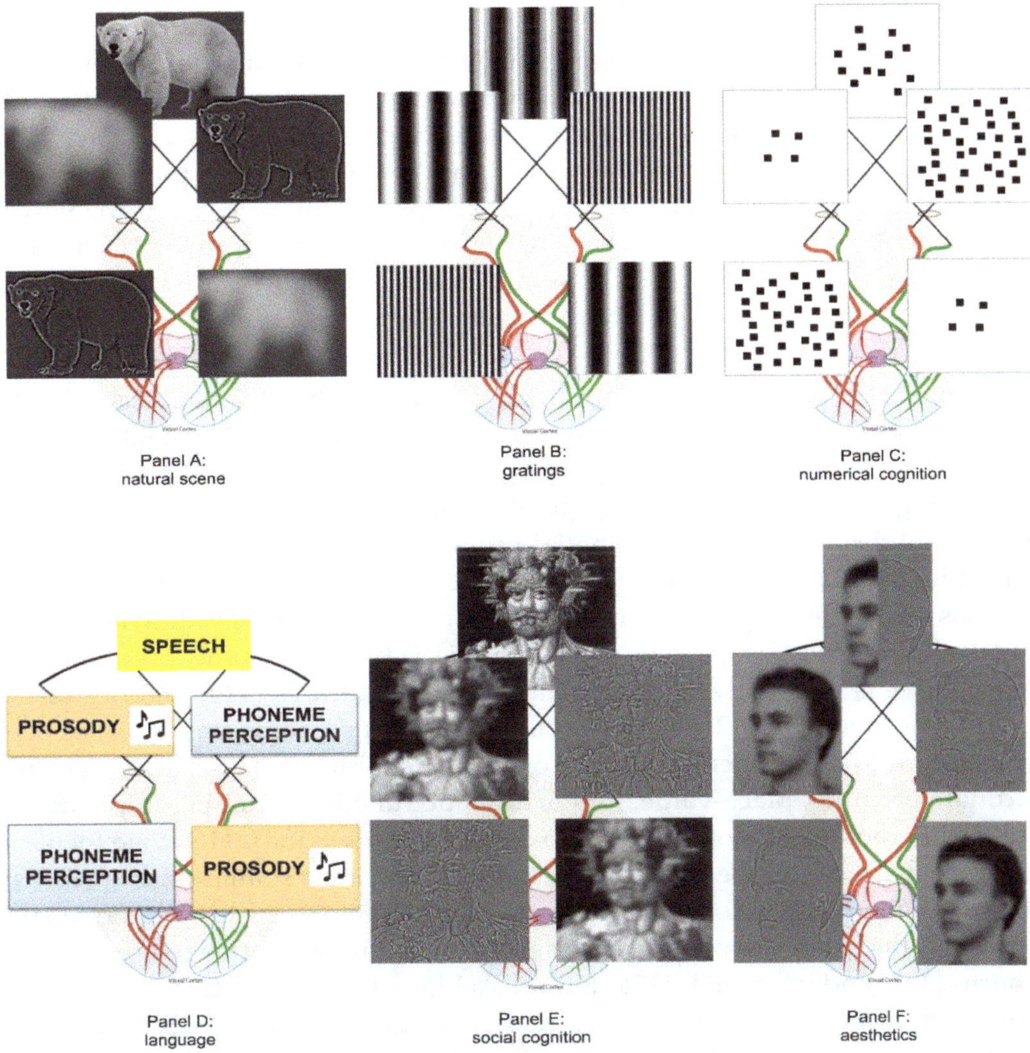

Figure 2. Components and implications of the Brain's Asymmetric Frequency Tuning (BAFT) model. All panels depict the BAFT principle postulating that, for a given percept (top row), the left/right hemisphere preferentially processes the high/low frequencies (bottom row), thus, leading to representation of detail/coarse elements on the right/left hemi-field (middle row), respectively. Panels **A,B** display applications of the BAFT principle to a visual scene (panel **A**) and to Spatial Frequency (SF) defined contrast gratings (Panel **B**), respectively. For a given percept that contains SFs in the middle range, the left/right hemisphere preferentially filters more/less dark and light cycles per degree of the visual angle and entails creation of a high/low SF percept in the contralateral hemi-field. Panels **C–F** represent implications of BAFT for domains of numerical cognition, language, social cognition, and aesthetics, respectively. They explain and illustrate specific predictions of BAFT: an association of small numerosities with left space and of large numerosities with a right space (Panel **C**). The left lateralization for high spatial/temporal linguistic features, such as syllable and phoneme processing, and right lateralization for low spatial/temporal modulation of language, such as sentence processing and prosody (Panel **D**). Hemispheric tuning for local/global processing involved in object/face recognition in ambiguous portraits such as those by Arcimboldo (Panel **E**), and more attractiveness for faces showing the left-cheek (Panel **F**). Notes: The polar bear scenes of Panel A are adapted from Figure 3 of Reference [115], licensed under CC-BY, version 4.0. The painting 'Vertumnus' by Guiseppe Arcimboldo of Panel E is filtered from https://commons.wikimedia.org/wiki/File:Vertumnus_årstidernas_gud_målad_av_Giuseppe_Arcimboldo_1591_-_Skoklosters_slott_-_91503.tiff; public domain. The model's photo of Panel F is filtered and adapted from Figure 1 of Reference [116], licensed under the Copyright Clearance Center. The anatomy of visual pathways is redrawn after Figure 1 of Reference [117], licensed under CC-BY, version 4.0.

4. Extending BAFT to Other Cognitive Domains

In the first part of this paper, we reviewed a wide range of asymmetries in behavior that can be explained as resulting from functional perceptual asymmetries. In the second part, we described several models of asymmetrical perceptual processing that can account for these observations. We ended that second section with the introduction of BAFT, which is a recently developed proposal that relies on the principle of asymmetrical SF processing (see Figure 2, especially panels A and B). Now we explain how BAFT can account for processing biases in higher-level cognitive domains, including numerical cognition, reading difficulties, social interactions, and aesthetic preferences (see Figure 2, panels C–F).

4.1. Numerical Cognition and Dyscalculia

Our ability to process and compare quantities is evolutionarily advantageous. Clearly, when the visual angle is constant, then a larger numerosity is related to a higher SF content. Therefore, our first extension of BAFT is to the domain of visual quantities and their asymmetrical processing. In numerical cognition, we distinguish numerosities (i.e., quantities of objects) from numbers (i.e., the symbols denoting these quantities). Asymmetrical spatial-numerical associations (SNAs) were an important discovery, reflecting the ubiquitous tendency to associate numbers with space [118]. This frequently replicated fact has suggested a spatial representation of numerical information along a horizontally oriented *mental number line* (for review, see Reference [119]). Mapping numbers (as symbolic quantities) onto space is a cognitive strategy shared by all cultures [120] and not restricted to the human kingdom (See Reference [121] for review). Recently, a taxonomy on SNAs has been provided to account for the multi-componential nature of this phenomenon [122]. Different properties of numbers (ordinal, cardinal, place-value, and arithmetic functions) can be, implicitly or explicitly, associated with different aspects of the space (extension or direction). Here, we focus on mapping the cardinal information of numbers (small vs. large) to different spatial directions (left vs. right). While humans may learn this association between number symbols and horizontal space through cultural techniques, the presence of a similar association for non-symbolic numerosities already in human newborns [123] and in animals [124] requires a biological explanation.

The BAFT hypothesis postulates a non-numerical origin of horizontal SNAs by relying on the above-mentioned functional perceptual asymmetries. The typical behavioral bias reported by human newborns and non-human animals, when dealing with non-symbolic numerosities, can be explained by the hemispheric SF processing asymmetry described above. As shown by Felisatti et al. (2020) [111], patterns with few elements, containing more power on low SFs, would preferentially engage the right hemisphere, inducing a left-bias. Conversely, patterns with many elements, containing more power on high SFs, would preferentially engage the left hemisphere, inducing a right bias (see Figure 2, panel C). In addition, there is evidence for non-symbolic SNAs in adults that could reflect the influence of hemispheric spatial frequency tuning [125–127]. Importantly, as in SF processing, what determines the spatial bias is the relative SF range contained in the stimulus of interest with respect to the overall SF range defining the stimulus set [104,105]. Furthermore, in numerical cognition, the spatial mapping of numbers is not absolute but depends on the numerical range ([128], Exp. 3, [129]).

BAFT can be extended to other studies of early emerging non-symbolic SNAs. Specifically, Bulf and colleagues (2016) [130] provided evidence of horizontal space-quantity-associations in eight-to-nine-month-old infants by using a detection paradigm where the observers' attention was directed laterally by a cue before measuring the efficiency of sensory registration. Their attentional cue consisted of either non-symbolic numbers (two vs. nine dots) or X-shaped stimuli varying in size (small vs. large). The authors predicted that if small is associated with left and large with right, then small cues (a 2-dot pattern and small letter X) should facilitate detection of left-located target stimuli. Conversely, large cues (a 9-dot pattern and large letter X) should facilitate detection of right-located target stimuli, as reported in adults [131]. While the non-symbolic-number cues corroborated the hypothesis, the X-shaped cues revealed an opposite trend. The authors interpreted their results in terms of an automatic vs. acquired tendency to map numerical vs. non-numerical magnitude onto space, respectively. Instead, the BAFT account unfolds the apparently counterintuitive findings in light of SF processing. In addition, 2-dot as well as large X-shaped stimuli contain lower SFs with respect to 9-dot and small X-shaped stimuli, thus, resulting in a leftward bias. Together, the facts that we naturally apply frequency filtering to visual perception, and that this functional filter is shared by a wide range of non-human species, can explain how non-symbolic associations between quantities and space emerge as a result of the evolutionary developed, biological structure of our minds.

4.2. *Language, Dyslexia, and Music*

The notion of functional hemispheric specialization for low vs. high SFs is also an important approach for understanding deficits in the acquisition of reading skills, commonly referred to as Developmental Dyslexia (DD). DD can be defined as the inability to obtain, despite adequate training opportunities, an age-consistent level of reading competence, considering both reading speed and text comprehension. Depending on the specific criteria applied in the assessment of DD, between 5% and 17% of children can be considered dyslexic [132]. The condition can be inherited and affects more males than females [133]. Dyslexia is often comorbid with dyscalculia ([134–137], but see Reference [138]). Given that reading is a multi-componential task involving perceptual, cognitive, and oculo-motor processes, it is not easy to determine whether a dyslexia-causing deficit originates with stimulus encoding, or with phonological activation induced by successfully identified graphemes, or as a result of imprecise control over one's eye movements.

Ever more perceptual, language-specific cognitive and motor deficits have been reported in Developmentally Dyslexic children (DDs) over the decades. Although substantial evidence has converged on a phonological (awareness or discrimination) deficit at the core of DD [139,140], more recent studies have identified perceptual limitations as additional and, perhaps, more fundamental contributors to DD. Given our present focus on cognitive signatures induced by functional perceptual processing asymmetries, we selectively report this evidence here.

In his recent review of dyslexia research, Stein (2018) [141] points out that the two brain hemispheres must provide temporally structured input for cognition from all modalities, including stimulation from visual and auditory language. The brain's inability to relay this input in a timely manner seems to be the common denominator for the wide range of performance deficits observed in DDs. The deficit relates to the already-mentioned two neuro-biologically distinct processing pathways in each of the two brain hemispheres, which originate at the retinae and then connect through sub-cortical channels into cortical areas. To remind readers, the magnocellular pathway is characterized by relatively fast processing of coarse visual information feeding dorsal processing streams into the parietal lobes that resolve a spatial detail for action control. This view lines up with the low spatial frequency tuning previously described for right-hemispheric processing. Instead, the parvocellular pathway processes visual detail (i.e., higher spatial frequencies at slower speed, the ventral cortical streams receive a mix of magno-cellular and parvo-cellular input to support attention allocation for object identification (Stein, 2018). In this view, DD can be understood as reflecting a damaged magnocellular pathway that slows down information for all cognition.

In a recent series of experiments, Franceschini and colleagues (2017) [142] provided converging evidence for the view that the normal processing speed advantage of low over high SFs (the previously mentioned "global precedence," [4]) is not present in unselected samples of DDs. They showed instead local precedence, as indicated by interference from local on global visual elements in a task requiring the processing of hierarchical Navon stimuli (see Figure 1 above). This finding was interpreted as evidence for a selective processing deficit along the magnocellular dorsal stream, which is known to be specialized for low spatial frequencies and the provision of information on stimulus locations. The consequence of the resulting relative local precedence is that reading cannot rely on the initial classification of letter strings that normally precedes identification of individual elements (cf. [143]).

Additionally, acoustic information travels along two streams, extending from the cochleae to primary and non-primary auditory cortices. The dorsal pathway is confined to the left hemisphere and is responsible for transformation of time-dependent speech signals into a motor format. The ventral pathway is organized more bilaterally and converts complex auditory features (e.g., prosody) into time-invariant speech representations [144,145]. The stronger lateralization and frequency dependency of the dorsal route further supports the prediction of the magnocellular pathway involvement in the impaired perception and motor computation of speech with intact prosody in DD.

In his review, Stein (2018) [141] explains the rationale for identifying the perceptual, timing-related processing deficit of DDs that would extend BAFT: "*By exploiting the high contrast sensitivity of magno-cells at low luminances and high temporal frequencies, to which parvo-cells do not respond at all, we can selectively stimulate the subcortical magnocellular system in order to decide whether its impairment impacts on dorsal stream function as a whole*" ([141], page 5). Although Skottun (2015) [146] has cautioned against such a strict separability of processing, we believe that the idea of impaired high-speed temporal processing not only explains DD's problems with phonological and discrimination tasks but also the frequent co-morbidity of dyslexia and dyscalculia we mentioned earlier.

The apparent lack of the neuro-typical visual processing succession from global to local visual elements in dyslexics may also be the reason for further correlated cognitive deficits in this population, including attentional deficits, hyperactivity, or learning disabilities [147,148]. An implication of the view of dyslexia as caused by an SF processing imbalance is that this easily measurable encoding anomaly could be incorporated into personalized models of dyslexia, along with orthographic, phonological, and vocabulary knowledge as predictors of an individual's deficit [132].

Language and, especially, language production, is the textbook example of a lateralized brain function, and is usually left-lateralized, as exemplified by the canonical Wernicke-Geschwind model [52,149,150]. On the other hand, music is right-lateralized, which might explain why music and math are related (cf. [151]). Since music is a kind of communication, it is possible that the brain tries to keep the two communication systems as distinct as possible. "Amusical" individuals, who cannot sing in tune and often cannot detect out-of-tune melodies, are characterized by abnormalities in neural transmission between the auditory cortex and the inferior frontal gyrus in the right cerebral hemisphere [152]. Disorders of musical pitch occur in relative isolation from speech disorders [153].

Some aspects of music, such as the syntax of complex pieces, however, might be left-lateralized and, thus, be contributed by language-specialized areas, while the processing of most other features, such as pitch and rhythm, is right-lateralized. On the other hand, a few aspects of language processing such as rhythm and sentence-level prosody seem to be contributed by the right hemisphere [154]. This is exploited by "Melodic Intonation Therapy" [155], which is one of a few effective therapies for aphasia, based on the observation that patients can often sing words that they cannot speak. Training the singing of words seems to be effective in recovering language functioning, if only for more or less formulaic speech. Melodic Intonation Therapy also includes rhythmically stroking the left hand, which is intended to activate the right hemisphere.

A recent study sheds some light on how the differential hemispheric specialization to language and music might be related to different sensitivity to spatial and temporal frequencies. Albouy and colleagues (2020) [156] selectively manipulated temporal or spectral features in sung speech. They found that perception of speech decreases only with degradation of temporal information, whereas perception of melodies decreases only with spectral degradation. These results are consistent with observations that the temporal modulation rate found in speech samples from many languages is substantially higher than that of music samples across genres [106].

Again, in terms of BAFT, a high temporal modulation rate might correspond to detailed, local processing, whereas music perception might correspond to more global processing (see Figure 2, panel D). The two parallel systems of communication that humans have developed including one in each hemisphere, and the need to efficiently separate encoding of their respective preferred features, might actually be one of the prime driving forces of the brain's top-down modulation of frequency tuning.

4.3. *Social Cognition and Emotion*

Humans, like most animals, are inherently social and devote considerable neural resources to the identification, understanding, and prediction of the emotional and cognitive states of others. This capability encompasses a wide variety of different mental tasks from the basic perception of social cues to complex social learning and mimicry [157]. The mechanisms underlying social cognition include highly specialized processes that are seemingly developed specifically to support social interactions (e.g., dedicated cortical face processing areas) as well as more general cognitive areas in supporting roles (e.g., attentional cueing mechanisms). The network of regions with seemingly dedicated social functions, the "social brain," involves many distinct cortical and subcortical regions throughout the brain [158]. Several of these social functions exhibit not only some degree of hemispheric lateralization but also a special sensitivity to particular SF bands.

The detection, identification, and processing of face stimuli are important for many aspects of social cognition. Both the left and right fusiform gyri show a preference for face stimuli over non-face stimuli, albeit with strong activity typically found in the right [159,160]. However, more detailed studies with carefully controlled stimuli suggest a qualitative difference in the type of face information that is the focus of each hemisphere. In a detailed fMRI examination of face processing using both real faces and exceedingly face-like and non-face objects, Meng and colleagues (2012) [161] identified several systematic differences between the two hemispheres. Specifically, they noted that the activity of the left fusiform gyrus was faster and more influenced (with either inhibition or facilitation) by context than the slower, context agnostic activity of the right fusiform gyrus. Interestingly, while activity in the left hemisphere appeared to represent a more image-like representation, activity in the right hemisphere was closely correlated with the categorical decision of whether the stimulus was a face or non-face. Together, these findings were consistent with the left gyrus, representing a detail-focused representation of the stimulus and the right gyrus representing a more abstract representation.

In support of hemispheric tuning for local/global features involved in object/face processing, some studies considered the ambiguous portraits painted by Giuseppe Arcimboldo (see Figure 2, panel E). They deal with hierarchical stimuli reflecting single big faces when processed holistically, or many little objects when processed analytically. Caharel and colleagues (2013) [162] found that Arcimboldo stimuli elicited an N170 signal, which is an electrical signal of the brain that is sensitive to properties of faces. Its amplitude was comparable to faces over the right hemisphere but comparable to objects over the left hemisphere. Moreover, in 7-month-old to 8-month-old infants, Arcimboldo portraits are already recognized as faces but, unlike normal faces, they correlate with neural activity in the left hemisphere due to feature-driven elaboration [163].

Furthermore, face processing is known to be highly influenced by the spatial frequency information available [164,165]. A prominent theory of face processing, the Dual-route model [166], proposes that two interconnected pathways—one cortical and one subcortical—are critical to our face perception. The rapid, subcortical pathway is thought to operate on predominantly LSF information and enables rapid face classification subserving behavior, while the slower cortical pathway, modulated by the faster subcortical inputs, conveys mainly HSF facial information [167,168]. Thus, although not containing explicit hemispherical segmentation, the Dual-route model proposes a similar two-step process with rapid LSF processing preceding and influencing the detailed processing of HSF information. When both the detailed methodological studies on hemispherical differences and the spatial frequency findings are considered together, they align closely with the proposal outlined in BAFT.

Hemispherical differences also appear to play a role in emotion processing. Emotional facial expressions presented in the left visual field appear to be perceived more intensely than those in the right visual field [169], suggesting a right-brain dominance for general emotion processing [170]. However, there remains much debate about the origin of this lateralization. While the right hemisphere hypothesis suggests the right hemisphere specializes in general emotional processing [171], the valence hypothesis suggests that the right hemisphere processes negative emotions while the left hemisphere processes positive emotions [172,173]. Both have received support in the literature, depending on the paradigm and stimuli chosen, alongside more cognitive explanations in which the difference in hemispherical activity is interpreted as approach/avoidance or behavior activation/inactivation [174].

4.4. Aesthetics

Our hypothesis/assumption of functional asymmetry for the processing of SFs can easily be applied to account for some intriguing horizontal asymmetries in the domain of aesthetic preferences. Although mankind's interest in art is ancient, as is the aesthetic interest in symmetry, only more recently systematic spatial aesthetic biases were reported both at the perceptual level of aesthetic appreciation and at the behavioral level of aesthetic preferences.

Several comprehensive surveys of painted portraits found a tendency to paint the left cheek rather than the right one ([175–178], for review, see Reference [179]). Corresponding rightward head-turning biases, revealing one's left cheek to others, were found when participants posed for a portrait in an emotional context, in photography composition [180–183], when rating mirrored portraits [184], and, with clear preference for right-facing objects rather than left-facing ones [183,185]. Recently, Park, Spense, Ishii, and Togawa (2020) [116] reported that left-oriented faces were perceived as more attractive than right-oriented faces, even when stimuli were identical. The authors found the perceived prototypicality as the mediator but a closer inspection may identify in the brain's asymmetric frequency tuning the mechanism underlying apparently dissociable phenomena related to left-oriented faces: more fixations [186], ease of recognition [187], prototypicality, and attractiveness [116].

Nevertheless, the accumulated evidence for gender differences [188], a possible change of bias over the life span [189], the mood-dependency of aesthetic preferences [190–193], and the involvement of culturally acquired techniques, such as reading direction in aesthetic preferences ([194–197], for review see Reference [198]) all indicate against a simple explanation, such as innate asymmetry of hemisphere specialization. However, and although speculative, it may be the case that aesthetic preferences for portrait directionality, as well as for horizontal-facing objects, are also partially influenced by the brain's asymmetric frequency tuning (see Figure 2, panel F).

Our hypothesis calls for revisiting some other well-established horizontal perceptual asymmetries. For example, various asymmetries in spatial composition were found, such as:

(a) a preference to place content of greater interest ('weight') on the right compared to the left side (the Right Bias), at least in right-handed participants [199,200],
(b) similar asymmetrical spatial preferences for larger salient content on the right side of paintings [199],
(c) the scanning motion bias, according to which we tend to scan our perceptual field left-to-right [201, 202], which is in accordance with a preference for stimuli with left-to-right directionality [203]. Moreover, Maass, Pagani, and Berta (2007) [204] found that left-to-right readers rated movie clips of lateral actions as stronger, faster, and more beautiful when actions had left-to-right directionality, while right-to-left readers showed the reverse pattern (see Reference [205]),
(d) a leftward attractiveness bias, according to which participants judge the left side of abstract visual patterns as more attractive than the right side [206].

The lack of comprehensive cross-cultural studies makes it hard to decide the possibility of a biological origin of these effects. The current results from cross-cultural studies seem to favor a view that the aesthetic preference bias is grounded in hemispheric specialization, but its strength is modulated by learned scanning habits such as reading direction [205].

5. Implications and Outstanding Questions—Experimental Avenues

It is clear that human behavior consists of a wide range of asymmetrical activities that span the perceptual, cognitive, and motor domains. We have previously reviewed the empirical evidence and described theoretical accounts for asymmetric signatures. One main message was that the idea of spatial frequency tuning of the brain's hemispheres can be considered as a broad principle from which most of these asymmetries can be explained. Moreover, the same principle can be extended to also cover a higher level of cognitive biases. In this final section, we make some suggestions for future research that could help to develop our proposal further.

Consider first the visual processing. The majority of literature focuses on what happens at fixation. However, humans presumably spend considerable time attending to objects in their visual periphery through covert attention, e.g., to plan forthcoming eye movements that target objects of detailed interest. Given the SF tuning of the two hemispheres and resulting asymmetry, peripheral signals will be differentially represented when located in the left vs. right hemifield. This has implications for reading research and scene perception studies, where our understanding of the use of parafoveal previews can distinguish between competing models (cf. [85,207–213]). It also affects our everyday life, ranging from design decisions for classroom setups (where emotions are differently interpreted by different hemispheres) to driving regulations (where obstacles must be processed and responded to) and to aesthetic judgement and marketing communication (where spatial orientation influences product evaluation).

Now, consider the foundational domain of numerical cognition. According to the BAFT hypothesis, the functional link between SF processing and space-quantity associations described previously could predict the link between impaired number acuity (i.e., the ability to discriminate visual numerosities) and the propensity to develop *dyscalculia*, which is a developmental disability affecting numerical and mathematical learning [214]. Dyscalculia might be the anatomical expression of asymmetric inhibitory control between the two brain hemispheres [44,45].

An informative experiment would consist of manipulating the SF content of numerical stimuli. Furthermore, if functional lateralization for SF processing establishes our tendency to map numbers onto space, it would be expected that, in healthy infants, but not in developmental dyscalculics, spatial-numerical associations will emerge, even when using different SF contents for the same number.

Given the large heterogeneity in lateralization in the population, this has implications for how individuals may vary. Future work should measure differences in anatomical and functional lateralization and see how this predicts performance in numerical vs. non-numerical tasks. Particularly, the diagnostic would also be a consideration of brain lateralization, and of the BAFT mechanism in particular, in artificial neural network models. Computational modelling has already provided evidence in support of an emergentist perspective, according to which our intuitive number sense would originate from contributions by evolutionary and learning constraints on perception and cognition [215].

BAFT can also be extended to the auditory perceptual domain, motivated by the following considerations. First, there is a close analogy between visual and auditory signal decomposition into frequency components (Fourier analysis). Second, a similar analogy exists between the functional asymmetric frequency processing of visual and auditory stimuli [92,93]. As a consequence, in analogy to the hemispheric spatial frequency tuning for visual stimuli, a hemispheric temporal frequency tuning could be expected for auditory stimuli. This view offers a re-interpretation of the findings reported by de Hevia and colleagues (2017) [216]. Human infants exhibit leftward/rightward behavioral biases after presentation of a few/many syllables, respectively. Specifically, for a given overall duration, few syllables are conveyed through lower temporal frequencies with respect to many syllables, thus, resulting in more engagement of the right hemisphere and leftward behavioral bias (see Reference [216], Experiment 4). Instead, when syllable durations remain constant, presenting few syllables after familiarization with many syllables triggers fine-to-coarse processing and involves the right hemisphere preferentially, with consequent leftward behavioral bias (see Reference [216], Experiment 5).

A final domain of study where we expect valuable insights through the BAFT perspective is neuropsychology with a focus on rehabilitation procedures. Specifically, it may be possible to reduce the impact of cortical damage by careful design and presentation of SF-filtered stimuli. Especially with the emergence of AR and VR devices, where stimuli can be preferentially presented to specific eyes, this could be used to try to drive processing toward the desirable hemisphere for different tasks.

However, before BAFT can be applied, certain challenges have to be addressed. For instance, usually the task to assess spatial attention biases is the landmark task, in which subjects have to indicate whether a line is transected to the left or right of its midpoint. Recent work looking at a variety of different spatial bias measures (see Reference [217]) demonstrated a profound (and replicated) lack of inter-task correlations. This suggests that these different measures of spatial attention bias are themselves tapping into different mechanisms. Notably, these tasks differ in how they utilize spatial frequency information alongside attentional biases. The spatial attentional biases most relevant to the BAFT theory are those in which there is competition for attention allocation to either the left or right visual field. With regard to the various implications of BAFT that we outlined (be it numerosity or aesthetic judgements), these are situations in which there is competition of the allocation of attention to the left or right visual field. The efficiency with which different information (at different spatial frequencies) is processed in the left and right hemifield will influence their relative salience and the biasing in orientating behaviour. This effect may be further supplemented by generalized spatial attention biases (see Reference [17]). However, with more complex stimuli (beyond a simple uniform line) that convey different (when images that are not horizontally mirrored) information at multiple different spatial frequencies, hemispherical competition in spatial orientating is much more subject to the saliency of image and its spatial frequency properties.

In conclusion, the BAFT hypothesis does not argue for an exclusive role of evolutionary predisposition to perceptual, cognitive, and motor spatial biases. As we already discussed above, recently accumulated evidence highlights the contributions of both embodied cultural habits and situated experiences to behavioral spatial asymmetries. We call for revisiting previously found asymmetric behavior in various domains, considering brain asymmetric frequency tuning, which can be later shaped by spatial habits and recent temporary events.

Author Contributions: Conceptualization, A.F., D.A.-M. and M.H.F.; writing—original draft preparation, A.F., D.A.-M., J.L., S.S., M.H.F.; writing—review and editing, A.F., D.A.-M., J.L., S.S., M.H.F.; supervision, M.H.F.; funding acquisition, A.F. and M.H.F. All authors have read and agreed to the published version of the manuscript.

Abbreviations

BAFT	Brain's Asymmetric Frequency Tuning
CTF	Coarse-To-Fine
DD	Developmental Dyslexia
DDs	Developmental Dyslexics
DFF	Dual Filtering by Frequency
HSFs	High Spatial Frequencies
LSFs	Low Spatial Frequencies
RHT	Reverse Hierarchy Theory
SFs	Spatial Frequencies
SNAs	Spatial Numerical Associations
TFs	Temporal Frequencies

References

1. Sergent, J. The cerebral balance of power: Confrontation or cooperation? *J. Exp. Psychol. Human Percept. Perform.* **1982**, *8*, 253–272. [CrossRef]
2. Hellige, J.B. Hemispheric asymmetry for visual information processing. *Acta Neurobiol. Exp.* **1969**, *56*, 485–497.
3. Kauffmann, L.; Ramanoël, S.; Peyrin, C. The neural bases of spatial frequency processing during scene perception. *Front. Integr. Neurosci.* **2014**, *8*. [CrossRef] [PubMed]
4. Navon, D. Forest before trees: The precedence of global features in visual perception. *Cogn. Psychol.* **1977**, *9*, 353–383. [CrossRef]

5. Van Kleeck, M.H. Hemispheric differences in global versus local processing of hierarchical visual stimuli by normal subjects: New data and a meta-analysis of previous studies. *Neuropsychologia* **1989**, *27*, 1165–1178. [CrossRef]
6. Sergent, J.; Hellige, J.B. Role of input factors in visual-field asymmetries. *Brain Cogn.* **1986**, *5*, 174–199. [CrossRef]
7. Kitterle, F.L.; Christman, S.; Hellige, J.B. Hemispheric differences are found in the identification, but not the detection, of low versus high spatial frequencies. *Percept. Psychophys.* **1990**, *48*, 297–306. [CrossRef]
8. Christman, S.; Kitterle, F.L.; Hellige, J. Hemispheric asymmetry in the processing of absolute versus relative spatial frequency. *Brain Cogn.* **1991**, *16*, 62–73. [CrossRef]
9. Peyrin, C.; Chauvin, A.; Chokron, S.; Marendaz, C. Hemispheric specialization for spatial frequency processing in the analysis of natural scenes. *Brain Cogn.* **2003**, *53*, 278–282. [CrossRef]
10. Peyrin, C.; Chokron, S.; Guyader, N.; Gout, O.; Moret, J.; Marendaz, C. Neural correlates of spatial frequency processing: A neuropsychological approach. *Brain Res.* **2006**, *1073–1074*, 1–10. [CrossRef] [PubMed]
11. Piazza, E.A.; Silver, M.A. Persistent Hemispheric Differences in the Perceptual Selection of Spatial Frequencies. *J. Cogn. Neurosci.* **2014**, *26*, 2021–2027. [CrossRef] [PubMed]
12. Guiard, Y. Asymmetric Division of Labor in Human Skilled Bimanual Action: The Kinematic Chain as a Model. *J. Mot. Behav.* **1987**, *19*, 486–517. [CrossRef] [PubMed]
13. Stanković, M.; Nešić, M. Contralateral Hemisphere Activation by Unilateral Hand Contraction: ReExamining of Global and Local Attention. *Percept. Mot. Ski.* **2018**. [CrossRef] [PubMed]
14. Behrmann, M.; Plaut, D.C. A vision of graded hemispheric specialization: Graded hemispheric specialization. *Ann. N. Y. Acad. Sci.* **2015**, *1359*, 30–46. [CrossRef]
15. Brederoo, S.G.; Nieuwenstein, M.R.; Cornelissen, F.W.; Lorist, M.M. Reproducibility of visual-field asymmetries: Nine replication studies investigating lateralization of visual information processing. *Cortex* **2019**, *111*, 100–126. [CrossRef]
16. Vingerhoets, G. Phenotypes in hemispheric functional segregation? Perspectives and challenges. *Phys. Life Rev.* **2019**, *30*, 1–18. [CrossRef]
17. Brederoo, S.G.; Van der Haegen, L.; Brysbaert, M.; Nieuwenstein, M.R.; Cornelissen, F.W.; Lorist, M.M. Towards a unified understanding of lateralized vision: A large-scale study investigating principles governing patterns of lateralization using a heterogeneous sample. *Cortex* **2020**, *133*, 201–214. [CrossRef]
18. Ventura, P.; Delgado, J.; Ferreira, M.; Farinha-Fernandes, A.; Guerreiro, J.C.; Faustino, B.; Leite, I.; Wong, A.C.-N. Hemispheric asymmetry in holistic processing of words. *Laterality Asymmetries Body Brain Cogn.* **2019**, *24*, 98–112. [CrossRef]
19. Dundas, E.M.; Plaut, D.C.; Behrmann, M. Variable Left-hemisphere Language and Orthographic Lateralization Reduces Right-hemisphere Face Lateralization. *J. Cogn. Neurosci.* **2015**, *27*, 913–925. [CrossRef]
20. Karlsson, E.M.; Johnstone, L.T.; Carey, D.P. The depth and breadth of multiple perceptual asymmetries in right handers and non-right handers. *Laterality Asymmetries Body Brain Cogn.* **2019**, *24*, 707–739. [CrossRef]
21. Gerrits, R.; Van der Haegen, L.; Brysbaert, M.; Vingerhoets, G. Laterality for recognizing written words and faces in the fusiform gyrus covaries with language dominance. *Cortex* **2019**, *117*, 196–204. [CrossRef] [PubMed]
22. Gerrits, R.; Verhelst, H.; Vingerhoets, G. Mirrored brain organization: Statistical anomaly or reversal of hemispheric functional segregation bias? *Proc. Natl. Acad. Sci. USA* **2020**, *117*, 14057–14065. [CrossRef] [PubMed]
23. Jewell, G.; McCourt, M.E. Pseudoneglect: A review and meta-analysis of performance factors in line bisection tasks. *Neuropsychologia* **2000**, *38*, 93–110. [CrossRef]
24. Fischer, M.H. Cognition in the bisection task. *Trends Cogn. Sci.* **2001**, *5*, 460–462. [CrossRef]
25. Fischer, M.H. Bisection performance indicates spatial word representation. *Cogn. Brain Res.* **1996**, *4*, 163–170. [CrossRef]
26. Fischer, M.H. Word Centre is Misperceived. *Perception* **2000**, *29*, 337–354. [CrossRef] [PubMed]
27. Fischer, M. Orthographic contributions to perceived word center. *Brain Lang.* **2004**, *88*, 321–330. [CrossRef]
28. Fischer, M.H. Number processing induces spatial performance biases. *Neurology* **2001**, *57*, 822–826. [CrossRef]
29. Girelli, L.; Marinelli, C.V.; Grossi, G.; Arduino, L.S. Cultural and biological factors modulate spatial biases over development. *Laterality Asymmetries Body Brain Cogn.* **2017**, *22*, 725–739. [CrossRef]

30. Rinaldi, L.; Di Luca, S.; Henik, A.; Girelli, L. Reading direction shifts visuospatial attention: An Interactive Account of attentional biases. *Acta Psychol.* **2014**, *151*, 98–105. [CrossRef]
31. Maass, A.; Suitner, C.; Nadhmi, F. What drives the spatial agency bias? An Italian-Malagasy-Arabic comparison study. *J. Exp. Psychol. Gen.* **2014**, *143*, 991–996. [CrossRef] [PubMed]
32. Rosenich, E.; Shaki, S.; Loetscher, T. Unstable world: Recent experience affects spatial perception. *Psychon. Bull. Rev.* **2020**, *27*, 286–292. [CrossRef] [PubMed]
33. McManus, I.C.; Edmondson, D.; Rodger, J. Balance in pictures. *Br. J. Psychol.* **1985**, *76*, 311–324. [CrossRef]
34. Robertson, L.C.; Lamb, M.R. Neuropsychological contributions to theories of part/whole organization. *Cogn. Psychol.* **1991**, *23*, 299–330. [CrossRef]
35. Bowers, D.; Heilman, K.M. Pseudoneglect: Effects of hemispace on a tactile line bisection task. *Neuropsychologia* **1980**, *18*, 491–498. [CrossRef]
36. Cazzoli, D.; Chechlacz, M. A matter of hand: Causal links between hand dominance, structural organization of fronto-parietal attention networks, and variability in behavioural responses to transcranial magnetic stimulation. *Cortex* **2017**, *86*, 230–246. [CrossRef]
37. Thiebaut de Schotten, M.; Dell'Acqua, F.; Forkel, S.; Simmons, A.; Vergani, F.; Murphy, D.G.M.; Catani, M. A Lateralized Brain Network for Visuo-Spatial Attention. *Nat. Prec.* **2011**. [CrossRef]
38. Dos Santos, N.A.; Andrade, S.M.; Fernandez Calvo, B. Detection of spatial frequency in brain-damaged patients: Influence of hemispheric asymmetries and hemineglect. *Front. Hum. Neurosci.* **2013**, *7*. [CrossRef]
39. Chechlacz, M.; Mantini, D.; Gillebert, C.R.; Humphreys, G.W. Asymmetrical white matter networks for attending to global versus local features. *Cortex* **2015**, *72*, 54–64. [CrossRef]
40. Berardi, N.; Bodis-Wollner, I.; Fiorentini, A.; Giuffré, G.; Morelli, M. Electrophysiological evidence for interhemispheric transmission of visual information in man. *J. Physiol.* **1989**, *411*, 207–225. [CrossRef]
41. Nowicka, A.; Grabowska, A.; Fersten, E. Interhemispheric transmission of information and functional asymmetry of the human brain. *Neuropsychologia* **1996**, *34*, 147–151. [CrossRef]
42. Robertson, L.C.; Lamb, M.R.; Zaidel, E. Interhemispheric relations in processing hierarchical patterns: Evidence from normal and commissurotomized subjects. *Neuropsychology* **1993**, *7*, 325–342. [CrossRef]
43. Kleinman, J.T.; Gupta, A. The Right Hand Draws the Trees, But the Left Draws the Forest? *Behav. Neurol.* **2008**, *20*, 55–60. [CrossRef] [PubMed]
44. Putnam, M.C.; Steven, M.S.; Doron, K.W.; Riggall, A.C.; Gazzaniga, M.S. Cortical Projection Topography of the Human Splenium: Hemispheric Asymmetry and Individual Differences. *J. Cogn. Neurosci.* **2010**, *22*, 1662–1669. [CrossRef]
45. Koch, G.; Cercignani, M.; Bonni, S.; Giacobbe, V.; Bucchi, G.; Versace, V.; Caltagirone, C.; Bozzali, M. Asymmetry of Parietal Interhemispheric Connections in Humans. *J. Neurosci.* **2011**, *31*, 8967–8975. [CrossRef]
46. Warrington, E.K.; Broadbent, D.E.; Weiskrantz, L. Neuropsychological studies of object recognition. *Philos. Trans. R. Soc. Lond. B Biol. Sci.* **1982**, *298*, 15–33. [CrossRef]
47. Damasio, A.R. Prosopagnosia. *Trends Neurosci.* **1985**, *8*, 132–135. [CrossRef]
48. Farah, M.J. Cognitive Neuropsychology: Patterns of Co-occurrence Among the Associative Agnosias: Implications for Visual Object Representation. *Cogn. Neuropsychol.* **1991**, *8*, 1–19. [CrossRef]
49. Musel, B.; Bordier, C.; Dojat, M.; Pichat, C.; Chokron, S.; Le Bas, J.-F.; Peyrin, C. Retinotopic and Lateralized Processing of Spatial Frequencies in Human Visual Cortex during Scene Categorization. *J. Cogn. Neurosci.* **2013**, *25*, 1315–1331. [CrossRef]
50. Woodhead, Z.V.J.; Wise, R.J.S.; Sereno, M.; Leech, R. Dissociation of Sensitivity to Spatial Frequency in Word and Face Preferential Areas of the Fusiform Gyrus. *Cereb. Cortex* **2011**, *21*, 2307–2312. [CrossRef]
51. Ocklenburg, S.; Güntürkün, O. Hemispheric Asymmetries: The Comparative View. *Front. Psychol.* **2012**, *3*. [CrossRef] [PubMed]
52. Corballis, M.C. What's left in language? Beyond the classical model: What's left in language? *Ann. N. Y. Acad. Sci.* **2015**, *1359*, 14–29. [CrossRef] [PubMed]
53. Vogel, J.J.; Bowers, C.A.; Vogel, D.S. Cerebral lateralization of spatial abilities: A meta-analysis. *Brain Cogn.* **2003**, *52*, 197–204. [CrossRef]
54. Concha, M.L.; Bianco, I.H.; Wilson, S.W. Encoding asymmetry within neural circuits. *Nat. Rev. Neurosci.* **2012**, *13*, 832–843. [CrossRef] [PubMed]
55. Rogers, L.J. A Matter of Degree: Strength of Brain Asymmetry and Behaviour. *Symmetry* **2017**, *9*, 57. [CrossRef]

56. Karenina, K.; Giljov, A.; Ivkovich, T.; Malashichev, Y. Evidence for the perceptual origin of right-sided feeding biases in cetaceans. *Anim. Cogn.* **2016**, *19*, 239–243. [CrossRef] [PubMed]
57. Robins, A.; Rogers, L.J. Lateralized prey-catching responses in the cane toad, Bufo marinus: Analysis of complex visual stimuli. *Anim. Behav.* **2004**, *68*, 767–775. [CrossRef]
58. Andrew, R.J.; Tommasi, L.; Ford, N. Motor Control by Vision and the Evolution of Cerebral Lateralization. *Brain Lang.* **2000**, *73*, 220–235. [CrossRef]
59. Rogers, L.J. Lateralization in vertebrates: Its early evolution, general pattern, and development. In *Advances in the Study of Behavior*; Elsevier: Amsterdam, The Netherlands, 2002; Volume 31, pp. 107–161, ISBN 978-0-12-004531-0.
60. Vallortigara, G. The evolutionary psychology of left and right: Costs and benefits of lateralization. *Dev. Psychobiol.* **2006**, *48*, 418–427. [CrossRef]
61. Koboroff, A.; Kaplan, G.; Rogers, L.J. Hemispheric specialization in Australian magpies (*Gymnorhina tibicen*) shown as eye preferences during response to a predator. *Brain Res. Bull.* **2008**, *76*, 304–306. [CrossRef]
62. Sovrano, V.A. Visual lateralization in response to familiar and unfamiliar stimuli in fish. *Behav. Brain Res.* **2004**, *152*, 385–391. [CrossRef] [PubMed]
63. MacNeilage, P.F.; Rogers, L.J.; Vallortigara, G. Origins of the left & right brain. *Sci. Am.* **2009**, *301*, 60–67. [PubMed]
64. Vallortigara, G.; Chiandetti, C.; Sovrano, V.A. Brain asymmetry (animal): Brain asymmetry. *WIREs Cogn. Sci.* **2011**, *2*, 146–157. [CrossRef] [PubMed]
65. Vallortigara, G.; Rogers, L.J. Survival with an asymmetrical brain: Advantages and disadvantages of cerebral lateralization. *Behav. Brain Sci.* **2005**, *28*, 575–589. [CrossRef]
66. Güntürkün, O.; Diekamp, B.; Manns, M.; Nottelmann, F.; Prior, H.; Schwarz, A.; Skiba, M. Asymmetry pays: Visual lateralization improves discrimination success in pigeons. *Curr. Biol.* **2000**, *10*, 1079–1081. [CrossRef]
67. Rogers, L.J.; Zucca, P.; Vallortigara, G. Advantages of having a lateralized brain. *Proc. R. Soc. Lond. B* **2004**, *271*, S420–S422. [CrossRef]
68. Rezvani, Z.; Katanforoush, A.; Pouretemad, H. Global precedence changes by environment: A systematic review and meta-analysis on effect of perceptual field variables on global-local visual processing. *Atten. Percept. Psychophys.* **2020**, *82*, 2348–2359. [CrossRef]
69. Campbell, F.W.; Maffei, L. Contrast and Spatial Frequency. *Sci. Am.* **1974**, *231*, 106–115. [CrossRef]
70. Lamb, M.R.; Yund, E.W. The role of spatial frequency in the processing of hierarchically organized stimuli. *Percept. Psychophys.* **1993**, *54*, 773–784. [CrossRef]
71. Shulman, G.L.; Sullivan, M.A.; Gish, K.; Sakoda, W.J. The Role of Spatial-Frequency Channels in the Perception of Local and Global Structure. *Perception* **1986**, *15*, 259–273. [CrossRef]
72. Shulman, G.L.; Wilson, J. Spatial Frequency and Selective Attention to Local and Global Information. *Perception* **1987**, *16*, 89–101. [CrossRef] [PubMed]
73. LeCun, Y.; Boser, B.; Denker, J.S.; Henderson, D.; Howard, R.E.; Hubbard, W.; Jackel, L.D. Backpropagation Applied to Handwritten Zip Code Recognition. *Neural Comput.* **1989**, *1*, 541–551. [CrossRef]
74. LeCun, Y.; Bengio, Y.; Hinton, G. Deep learning. *Nature* **2015**, *521*, 436–444. [CrossRef] [PubMed]
75. Yamins, D.L.K.; Hong, H.; Cadieu, C.F.; Solomon, E.A.; Seibert, D.; DiCarlo, J.J. Performance-optimized hierarchical models predict neural responses in higher visual cortex. *Proc. Natl. Acad. Sci. USA* **2014**, *111*, 8619–8624. [CrossRef]
76. Dreher, B.; Fukada, Y.; Rodieck, R.W. Identification, classification and anatomical segregation of cells with X-like and Y-like properties in the lateral geniculate nucleus of old-world primates. *J. Physiol.* **1976**, *258*, 433–452. [CrossRef]
77. Lawton, T.; Shelley-Tremblay, J. Training on Movement Figure-Ground Discrimination Remediates Low-Level Visual Timing Deficits in the Dorsal Stream, Improving High-Level Cognitive Functioning, Including Attention, Reading Fluency, and Working Memory. *Front. Hum. Neurosci.* **2017**, *11*, 236. [CrossRef]
78. Bullier, J. Integrated model of visual processing. *Brain Res. Rev.* **2001**, *36*, 96–107. [CrossRef]
79. Bar, M. A Cortical Mechanism for Triggering Top-Down Facilitation in Visual Object Recognition. *J. Cogn. Neurosci.* **2003**, *15*, 600–609. [CrossRef]
80. Peyrin, C.; Michel, C.M.; Schwartz, S.; Thut, G.; Seghier, M.; Landis, T.; Marendaz, C.; Vuilleumier, P. The Neural Substrates and Timing of Top-Down Processes during Coarse-to-Fine Categorization of Visual Scenes: A Combined fMRI and ERP Study. *J. Cogn. Neurosci.* **2010**, *22*, 2768–2780. [CrossRef]

81. Musel, B.; Kauffmann, L.; Ramanoël, S.; Giavarini, C.; Guyader, N.; Chauvin, A.; Peyrin, C. Coarse-to-fine Categorization of Visual Scenes in Scene-selective Cortex. *J. Cogn. Neurosci.* **2014**, *26*, 2287–2297. [CrossRef]
82. Goodale, M.A.; Milner, A.D. Separate visual pathways for perception and action. *Trends Neurosci.* **1992**, *15*, 20–25. [CrossRef]
83. Larson, A.M.; Loschky, L.C. The contributions of central versus peripheral vision to scene gist recognition. *J. Vis.* **2009**, *9*. [CrossRef] [PubMed]
84. Findlay, J.M.; Gilchrist, I.D. *Active Vision: The Psychology of Looking and Seeing*; Oxford University Press: Oxford, UK, 2003; ISBN 978-0-19-852479-3.
85. Laubrock, J.; Cajar, A.; Engbert, R. Control of fixation duration during scene viewing by interaction of foveal and peripheral processing. *J. Vis.* **2013**, *13*, 11. [CrossRef] [PubMed]
86. Stevens, W.D.; Kahn, I.; Wig, G.S.; Schacter, D.L. Hemispheric Asymmetry of Visual Scene Processing in the Human Brain: Evidence from Repetition Priming and Intrinsic Activity. *Cereb. Cortex* **2012**, *22*, 1935–1949. [CrossRef] [PubMed]
87. Pisella, L.; Alahyane, N.; Blangero, A.; Thery, F.; Blanc, S.; Pelisson, D. Right-hemispheric dominance for visual remapping in humans. *Phil. Trans. R. Soc. B* **2011**, *366*, 572–585. [CrossRef]
88. Sheremata, S.L.; Bettencourt, K.C.; Somers, D.C. Hemispheric Asymmetry in Visuotopic Posterior Parietal Cortex Emerges with Visual Short-Term Memory Load. *J. Neurosci.* **2010**, *30*, 12581–12588. [CrossRef]
89. Stephan, K.E.; Marshall, J.C.; Penny, W.D.; Friston, K.J.; Fink, G.R. Interhemispheric Integration of Visual Processing during Task-Driven Lateralization. *J. Neurosci.* **2007**, *27*, 3512–3522. [CrossRef]
90. Robertson, L.C.; Ivry, R. Hemispheric Asymmetries: Attention to Visual and Auditory Primitives. *Curr. Dir. Psychol. Sci.* **2000**, *9*, 59–63. [CrossRef]
91. Poeppel, D. The analysis of speech in different temporal integration windows: Cerebral lateralization as 'asymmetric sampling in time'. *Speech Commun.* **2003**, *41*, 245–255. [CrossRef]
92. Flinker, A.; Doyle, W.K.; Mehta, A.D.; Devinsky, O.; Poeppel, D. Spectrotemporal modulation provides a unifying framework for auditory cortical asymmetries. *Nat. Hum. Behav.* **2019**, *3*, 393–405. [CrossRef]
93. Telkemeyer, S.; Rossi, S.; Koch, S.P.; Nierhaus, T.; Steinbrink, J.; Poeppel, D.; Obrig, H.; Wartenburger, I. Sensitivity of Newborn Auditory Cortex to the Temporal Structure of Sounds. *J. Neurosci.* **2009**, *29*, 14726–14733. [CrossRef] [PubMed]
94. Ouimet, T.; Foster, N.E.V.; Tryfon, A.; Hyde, K.L. Auditory-musical processing in autism spectrum disorders: A review of behavioral and brain imaging studies. *Ann. N. Y. Acad. Sci.* **2012**, *1252*, 325–331. [CrossRef] [PubMed]
95. Bouvet, L.; Simard-Meilleur, A.-A.; Paignon, A.; Mottron, L.; Donnadieu, S. Auditory local bias and reduced global interference in autism. *Cognition* **2014**, *131*, 367–372. [CrossRef] [PubMed]
96. Haigh, S.M. Variable sensory perception in autism. *Eur. J. Neurosci.* **2018**, *47*, 602–609. [CrossRef] [PubMed]
97. Di Lollo, V. Hemispheric symmetry in duration of visible persistence. *Percept. Psychophys.* **1981**, *29*, 21–25. [CrossRef] [PubMed]
98. Grabowska, A.; Nowicka, A. Visual-spatial-frequency model of cerebral asymmetry: A critical survey of behavioral and electrophysiological studies. *Psychol. Bull.* **1996**, *120*, 434–449. [CrossRef]
99. Ivry, R.B.; Robertson, L.C.; Robertson, L.C. *The Two Sides of Perception*; MIT Press: Cambridge, MA, USA, 1998; ISBN 978-0-262-09034-6.
100. Hochstein, S.; Ahissar, M. View from the Top: Hierarchies and Reverse Hierarchies in the Visual System. *Neuron* **2002**, *36*, 791–804. [CrossRef]
101. Ahissar, M.; Hochstein, S. The reverse hierarchy theory of visual perceptual learning. *Trends Cogn. Sci.* **2004**, *8*, 457–464. [CrossRef]
102. Ahissar, M.; Nahum, M.; Nelken, I.; Hochstein, S. Reverse hierarchies and sensory learning. *Phil. Trans. R. Soc. B* **2009**, *364*, 285–299. [CrossRef]
103. Hegde, J. Time course of visual perception: Coarse-to-fine processing and beyond. *Prog. Neurobiol.* **2008**, *84*, 405–439. [CrossRef]
104. Flevaris, A.V.; Robertson, L.C. Spatial frequency selection and integration of global and local information in visual processing: A selective review and tribute to Shlomo Bentin. *Neuropsychologia* **2016**, *83*, 192–200. [CrossRef] [PubMed]

105. Piazza, E.A.; Silver, M.A. Relative Spatial Frequency Processing Drives Hemispheric Asymmetry in Conscious Awareness. *Front. Psychol.* **2017**, *8*. [CrossRef] [PubMed]
106. Ding, S.; Cueva, C.J.; Tsodyks, M.; Qian, N. Visual perception as retrospective Bayesian decoding from high- to low-level features. *Proc. Natl. Acad. Sci. USA* **2017**, *114*, E9115–E9124. [CrossRef] [PubMed]
107. Barsalou, L.W. Grounded Cognition. *Annu. Rev. Psychol.* **2008**, *59*, 617–645. [CrossRef] [PubMed]
108. Matheson, H.E.; Barsalou, L.W. Embodiment and Grounding in Cognitive Neuroscience. In *Stevens' Handbook of Experimental Psychology and Cognitive Neuroscience*; Wixted, J.T., Ed.; John Wiley & Sons, Inc.: Hoboken, NJ, USA, 2018; pp. 1–27, ISBN 978-1-119-17016-7.
109. Fischer, M.H.; Coello, Y.E. *Foundations of Embodied Cognition: Conceptual and Interactive Embodiment*; Routledge/Taylor & Francis Group: New York, NY, USA, 2016; ISBN 978-1-138-80582-8.
110. Newen, A.; Bruin, L.D.; Gallagher, S. *The Oxford Handbook of 4E Cognition*; Oxford University Press: Oxford, UK, 2018; ISBN 978-0-19-105435-8.
111. Felisatti, A.; Laubrock, J.; Shaki, S.; Fischer, M.H. A biological foundation for spatial–numerical associations: The brain's asymmetric frequency tuning. *Ann. N. Y. Acad. Sci.* **2020**. [CrossRef] [PubMed]
112. Fischer, M.H. A hierarchical view of grounded, embodied, and situated numerical cognition. *Cogn. Process.* **2012**, *13*, 161–164. [CrossRef] [PubMed]
113. Pezzulo, G.; Barsalou, L.W.; Cangelosi, A.; Fischer, M.H.; McRae, K.; Spivey, M.J. Computational Grounded Cognition: A new alliance between grounded cognition and computational modeling. *Front. Psychol.* **2013**, *3*. [CrossRef]
114. Myachykov, A.; Scheepers, C.; Fischer, M.H.; Kessler, K. TEST: A Tropic, Embodied, and Situated Theory of Cognition. *Top Cogn. Sci.* **2014**, *6*, 442–460. [CrossRef]
115. Panichello, M.F.; Cheung, O.S.; Bar, M. Predictive Feedback and Conscious Visual Experience. *Front. Psychol.* **2013**, *3*. [CrossRef]
116. Park, J.; Spence, C.; Ishii, H.; Togawa, T. Turning the other cheek: Facial orientation influences both model attractiveness and product evaluation. *Psychol. Mark.* **2020**. [CrossRef]
117. Larsson, M.L. Binocular vision, the optic chiasm, and their associations with vertebrate motor behavior. *Front. Ecol. Evol.* **2015**, *3*. [CrossRef]
118. Shaki, S.; Fischer, M.H. Systematic spatial distortion of quantitative estimates. *Psychol. Res.* **2020**. [CrossRef] [PubMed]
119. Fischer, M.H.; Shaki, S. Spatial Associations in Numerical Cognition—From Single Digits to Arithmetic. *Q. J. Exp. Psychol.* **2014**, *67*, 1461–1483. [CrossRef] [PubMed]
120. Göbel, S.M.; Shaki, S.; Fischer, M.H. The Cultural Number Line: A Review of Cultural and Linguistic Influences on the Development of Number Processing. *J. Cross-Cult. Psychol.* **2011**, *42*, 543–565. [CrossRef]
121. Rugani, R.; de Hevia, M.-D. Number-space associations without language: Evidence from preverbal human infants and non-human animal species. *Psychon. Bull. Rev.* **2017**, *24*, 352–369. [CrossRef]
122. Cipora, K.; Schroeder, P.A.; Soltanlou, M.; Nuerk, H.-C. More Space, Better Mathematics: Is Space a Powerful Tool or a Cornerstone for Understanding Arithmetic? In *Visualizing Mathematics*; Mix, K.S., Battista, M.T., Eds.; Research in Mathematics Education; Springer International Publishing: Cham, Switzerland, 2018; pp. 77–116, ISBN 978-3-319-98766-8.
123. Di Giorgio, E.; Lunghi, M.; Rugani, R.; Regolin, L.; Dalla Barba, B.; Vallortigara, G.; Simion, F. A mental number line in human newborns. *Dev. Sci.* **2019**, *22*. [CrossRef]
124. Rugani, R.; Vallortigara, G.; Priftis, K.; Regolin, L. Number-space mapping in the newborn chick resembles humans' mental number line. *Science* **2015**, *347*, 534–536. [CrossRef]
125. Nemeh, F.; Humberstone, J.; Yates, M.J.; Reeve, R.A. Non-symbolic magnitudes are represented spatially: Evidence from a non-symbolic SNARC task. *PLoS ONE* **2018**, *13*, e0203019. [CrossRef]
126. Zhou, X.; Shen, C.; Li, L.; Li, D.; Cui, J. Mental Numerosity Line in the Human's Approximate Number System. *Exp. Psychol.* **2016**, *63*, 169–179. [CrossRef]
127. Mitchell, T.; Bull, R.; Cleland, A.A. Implicit response-irrelevant number information triggers the SNARC effect: Evidence using a neural overlap paradigm. *Q. J. Exp. Psychol.* **2012**, *65*, 1945–1961. [CrossRef]
128. Dehaene, S.; Bossini, S.; Giraux, P. The mental representation of parity and number magnitude. *J. Exp. Psychol. Gen.* **1993**, *122*, 371–396. [CrossRef]
129. Rugani, R.; Vallortigara, G.; Priftis, K.; Regolin, L. Numerical magnitude, rather than individual bias, explains spatial numerical association in newborn chicks. *eLife* **2020**, *9*, e54662. [CrossRef] [PubMed]

130. Bulf, H.; de Hevia, M.D.; Cassia, V.M. Small on the left, large on the right: Numbers orient visual attention onto space in preverbal infants. *Dev. Sci.* **2016**, *19*, 394–401. [CrossRef] [PubMed]
131. Bulf, H.; Cassia, V.M.; de Hevia, M.D. Are Numbers, Size and Brightness Equally Efficient in Orienting Visual Attention? Evidence from an Eye-Tracking Study. *PLoS ONE* **2014**, *9*, e99499. [CrossRef] [PubMed]
132. Perry, C.; Zorzi, M.; Ziegler, J.C. Understanding Dyslexia Through Personalized Large-Scale Computational Models. *Psychol. Sci.* **2019**, *30*, 386–395. [CrossRef] [PubMed]
133. Arnett, A.B.; Pennington, B.F.; Peterson, R.L.; Willcutt, E.G.; DeFries, J.C.; Olson, R.K. Explaining the sex difference in dyslexia. *J. Child Psychol. Psychiatr.* **2017**, *58*, 719–727. [CrossRef]
134. Badian, N.A. Persistent arithmetic, reading, or arithmetic and reading disability. *Ann. Dyslexia* **1999**, *49*, 43–70. [CrossRef]
135. Barbaresi, W.J.; Katusic, S.K.; Colligan, R.C.; Weaver, A.L.; Jacobsen, S.J. Math Learning Disorder: Incidence in a Population-Based Birth Cohort, 1976–82, Rochester, Minn. *Ambul. Pediatrics* **2005**, *5*, 281–289. [CrossRef]
136. Dirks, E.; Spyer, G.; van Lieshout, E.C.D.M.; de Sonneville, L. Prevalence of Combined Reading and Arithmetic Disabilities. *J. Learn. Disabil.* **2008**, *41*, 460–473. [CrossRef]
137. Lewis, C.; Hitch, G.J.; Walker, P. The Prevalence of Specific Arithmetic Difficulties and Specific Reading Difficulties in 9- to 10-year-old Boys and Girls. *J. Child Psychol. Psychiat.* **1994**, *35*, 283–292. [CrossRef]
138. Landerl, K.; Fussenegger, B.; Moll, K.; Willburger, E. Dyslexia and dyscalculia: Two learning disorders with different cognitive profiles. *J. Exp. Child Psychol.* **2009**, *103*, 309–324. [CrossRef] [PubMed]
139. Bradley, L.; Bryant, P.E. Categorizing sounds and learning to read—A causal connection. *Nature* **1983**, *301*, 419–421. [CrossRef]
140. Boets, B.; de Beeck, H.P.O.; Vandermosten, M.; Scott, S.K.; Gillebert, C.R.; Mantini, D.; Bulthe, J.; Sunaert, S.; Wouters, J.; Ghesquiere, P. Intact But Less Accessible Phonetic Representations in Adults with Dyslexia. *Science* **2013**, *342*, 1251–1254. [CrossRef] [PubMed]
141. Stein, J. What is Developmental Dyslexia? *Brain Sci.* **2018**, *8*, 26. [CrossRef] [PubMed]
142. Franceschini, S.; Bertoni, S.; Gianesini, T.; Gori, S.; Facoetti, A. A different vision of dyslexia: Local precedence on global perception. *Sci. Rep.* **2017**, *7*, 17462. [CrossRef]
143. Franceschini, S.; Bertoni, S.; Puccio, G.; Mancarella, M.; Gori, S.; Facoetti, A. Local perception impairs the lexical reading route. *Psychol. Res.* **2020**. [CrossRef]
144. Hickok, G.; Poeppel, D. The cortical organization of speech processing. *Nat. Rev. Neurosci.* **2007**, *8*, 393–402. [CrossRef]
145. Sammler, D.; Grosbras, M.-H.; Anwander, A.; Bestelmeyer, P.E.G.; Belin, P. Dorsal and Ventral Pathways for Prosody. *Curr. Biol.* **2015**, *25*, 3079–3085. [CrossRef]
146. Skottun, B.C. On the use of spatial frequency to isolate contributions from the magnocellular and parvocellular systems and the dorsal and ventral cortical streams. *Neurosci. Biobehav. Rev.* **2015**, *56*, 266–275. [CrossRef]
147. Grinter, E.J.; Maybery, M.T.; Badcock, D.R. Vision in developmental disorders: Is there a dorsal stream deficit? *Brain Res. Bull.* **2010**, *82*, 147–160. [CrossRef]
148. Van der Hallen, R.; Evers, K.; Brewaeys, K.; Van den Noortgate, W.; Wagemans, J. Global processing takes time: A meta-analysis on local–global visual processing in ASD. *Psychol. Bull.* **2015**, *141*, 549–573. [CrossRef] [PubMed]
149. Geschwind, N. Disconnexion Syndromes in Animals and Man. *Brain* **1965**, *88*, 585. [CrossRef] [PubMed]
150. Gazzaniga, M.S. Right hemisphere language following brain bisection: A 20-year perspective. *Am. Psychol.* **1983**, *38*, 525–537. [CrossRef] [PubMed]
151. Hofstadter, D.R. *Gödel, Escher, Bach: An Eternal Golden Braid*; Penguin Books Ltd.: Middlesex, UK, 1979.
152. Peretz, I. Neurobiology of Congenital Amusia. *Trends Cogn. Sci.* **2016**, *20*, 857–867. [CrossRef] [PubMed]
153. Peretz, I.; Hyde, K.L. What is specific to music processing? Insights from congenital amusia. *Trends Cogn. Sci.* **2003**, *7*, 362–367. [CrossRef]
154. Friederici, A.D.; Alter, K. Lateralization of auditory language functions: A dynamic dual pathway model. *Brain Lang.* **2004**, *89*, 267–276. [CrossRef]
155. Norton, A.; Zipse, L.; Marchina, S.; Schlaug, G. Melodic Intonation Therapy: Shared Insights on How It Is Done and Why It Might Help. *Ann. N. Y. Acad. Sci.* **2009**, *1169*, 431–436. [CrossRef]
156. Albouy, P.; Benjamin, L.; Morillon, B.; Zatorre, R.J. Distinct sensitivity to spectrotemporal modulation supports brain asymmetry for speech and melody. *Science* **2020**, *367*, 1043–1047. [CrossRef]

157. Happé, F.; Cook, J.L.; Bird, G. The Structure of Social Cognition: In(ter)dependence of Sociocognitive Processes. *Annu. Rev. Psychol.* **2017**, *68*, 243–267. [CrossRef]
158. Kennedy, D.P.; Adolphs, R. The social brain in psychiatric and neurological disorders. *Trends Cogn. Sci.* **2012**, *16*, 559–572. [CrossRef]
159. McCarthy, G.; Puce, A.; Gore, J.C.; Allison, T. Face-Specific Processing in the Human Fusiform Gyrus. *J. Cogn. Neurosci.* **1997**, *9*, 605–610. [CrossRef] [PubMed]
160. Gazzaniga, M.S.; Smylie, C.S. Facial recognition and brain asymmetries: Clues to underlying mechanisms. *Ann. Neurol.* **1983**, *13*, 536–540. [CrossRef] [PubMed]
161. Meng, M.; Cherian, T.; Singal, G.; Sinha, P. Lateralization of face processing in the human brain. *Proc. R. Soc. B* **2012**, *279*, 2052–2061. [CrossRef] [PubMed]
162. Caharel, S.; Leleu, A.; Bernard, C.; Viggiano, M.-P.; Lalonde, R.; Rebaï, M. Early holistic face-like processing of Arcimboldo paintings in the right occipito-temporal cortex: Evidence from the N170 ERP component. *Int. J. Psychophysiol.* **2013**, *90*, 157–164. [CrossRef] [PubMed]
163. Kobayashi, M.; Otsuka, Y.; Nakato, E.; Kanazawa, S.; Yamaguchi, M.K.; Kakigi, R. Do infants recognize the Arcimboldo images as faces? Behavioral and near-infrared spectroscopic study. *J. Exp. Child Psychol.* **2012**, *111*, 22–36. [CrossRef] [PubMed]
164. Goffaux, V.; Rossion, B. Faces are "spatial"—Holistic face perception is supported by low spatial frequencies. *J. Exp. Psychol. Human Percept. Perform.* **2006**, *32*, 1023–1039. [CrossRef]
165. Stein, T.; Seymour, K.; Hebart, M.N.; Sterzer, P. Rapid Fear Detection Relies on High Spatial Frequencies. *Psychol. Sci.* **2014**, *25*, 566–574. [CrossRef]
166. Johnson, M.H. Subcortical face processing. *Nat. Rev. Neurosci.* **2005**, *6*, 766–774. [CrossRef]
167. Öhman, A. The role of the amygdala in human fear: Automatic detection of threat. *Psychoneuroendocrinology* **2005**, *30*, 953–958. [CrossRef]
168. Tamietto, M.; de Gelder, B. Neural bases of the non-conscious perception of emotional signals. *Nat. Rev. Neurosci.* **2010**, *11*, 697–709. [CrossRef]
169. Blom, S.S.A.H.; Aarts, H.; Semin, G.R. Lateralization of facial emotion processing and facial mimicry. *Laterality* **2020**, *25*, 259–274. [CrossRef] [PubMed]
170. Bourne, V.J. How are emotions lateralised in the brain? Contrasting existing hypotheses using the Chimeric Faces Test. *Cogn. Emot.* **2010**, *24*, 903–911. [CrossRef]
171. Demaree, H.A.; Everhart, D.E.; Youngstrom, E.A.; Harrison, D.W. Brain Lateralization of Emotional Processing: Historical Roots and a Future Incorporating "Dominance". *Behav. Cogn. Neurosci. Rev.* **2005**, *4*, 3–20. [CrossRef] [PubMed]
172. Ahern, G.L.; Schwartz, G.E. Differential lateralization for positive and negative emotion in the human brain: EEG spectral analysis. *Neuropsychologia* **1985**, *23*, 745–755. [CrossRef]
173. Davidson, R.J. Well-being and affective style: Neural substrates and biobehavioural correlates. *Phil. Trans. R. Soc. Lond. B* **2004**, *359*, 1395–1411. [CrossRef]
174. Packheiser, J.; Rook, N.; Dursun, Z.; Mesenhöller, J.; Wenglorz, A.; Güntürkün, O.; Ocklenburg, S. Embracing your emotions: Affective state impacts lateralisation of human embraces. *Psychol. Res.* **2019**, *83*, 26–36. [CrossRef]
175. Gordon, I.E. Left and right in Goya's portraits. *Nature* **1974**, *249*, 197–198. [CrossRef]
176. Mcmanus, I.C.; Humphrey, N.K. Turning the Left Cheek. *Nature* **1973**, *243*, 271–272. [CrossRef]
177. Pérez González, C. Lateral organisation in nineteenth-century studio photographs is influenced by the direction of writing: A comparison of Iranian and Spanish photographs. *Laterality Asymmetries Body Brain Cogn.* **2012**, *17*, 515–532. [CrossRef]
178. Chahboun, S.; Flumini, A.; González, C.P.; McManus, I.C.; Santiago, J. Reading and writing direction effects on the aesthetic appreciation of photographs. *Laterality Asymmetries Body Brain Cogn.* **2017**, *22*, 313–339. [CrossRef] [PubMed]
179. Powell, W.R.; Schirillo, J.A. Asymmetrical facial expressions in portraits and hemispheric laterality: A literature review. *Laterality Asymmetries Body Brain Cogn.* **2009**, *14*, 545–572. [CrossRef] [PubMed]
180. Lindell, A.K. The silent social/emotional signals in left and right cheek poses: A literature review. *Laterality Asymmetries Body Brain Cogn.* **2013**, *18*, 612–624. [CrossRef] [PubMed]
181. Lindell, A.K. Consistently Showing Your Best Side? Intra-individual Consistency in# Selfie Pose Orientation. *Front. Psychol.* **2017**, *8*, 26. [CrossRef]

182. Manovich, L.; Ferrari, V.; Bruno, N. Selfie-Takers Prefer Left Cheeks: Converging Evidence from the (Extended) selfiecity Database. *Front. Psychol.* **2017**, *8*, 1460. [CrossRef]
183. Wickens, T.; Palmer, S.; Gardner, J. Aesthetic issues in spatial composition: Effects of position and direction on framing single objects. *Spat. Vis.* **2008**, *21*, 421–449. [CrossRef]
184. Benjafield, J.; Segalowitz, S.J. Left and Right in Leonardo's Drawings of Faces. *Empir. Stud. Arts* **1993**, *11*, 25–32. [CrossRef]
185. Christman, S.; Pinger, K. Lateral Biases in Aesthetic Preferences: Pictorial Dimensions and Neural Mechanisms. *Laterality Asymmetries Body Brain Cogn.* **1997**, *2*, 155–175. [CrossRef]
186. Busin, Y.; Lukasova, K.; Asthana, M.K.; Macedo, E.C. Hemiface Differences in Visual Exploration Patterns When Judging the Authenticity of Facial Expressions. *Front. Psychol.* **2018**, *8*, 2332. [CrossRef]
187. Yamamoto, M.; Kowatari, Y.; Ueno, S.; Yamane, S.; Kitazawa, S. Accelerated recognition of left oblique views of faces. *Exp. Brain Res.* **2005**, *161*, 27–33. [CrossRef]
188. Hayes, T.; Muday, J.A.; Schirillo, J.A. Portrait hemispheric laterality measured using pupil diameter and aesthetic judgments. *Psychol. Aesthet. Creat. Arts* **2013**, *7*, 276–284. [CrossRef]
189. Grüsser, O.-J.; Selke, T.; Zynda, B. Cerebral Lateralization and Some Implications for Art, Aesthetic Perception, and Artistic Creativity. In *Beauty and the Brain: Biological Aspects of Aesthetics*; Rentschler, I., Herzberger, B., Epstein, D., Eds.; Birkhäuser: Basel, Switzerland, 1988; pp. 257–293, ISBN 978-3-0348-6350-6.
190. Lindell, A.K.; Savill, N.J. Time to turn the other cheek? The influence of left and right poses on perceptions of academic specialisation. *Laterality Asymmetries Body Brain Cogn.* **2010**, *15*, 639–650. [CrossRef] [PubMed]
191. Nicholls, M.E.R.; Clode, D.; Wood, S.J.; Wood, A.G. Laterality of expression in portraiture: Putting your best cheek forward. *Proc. R. Soc. Lond. B* **1999**, *266*, 1517–1522. [CrossRef] [PubMed]
192. Nicholls, M.E.; Roberts, G.R. Can Free-Viewing Perceptual Asymmetries be Explained by Scanning, Pre-Motor or Attentional Biases? *Cortex* **2002**, *38*, 113–136. [CrossRef]
193. Roether, C.L.; Omlor, L.; Giese, M.A. Lateral asymmetry of bodily emotion expression. *Curr. Biol.* **2008**, *18*, R329–R330. [CrossRef] [PubMed]
194. Chokron, S.; De Agostini, M. Reading habits influence aesthetic preference. *Cogn. Brain Res.* **2000**, *10*, 45–49. [CrossRef]
195. Friedrich, T.E.; Elias, L.J. The write bias: The influence of native writing direction on aesthetic preference biases. *Psychol. Aesthet. Creat. Arts* **2016**, *10*, 128–133. [CrossRef]
196. Nachson, I.; Argaman, E.; Luria, A. Effects of Directional Habits and Handedness on Aesthetic Preference for Left and Right Profiles. *J. Cross-Cult. Psychol.* **1999**, *30*, 106–114. [CrossRef]
197. Smith, A.K.; Duerksen, K.N.; Gutwin, C.; Elias, L.J. Lateral biases in aesthetic and spatial location judgments: Differences between tasks and native reading directions. *Laterality* **2020**, *25*, 5–21. [CrossRef]
198. Page, A.G.; McManus, C.; González, C.P.; Chahboun, S. Is Beauty in the Hand of the Writer? Influences of Aesthetic Preferences through Script Directions, Cultural, and Neurological Factors: A Literature Review. *Front. Psychol.* **2017**, *8*, 1325. [CrossRef]
199. Beaumont, J.G. Lateral organization and aesthetic preference: The importance of peripheral visual asymmetries. *Neuropsychologia* **1985**, *23*, 103–113. [CrossRef]
200. Levy, J. Lateral dominance and aesthetic preference. *Neuropsychologia* **1976**, *14*, 431–445. [CrossRef]
201. Gaffron, M. Left and right in pictures. *Art Q.* **1950**, *13*, 312–321.
202. Kliegl, R.; Laubrock, J.; Köstler, A. Augenblicke bei der Bildbetrachtung. Eine kognitionswissenschaftliche Spekulation zum Links und Rechts im Bild. In *Räume-Bilder-Kulturen*; Lepper, V.M., Deuflhard, P., Markschies, C., Eds.; de Gruyter: Berlin, Germany, 2015; pp. 77–90.
203. Mead, A.M.; McLaughlin, J.P. The roles of handedness and stimulus asymmetry in aesthetic preference. *Brain Cogn.* **1992**, *20*, 300–307. [CrossRef]
204. Maass, A.; Pagani, D.; Berta, E. How Beautiful is the Goal and How Violent is the Fistfight? Spatial Bias in the Interpretation of Human Behavior. *Soc. Cogn.* **2007**, *25*, 833–852. [CrossRef]
205. Flath, M.E.; Smith, A.K.; Elias, L.J. Cultural differences in lateral biases on aesthetic judgments: The effect of native reading direction. *Cult. Brain* **2019**, *7*, 57–66. [CrossRef]
206. Rodway, P.; Schepman, A.; Crossley, B.; Lee, J. A leftward perceptual asymmetry when judging the attractiveness of visual patterns. *Laterality Asymmetries Body Brain Cogn.* **2019**, *24*, 1–25. [CrossRef]
207. Cajar, A.; Engbert, R.; Laubrock, J. How spatial frequencies and color drive object search in real-world scenes: A new eye-movement corpus. *J. Vis.* **2020**, *20*, 8. [CrossRef]

208. Cajar, A.; Engbert, R.; Laubrock, J. Spatial frequency processing in the central and peripheral visual field during scene viewing. *Vis. Res.* **2016**, *127*, 186–197. [CrossRef]
209. Cajar, A.; Schneeweiß, P.; Engbert, R.; Laubrock, J. Coupling of attention and saccades when viewing scenes with central and peripheral degradation. *J. Vis.* **2016**, *16*, 8. [CrossRef]
210. Engbert, R.; Nuthmann, A.; Richter, E.M.; Kliegl, R. SWIFT: A Dynamical Model of Saccade Generation during Reading. *Psychol. Rev.* **2005**, *112*, 777–813. [CrossRef]
211. Kliegl, R.; Risse, S.; Laubrock, J. Preview benefit and parafoveal-on-foveal effects from word n + 2. *J. Exp. Psychol. Human Percept. Perform.* **2007**, *33*, 1250–1255. [CrossRef] [PubMed]
212. Pan, J.; Yan, M.; Laubrock, J. Semantic preview benefit and cost: Evidence from parafoveal fast-priming paradigm. *Cognition* **2020**, *205*, 104452. [CrossRef] [PubMed]
213. Reichle, E.D.; Pollatsek, A.; Fisher, D.L.; Rayner, K. Toward a Model of Eye Movement Control in Reading. *Psychol. Rev.* **1998**, *105*, 125. [CrossRef] [PubMed]
214. Piazza, M.; Facoetti, A.; Trussardi, A.N.; Berteletti, I.; Conte, S.; Lucangeli, D.; Dehaene, S.; Zorzi, M. Developmental trajectory of number acuity reveals a severe impairment in developmental dyscalculia. *Cognition* **2010**, *116*, 33–41. [CrossRef]
215. Zorzi, M.; Testolin, A. An emergentist perspective on the origin of number sense. *Phil. Trans. R. Soc. B* **2018**, *373*. [CrossRef]
216. De Hevia, M.D.; Veggiotti, L.; Streri, A.; Bonn, C.D. At Birth, Humans Associate "Few" with Left and "Many" with Right. *Curr. Biol.* **2017**, *27*, 3879–3884. [CrossRef]
217. Märker, G.; Learmonth, G.; Thut, G.; Harvey, M. Intra- and inter-task reliability of spatial attention measures in healthy older adults. *PLoS ONE* **2019**, *14*, e0226424. [CrossRef]

2

Major Depression and Brain Asymmetry in a Decision-Making Task with Negative and Positive Feedback

Almira Kustubayeva [1,2], Altyngul Kamzanova [1,2], Sandugash Kudaibergenova [2], Veronika Pivkina [2] and Gerald Matthews [3,*]

1 Center for Cognitive Neuroscience, Department of Biophysics, Biomedicine, and Neuroscience, Al-Farabi Kazakh National University, Almaty 050040, Kazakhstan; almkusto@kaznu.kz (A.K.); kamzanova.altyngul@kaznu.kz (A.K.)
2 Center for Cognitive Neuroscience, Department of Psychology, Al-Farabi Kazakh National University, Almaty 050040, Kazakhstan; sandugash.kudaibergenova@kaznu.kz (S.K.); pivkina_veronika@live.kaznu.kz (V.P.)
3 Institute for Simulation and Training, University of Central Florida, Orlando, FL 32826, USA
* Correspondence: gmatthews@ist.ucf.edu

Abstract: Depressed patients are characterized by hypoactivity of the left and hyperactivity of the right frontal areas during the resting state. Depression is also associated with impaired decision-making, which reflects multiple cognitive, affective, and attentional processes, some of which may be lateralized. The aim of this study was to investigate brain asymmetry during a decision-making task performed in negative and positive feedback conditions in patients with Major Depressive Disorder (MDD) in comparison to healthy control participants. The electroencephalogram (EEG) was recorded from 60 MDD patients and 60 healthy participants while performing a multi-stage decision-making task. Frontal, central, and parietal alpha asymmetry were analyzed with EEGlab/ERPlab software. Evoked potential responses (ERPs) showed general lateralization suggestive of an initial right dominance developing into a more complex pattern of asymmetry across different scalp areas as information was processed. The MDD group showed impaired mood prior to performance, and decreased confidence during performance in comparison to the control group. The resting state frontal alpha asymmetry showed lateralization in the healthy group only. Task-induced alpha power and ERP P_{100} and P_{300} amplitudes were more informative biomarkers of depression during decision making. Asymmetry coefficients based on task alpha power and ERP amplitudes showed consistency in the dynamical changes during the decision-making stages. Depression was characterized by a lack of left dominance during the resting state and left hypoactivity during the task baseline and subsequent decision-making process. Findings add to understanding of the functional significance of lateralized brain processes in depression.

Keywords: EEG; brain asymmetry; lateralization; alpha rhythm; event related potential; depression; decision-making

---

1. Introduction

Many studies have explored relationships between brain asymmetry and clinical depression, using methods including electroencephalography (EEG) and brain-imaging [1]. Depression relates to resting alpha asymmetry [2], but the functional significance of resting state asymmetry for cognitive processing during task performance requires further investigation [3]. Diminished ability to think or concentrate is a diagnostic criterion for depression in the Fifth Edition of the Diagnostic and Statistical

Manual of Mental Disorders (DSM-5) [4]. Experimental studies have confirmed decision-making deficits in depressed patients, although findings vary somewhat across different tasks [5]. Lateralized processing such as use of language, regulation of attention, and computation of costs and benefits may contribute to depression effects on decision-making [6], but direct evidence is lacking. The present study aimed to test whether patients with major depressive disorder (MDD) differed from controls in lateralized brain responses during a decision-making task, assessed using event related potentials (ERPs) and alpha power measures.

1.1. *Lateralization in the Resting Frontal EEG as a Marker of Depression*

Lateralization in frontal EEG activity has been extensively studied as a diagnostic measurement of depression [2–9]. Resting frontal alpha asymmetry (FAA) implies differentiation between depressed and healthy participants. Depressed patients were characterized by greater alpha power over the left frontal brain area in comparison to the right hemisphere, meaning hypoactivity of the left and hyperactivity of the right hemisphere [10–14]. Moreover, frontal and parietal asymmetry both served as predictive markers of the treatment effect by antidepressants or characteristic of non-responders [7,14,15]. However, FAA does not always discriminate MDD patients from control participants [16]. Indeed, a meta-analysis of 16 studies comparing frontal asymmetry during resting state in MDD patients (1883) and controls (2161) showed non-significance in the grand mean effect size [8] and raised doubts about its diagnostic capability. The authors highlighted that heterogeneity related to gender, age, and depression severity should be considered in future research. It is also unclear whether abnormality in FAA is best considered as an index of vulnerability to depression [17,18] or as a marker of brain functional state during task performance in acute depression or remission state [7,19].

1.2. *Resting Frontal Asymmetry as a Trait-Like or State-Like Measurement*

Anatomical differences may underlie stability of the EEG resting frontal asymmetry, supporting an idea of a trait-like alpha asymmetry [12,20]. From the trait perspective, FAA can be linked to the balance between the behavioral inhibition system (BIS) and the behavioral activity system (BAS) [21]. Right hemisphere hyperactivity represents inhibition, avoidance, and withdrawal whereas left hemisphere hyperactivity is associated with approach motivations. High trait BIS score and low BAS score are risk factors for depression and anxiety [22,23]. Similarly, the FAA characteristic of depression represents an affective style that is associated with deficient emotion regulation, negative affect, and low sociability and positive affect [18,24–27]. FAA was suggested as a measurement of "affective style" with moderating influences on the type of responses to emotional stimuli [2].

Alternatively, FAA may represent a transient state of brain activity that reflects situational factors including reward and punishment signals and immediate task demands as well as stable traits [18]. Consistent with the state perspective, indices of FAA may change dynamically during the resting measurement period [28]. The state perspective supports examination of asymmetry during task performance as well as at rest. FAA measurements during emotional tasks showed more powerful differences between depressed patients and controls than the resting state measure [19,29–32]. Alpha asymmetry measured during performance might contribute to understanding how disorganization of the right hemisphere contributes to deficits on a range of cognitive and emotional tasks [33]. States of asymmetry may also be associated with EEG responses to reward and punishment signals [34]. Care is necessary in determining whether states should be conceptualized as predictors, outcomes, mediators, or moderators [28].

1.3. *Decision Making in Depression and Brain Asymmetry*

Decision-making tasks involve multiple stages associated with diverse brain areas, responsible for mental functions including information processing, estimation of future results, attention to stimuli, comparison to previous experience stored in memory, evaluating future outcomes, making a choice after weighting cost/benefits, processing feedback, and comparison with estimation. Reviews of depression and decision [35,36] have, broadly, distinguished two types of mechanisms for depression effects. First, diminished energy and drive are central to depression. These motivational aspects may be associated with deficits in attention and executive control [37], deficits in effortful cognitive processing [38], and underestimation of the expected utility or value of processing effort [35,36]. Depressed patients are unwilling to expend efforts to obtain rewards, a deficit that may be associated with reduced decreased mesolimbic dopaminergic function [39,40]. Such deficits may contribute to general impairments in decision-making competence [41] and speed [37,42] observed in depressed patients.

Second, depression may be systematically related to biases in processing of rewards and threats, such as overly negative interpretations of the decision-making space [36] and underestimation of future rewards and outcomes [35,43]. A study with a battery of 10 decision-making tasks highlighted that MDD patients differed from the control group in reward and punishment learning and probability judgment tasks, as well as in pessimism bias in future expectations [44]. Impaired decision making in depression has been related to attentional bias toward negative stimuli as well as altered sensitivity to reward [37,45]. Approach and avoidance motivations are linked to congruent processing biases such as increased attention to reward and threat stimuli respectively [46]. Depression may be associated with lateralized processing biases as well as with approach/avoidance motivational tendencies.

Existing studies of the neuropsychology of decision-making provide complex findings on lateralization. A meta-analysis of functional magnetic resonance imaging (fMRI) studies [47] reported right hemisphere lateralization for some areas (e.g., prefrontal cortex, frontal eyefield) and left lateralization for others (e.g., intraparietal sulcus, basal forebrain). Lateralization is likely to be dependent on the specific cognitive processes engaged by the decision-making task, such as right hemisphere control of spatial cognition and left lateralization of language-based tasks [47]. Attentional processes contribute to a variety of tasks. A predominantly right-hemisphere frontoparietal network supports alertness and readiness [48], although other attentional networks may not be strongly lateralized [49,50]. Evidence from ERP studies on lateralization during decision-making is limited. The P_{300} has been used to investigate feedback processing in gambling tasks [51] but lateralization is not typically the major focus for such studies. Research that addresses lateralization explicitly has investigated alpha power asymmetry, most commonly in gambling-based paradigms [52]. For example, a bias towards reward on the Iowa Gambling Task, seen in high-BAS individuals, was associated with an increased left-hemisphere activity in response to losing [53]. It is largely unknown how depression might moderate asymmetry during decision-making.

1.4. ERPs in Depressed Patients

Previous EEG/ERP studies showed that ERP waves were sensitive to cognitive and emotional impairments in depression. Reviews of this literature [1,54] suggest that depression primarily impacts later waves with effects including reduced P_{300} amplitude and increased amplitude in the late positive potential (LPP). However, findings are not entirely consistent; effects on P_{300} may vary with factors including depressive subtype and the nature of the cognitive demands imposed by the task [54]. Effects on early ERPs appear to be relatively weak. The reviews cited found four studies in which N_{100} amplitude was reduced in depressed patients but larger numbers in which there was no depression effect. MDD patients also exhibit diminished brain activity and prolonged stimulus processing based on decreased peak amplitude and larger latency of P_{100} in cognitive tasks [55,56], but also at least one contrary finding is reported [57].

The effects of depression on ERPs may be modulated by affective factors. The general expectation is that depression will be associated with heightened sensitivity to stimuli of negative valence and reduced response to positive stimuli. Neuroimaging studies have tended to confirm that depressed patients show elevated brain activity to negative emotional stimuli [58,59]. Results from ERP studies are more complex. Bruder et al.'s [54] review cites studies showing reduced P_{300} response in depressives to both positive and negative stimuli. By contrast, other studies suggest mood-congruent effects associated with depressed individuals exhibiting increased P_{300} amplitude to negative stimuli including words of negative valence [60] and sad faces [61]. Monnart, Kornreich, Verbanck, and Campanella [62] reviewed studies using various attentional tasks to investigate inhibitory processes. Depression was associated with both increased and decreased P_{300} response to emotive stimuli in different task conditions, but results generally suggested that depression leads to dysfunctional inhibition of negative material. Comparable results have been found for earlier ERP components, including P_{100}, implying that depression influences multiple processing stages [62,63].

Depressed participants may be impaired in reinforcement learning processes, although depression does not appear to reliably affect the ability to learn from explicit positive and negative feedback [64]. ERP studies link depression to increased error related negativity (ERN), perhaps reflecting increased threat sensitivity or a negative cognitive bias [65], although effect sizes tend to be weak and heterogeneous [66]. Similarly, depressed participants were characterized by a larger feedback related negativity (FRN) ERP to negative feedback in comparison to the control group [25]. ERP studies have also confirmed that MDD patients are characterized by blunted reward sensitivity by using P_{300} amplitude measurements [67,68]. Another relevant indicator is the reward positivity (RewP) ERP component, which tends to be decreased in MDD patients, although results are rather mixed [66,67,69].

Bruder, Stewart, and McGrath [6] reviewed lateralization of brain function in depression through integration of findings from behavioral, electrophysiological, and brain imaging data. They concluded that the bulk of the evidence from these different sources is consistent with reduced left frontal and right parietotemporal function in depression. Consistent with this perspective, lower right-hemisphere P_{300} amplitude in depression has been observed in several studies [70]. This review [6] also discussed three studies in which depressed individuals showed reduced ERPs to emotional stimuli in the right parietal regions. Low resolution electromagnetic tomography (LORETA) has been used to infer sources of lateralization in several studies. Consistent with Bruder et al.'s [6] conclusions, Kawasaki et al. [71] reported lower P_{300} source activity in both left frontal and right temporoparietal areas, as well as bilateral prefrontal areas. Lower P_{300} source activity has been observed in the right frontal lobe, insula and limbic areas as well as in the right parietal and temporal lobes [70].

A challenge for further work in this area is that decision-making may reflect multiple brain processes that may be differentially related to depression. Many real-life decisions, like which house or a car to buy, can be taken on a rational basis, by weighing up the benefits and costs of each option. The unwillingness of depressed individuals to invest effort in demanding cognitive activity [35,36,39] leads to decision-making deficits. Biases in processing information on costs and benefits may also impair decision-making over and above insufficient effort. Depression promotes behavioral inhibition and avoidance motivation over behavioral activity and approach, which may be associated with deficits in effortful processing [72]. Such motivational deficits may be accompanied by cognitive biases that promote attention towards threat and away from reward [46]. Dysfunctional lateralization may be indexed by alpha power asymmetry [28], but ERPs may be better suited for investigating cognitive processing contributing to decision-making. Thus, for the present study, we utilized an explicit decision-making task that afforded manipulation of cost and benefit information, as well as positive and negative feedback on decisions.

1.5. Study Aims

The overall aim of the study was to test whether participants with MDD showed asymmetry in ERP responses during a cognitively demanding decision-making task, in comparison with healthy control subjects. We investigated the asymmetry of frontal, central, and parietal ERP amplitudes (P_{100} and P_{300}) and alpha spectrum power during both the resting state and performance. We anticipated that depressed patients would show asymmetries indicative of maladaptive avoidance-withdrawal tendencies [2]. We also investigated whether depression effects were moderated by different stages of processing and by affective factors.

The study utilized a decision-making task [73] that allowed ERPs to be recorded at different task stages. The task requires the participant to make a series of route choices in an Antarctic search-and-rescue scenario, in order to find the fastest route to a party of lost explorers. Choices can be made rationally by assessing the likely benefits and costs of each route, but it is demanding and effortful to do so. Previous studies confirmed the sensitivity of task performance to a range of affective factors, in nonclinical samples [73–75]. Task stages include 'Start' (initial preparedness), 'Hazard' and 'Benefit' text messages indicating potential losses and gains, 'Choice' (response selection), and 'Feedback' (positive or negative). The study also manipulated emotional context; half the participants experienced generally positive outcomes, whereas the remainder were exposed to negative outcomes. The following specific issues were investigated.

1. Lateralization of alpha during rest. Based on previous research we hypothesized that the MDD group would be characterized by lower right alpha power (i.e., right cortical hyperactivity) during the resting state.
2. Lateralization of decision-making stages. We anticipated a stronger right hemisphere response at the Start stage, reflecting the right-hemisphere frontoparietal network for alertness [48]. Processing verbal material describing costs and benefits should elicit a left hemisphere response, possibly modulated by a right-hemisphere negative emotional response to Hazard messages. However, these predictions were tentative, given the complexity of functional lateralization [47].
3. Emotional context and lateralization. We expected that emotional context would influence lateralization of ERPs. In the negative emotion condition, the experimental software was rigged so that participants' choices typically led to negative outcomes, leading to progressively diminishing likelihood of rescuing the explorers, and frequent negative feedback. We anticipated heightened right-hemisphere response amplitude in this condition, especially in response to hazard messages and negative feedback.
4. Impact of major depression. We expected that depression would be associated with resting alpha asymmetry [2,59], and we tested for this effect persisting during task performance. We also anticipated reduced right temporoparietal P_{300} amplitude in MDD patients [6,70]. We expected this effect of depression to be stronger in response to benefit messages and to feedback in the positive emotion condition, given evidence for reduced sensitivity to reward [6,67]. Findings with threat-related stimuli have been more equivocal; in some studies negative-valent stimuli evoke a stronger response in depressed individuals [60,61]. Most previous studies have investigated P_{300}, but we anticipated parallel effects for P_{100}, given that depression may also impair early attentional processes [62,63].
5. Relationships between task-induced alpha asymmetry and ERP amplitude. Previous studies have not investigated how ERP amplitude asymmetry during task performance is related to the asymmetry in alpha power. We measured the alpha response to the task stages for comparison with ERPs. As this was a supplementary analysis, we restricted it to frontal and parietal alpha in the time interval corresponding to P_{300}. These sites have been the main focus of previous studies of alpha asymmetry [2]. We expected that task-induced alpha would show depression effects on lateralization similar to the well-known FAA effect. To determine the equivalence of alpha and ERP measures of lateralization, we correlated measures of asymmetry in resting and task-induced alpha with measures of asymmetry in ERP response.

2. Method

2.1. Participants

Sixty volunteers who were diagnosed for the first time with major depressive disorder (MDD group: 30 males and 30 females: mean age = 26.62, SD = 7.45) and 60 healthy volunteers (control group: 30 males and 30 females: mean age = 25.35, SD = 6.42) participated. The study was approved by the Ethics Committee of the Faculty of Medicine and Health Care of the Al-Farabi Kazakh National University. Healthy participants were recruited by advertisement through social networks from the general public of Almaty city area and patients from Republican Scientific and Practical Center of

Mental Health. All participants were medication-free and had not started any treatment. They were right-handed and had normal or corrected vision. Volunteers with substance or alcohol abuse were excluded from the study. Women were excluded if they were having a menstrual period, or if they had been diagnosed with PMS (premenstrual syndrome). After signing the consent form all subjects completed the Inventory of Depressive Symptomatology I (IDS: Rush et al., 1996). Subjects who had an IDS score higher than 20 completed the Hamilton Rating Scale for Depression (HRSD, 1980). They were then interviewed by a clinical psychologist and by a psychiatrist for diagnosis (based on ICD-10, International Statistical Classification of Diseases and Related Health Problems).

2.2. *Design and Procedure*

The study utilized a 2 × 2 (group: healthy vs. depressed × feedback condition: positive vs. negative feedback) design, with repeated measures for feedback condition. Participants meeting the inclusion criteria initially completed the mood scale, and then viewed a detailed PowerPoint description of the decision-making task. Electrodes for EEG were attached and a 1-min baseline recording with eyes closed was obtained. Participants performed 30 trials on the decision-making task in each feedback condition, with order of conditions counterbalanced across participants. Mood and confidence ratings were obtained after every 10 trials. Finally, participants were debriefed.

2.3. *Questionnaire Measurements of Emotional State*

The first section of the Dundee Stress State Questionnaire (DSSQ) [76] assessed energetic arousal, tense arousal, hedonic tone, and frustration and anger before the decision-making task. Additionally, after every ten trials during task performance participants were asked "How much positive mood are you experiencing?" and "How confident are you about your ability to make the best choice?" (along with other questions). Participants responded on a 1–4 scale anchored by "Not at all" and "Very much".

2.4. *Decision-Making Task*

The "search-and-rescue" tactical decision-making task [73,75] was programmed in E-Prime 2.0 (Psychology Software Tools, Pittsburgh, PA, USA). It was adapted to the EEG/ERP experiment. The participant performed a rescue operation with a goal to find as fast as possible a lost party of explorers in the Antarctic and save their lives [75]. The participant was required to make 30 successive route choices (trials) to find the fastest route while driving a snowcat vehicle to the location of the lost party. Each trial presented a map of the terrain with two alternative color-coded routes and four icons for potential hazards and benefits on the routes (one hazard and one benefit on each route). A statement about probabilities of loss or gain and their percentage likelihoods in each route appeared to participants when they placed a cursor over icons, using the mouse. For example, a hazard might be a 20% chance of an avalanche that would cause a 40-min delay. After assessing the cost and benefit information, participants were prompted to make a route choice by clicking on one of two color-coded circles presented on the display. Information about the result of the choice was given after each route selection following each trial, which contained an image of the occurred event and a statement of time that had been lost or gained. The feedback screen described overall time lost or gained across all trials, with an image of either a contented or discontented explorer. EEG markers were added to the E-Prime task for the key events of each trial: start, benefits, hazards, choice of route, and feedback.

Each participant performed in positive and negative feedback conditions. The outcomes for each route choice were predetermined. In the positive feedback condition, benefits (time gains) were obtained on the majority of trials, whereas in the negative feedback condition, costs (time losses) predominated [75]. Thus, in the former condition, participants accumulated gains (with occasional losses) so that they became progressively further ahead of the schedule necessary to reach the lost party before the explorers expired. In the negative feedback condition, prospects of reaching the lost party became increasingly unlikely. Following the final trial, success or failure was confirmed according to feedback condition (Figure 1).

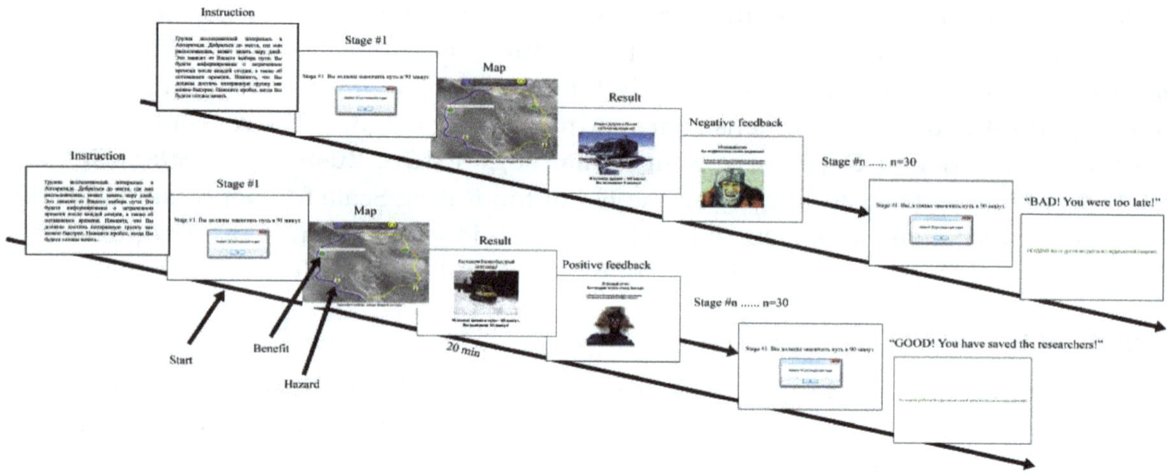

Figure 1. Decision-making task scheme and stimulus sequence in two feedback conditions. English statements above the final slides are translated from the original Russian.

Dependent measures were overall decision time, and the total time taken by the participant to inspect the hazard and benefit text descriptions ("inspection time")..

2.5. EEG Recording

EEG was recorded with a Neuron-Spectrum_4 system (Neurosoft Ltd., Ivanovo, Russia) in the following situations: baseline recording with closed eyes (1 min); performance of the decision-making task (40 min). Ag/AgCl electrodes were placed by using the 10–20% international system monopolar from the left and right frontal, parietal, occipital, and central areas (F_3, F_4, F_7, F_8, C_3, C_4, P_3, P_4, O_1, O_2, FP_z, F_z, FC_z, C_z, CP_z, P_z, O_z) using an electrode cap (Neurosoft) with an indifferent ear electrode. An additional two electrodes were used for vertical and horizontal electrooculogram recording. Electrode impedance was below 5 kOhm. EEG data were acquired with a sampling rate of 256 Hz. Synchronization between EEG and E-Prime software was programmed to elicit ERPs on the markers sent by the E-Prime task.

2.6. EEG Preprocessing

Spectral power density (SPD) was analyzed in Neuron-Spectrum NET software, version 3 for Windows (Neurosoft, 2019). Alpha SPD values were generated between 8–13 Hz from the right and left frontal (F_3, F_4) and parietal (P_3, P_4) electrodes, at rest and at each task stage. The alpha asymmetry coefficient was calculated by the formula ln[Right]-ln[Left] [77]. Data on reliability and validity of the coefficient are provided in [77]. ERP preprocessing was done in EEGLAB/ERPLAB toolbox [78,79] based on MATLAB R2019b [80]. The analysis included DC correction, epoching, baseline correction, artifact rejection (±75uV), and artifact removal by using ICA (independent component analysis). ICA identifies mutually independent component time courses in the spatially distributed recording [78]. Artifacts are independent from brain signals and may be presented as separate components that are easy to detect visually. EEGLAB performs ICA decomposition using the runica() algorithm, an automated and enhanced version of the infomax ICA algorithm [78]. ICA components with their time course were visually inspected. Frontal muscle tension artifacts usually appear at high frequencies (more then 20–50 Hz) and are localized spatially. Eyeblink artefacts can also be identified in a smoothly decreased EEG spectrum with far-frontal localization. Artifactual components were rejected on this basis. Rejected data were less than 10% overall. High bandpass 0.1 Hz filtering and low bandpass 30Hz filtering were applied in two steps to further reduce EMG artefact and to remove line noise during the entire recording. Artifact free EEG epochs between 200 ms pre-stimulus and 800 ms post-stimulus were extracted for the following events representing successive stages of decision-making:

Start. Participant clicks left mouse key following the presentation of the word "start" on the screen, initiating the next trial and displaying the routes on the map.

Hazards and Benefits. The map display includes warning triangle and smile icons for each route. The mouse is used to display a text box associated with the icon that states the probability of losing or gaining a fixed amount of time. The event for the ERP is the first occasion on which the participant accesses the hazards or benefits text. The participant chooses whether hazard or benefit information is accessed first but must access both.

Choice. The participant clicks on one of two colored circles on the map to make their route choice.

Feedback. The positive or negative feedback screen appears, showing overall progress relative to the time schedule for reaching the explorers.

P_{300} amplitude was measured as a peak between 200–500 ms, P_{100} as a peak between 50–150 ms at each stage for each electrode.

Additionally, ERP power spectrum for alpha frequency (8–13 Hz) was calculated for each category of stimulus during task performance, during the 200–500 ms interval after each event.

2.7. Statistical Analysis

The primary dependent variables from the EEG were P_{100} and P_{300} amplitudes. Mixed-model ANOVAs with two within-subject variables ('side': left (L) and right (R); 'feedback condition': positive and negative) and one between-subject variable ('group': MDD and Hth) were performed in SPSS for corresponding lateralized electrode pairs [81]. Supplementary analyses were conducted on alpha power. The dependent variable for analyses of alpha response during task performance indexed asymmetry of activity, measured at frontal (F_3–F_4) and parietal (P_3–P_4 sites). Effect sizes were quantified using the partial eta squared (η^2_p) statistic, defined as the ratio of the variability accounted for by an effect and the variability of that effect plus its associated error.

3. Results

3.1. Demographic Data

Demographic data and depression scores (IDS) for both groups are presented in Table 1. There was no difference in mean age between groups. Mean IDS score was significantly higher in the MDD group ($t = 14.834$, $p < 0.0005$) in comparison to Healthy participants.

Table 1. Demographic and clinical data.

Group	Gender	N	Age	IDS Score
MDD	Females	30	27.10, SD = 7.68	42.73 SD = 9.23
	Males	30	26.13, SD = 7.31	37.13 SD = 10.20
		60	26.62, SD = 7.45	39.93, SD = 10.05
Healthy	Females	30	24.6, SD = 7.07	17.90 SD = 6.43
	Males	30	26.10, SD = 5.71	15.40 SD = 7.12
		60	25.35, SD = 6.42	16.65, SD = 6.84

3.2. Mood Assessment

Pretask DSSQ parameters such as tense arousal ($t = 5.264$, $p < 0.0001$) and anger/frustration ($t = 5.146$, $p < 0.0001$) were significantly larger, whereas energetic arousal ($t = -5.759$, $p < 0.0001$) and hedonic tone ($t = -7.129$, $p < 0.0001$) showed lower scores in the MDD group in comparison to Hth group participants (Figure 2). Cronbach's alphas for DSSQ scores were as follows: tense arousal 0.796; anger/frustration 0.796; energetic arousal 0.564; hedonic tone 0.719. These data confirm the consistency of the translated questionnaire, except for energetic arousal.

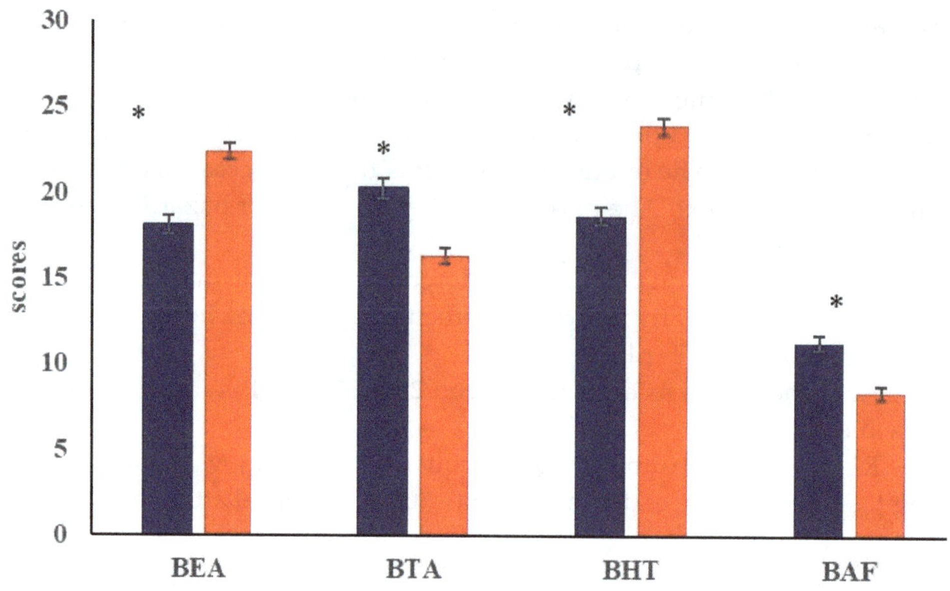

Figure 2. DSSQ scores before experiment: BEA—Energetic Arousal, BTA—Tense Arousal; BHT—Hedonic Tone; BAF—Anger/Frustration. MDD group in blue, Hth group in red. * $p < 0.05$.

The mood and confidence ratings obtained during the task were analyzed with $3 \times 2 \times 2$ (trial $\times$ feedback condition $\times$ group) mixed-model ANOVAs, where trial refers to ratings after 10, 20, and 30 trials. For mood, there was a significant main effect of condition ($F(1,118) = 17.694$, $p < 0.0001$, $\eta^2_p = 0.130$), with poorer mood in the negative condition (mean = 2.333, SE = 0.083) in comparison to the positive condition (mean = 2.625, SE = 0.092). A trend towards poorer mood in the MDD group failed to reach significance. There were no significant interactions. For confidence, there was a significant main effect of condition ($F(1,118) = 49.000$, $p < 0.0001$, $\eta^2_p = 0.293$), moderated by a condition $\times$ trial interaction ($F(2,236) = 8.149$, $p < 0.0001$, $\eta^2_p = 0.065$). Confidence was lower in the negative feedback condition, with the effect increasing across trials. At trial 10, confidence means were 2.883 (SE = 0.079) in the negative condition and 3.117 (SE = 0.066) in the positive condition. By trial 30, means were 2.583 (SD = 0.090) in the negative condition and 3.217 (SD = 0.074) in the positive condition. There was also a significant effect of group ($F(1,118) = 11.230$, $p < 0.01$, $\eta^2_p = 0.087$). Confidence was higher in the healthy group (M = 3.164, SE = 0.083) than in the depressed group (M = 2.772, SE = 0.083). There were no further significant interactions involving the group factor. Thus, it was confirmed that feedback condition influenced mood and confidence as expected, but depression was associated primarily with a decrease in confidence.

3.3. *Behavioral Results*

Table 2 shows behavioral data from the decision-making task. Overall decision time (DT) from the onset of the map stimulus to the time of the participant's choice of route was analyzed using a 2×2 (feedback condition $\times$ group) mixed-model ANOVA. There were no significant main effects or interaction.

The inspection times (ITs) for benefits and hazards refer to the total times during which the participant was using the mouse to display the text information on potential time gains and costs for each route. Data were analyzed with a $2 \times 2 \times 2$ (feedback condition $\times$ information type $\times$ group) mixed-model ANOVA, where information type contrasts benefits and hazards. The analysis showed a significant group effect ($F(1,118) = 7.067$, $p = 0.009$, $\eta^2_p = 0.057$) with longer ITs in MDD in comparison to Hth group participants (Figure 3). A significant information type effect ($F(1,118) = 12.284$, $p = 0.001$, $\eta^2_p = 0.094$; longer for hazard) provided evidence that participants attended more to negative than to positive information.

Table 2. Response time data for MDD and healthy groups as function of feedback condition.

Group	Condition	$DT_{decision\text{-}making}$, ms	IT $_{benefits}$, ms	IT $_{hazards}$, ms
MDD	Negative	15,548.74, SD = 3517.06	920.87, SD = 352.25	966.39, SD = 465.42
	Positive	14,954.47, SD = 4462.41	834.59, SD = 261.74	896.20, SD = 309.73
	Both conditions	14,639.11, SD = 3495.28	877.73, SD = 312.03	931.29, SD = 395.23
Healthy	Negative	14,854.67, SD = 3671.71	734.60, SD = 238.73	840.91, SD = 302.64
	Positive	14,046.56, SD = 3602.41	762.20, SD = 240.49	811.24, SD = 305.65
	Both conditions	14,450.61, SD = 3644.57	748.40, SD = 239.00	826.08, SD = 303.23

Note DT = Decision time, IT = Inspection time.

3.4. EEG Results

3.4.1. Lateralization in the Power of Resting Alpha

Two 2 × 2 (side × group) mixed-model ANOVAs were run to test the effects of the independent variables on resting alpha power at the paired frontal and parietal sites. The analysis showed a significant side effect ($F(1,118) = 7.590$, $p = 0.007$, $\eta^2_p = 0.060$) with higher alpha SPD in the right frontal F_4 (mean = 3.55, SE = 0.35) in comparison to F_3 (mean = 3.30, SE = 3.12) electrodes in all participants. There were no significant group effects or group × side interactions. Given the reliability of FAA differences in previous depression studies, we tested for side effects in each group separately, as planned comparisons, despite the lack of a significant interaction. There was a significant side effect only in the healthy group ($F(1,59) = 4.85$, $p = 0.032$, $\eta^2 = 0.076$, F_3: mean = 3.50, SE = 0.50; F_4: mean = 3.73, SE = 0.50). We observed lower alpha power in the left hemisphere in the healthy group but no asymmetry in the MDD group. The side effect was significant for alpha at parietal electrodes P_3 vs. P_4 ($F(1,118) = 6.644$, $p = 0.011$, $\eta^2_p = 0.053$), resulting from higher alpha power in the right hemisphere (mean = 8.30, SE = 1.04) in comparison to the left (mean = 7.14, SE = 0.96). However, there were no main or interactive effects involving group at parietal sites. Repeated-measures *t*-tests showed no significant group effects on the alpha asymmetry coefficient for either frontal or parietal electrodes.

3.4.2. Effects of Task Factors and Depression on ERP Amplitudes

Mixed-model 2 × 2 × 2 (side × feedback condition × group) ANOVAs were used to analyze factors influencing P_{100} and P_{300} amplitudes. Analyses were run separately for four lateralized electrode pairs, i.e., F_3 vs. F_4, F_7 vs. F_8, C_3 vs. C_4, and P_3 vs. P_4. Data were analyzed for ERPs to the key stages of the task: start of the trial, accessing hazard and benefit information, responding with a route choice, and receiving feedback.

Results from these analyses are presented in three subsections reflecting the aims of the study. First, we report the main effects of the side factor, which indicate the extent to which ERPs were generally lateralized during stages of decision-making. Second, we report the main effects of feedback condition and condition × side interactions, indicating the impact of emotional context and its effect on lateralization. Third, we report the main and interactive effects for the group factor, defining differences between healthy and depressed groups overall and in lateralization. Effects relevant to study aims are illustrated with amplitude plots and topographic maps as appropriate. The relevant cell means for each set of analyses are included in Supplementary Materials.

Lateralization of ERP Amplitudes during Decision-Making Task

The ANOVAs revealed significant ($p < 0.05$ or better) effects of side for responses at all task stages: Start (Figure 3), Hazard/Benefit (Figure 4), Choice (Figure 5), and Feedback (Figure 6). Analyses of P_{100} amplitude to Start revealed significant side effects in the central (C_3 vs. C_4, $F(1,118) = 18.177$, $p < 0.0001$, $\eta^2_p = 0.133$), and parietal (P_3 vs. P_4, $F(1,118) = 13.645$, $p < 0.0001$, $\eta^2_p = 0.104$) electrodes, with higher right response in both cases. P_{300} amplitude was higher in the right side in frontal (F_3 vs. F_4, $F(1,118) = 4.969$, $p = 0.028$, $\eta^2_p = 0.040$), and parietal (P_3 vs. P_4, $F(1,118) = 14.259$, $p < 0.0001$, $\eta^2_p = 0.108$) electrodes.

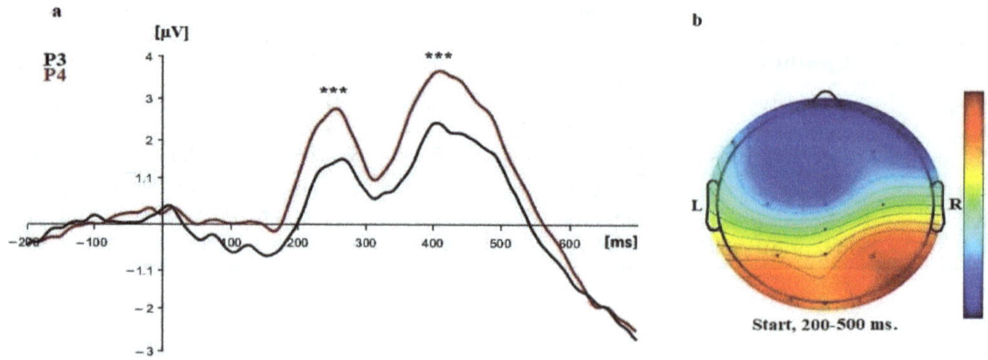

Figure 3. (**a**) ERPs for P300 to Start at P_3 (black line) and P_4 (red line) electrodes. (**b**) 2-d map of the mean P_{300} amplitude between 200–500 ms. *** $p < 0.001$.

Hazard and Benefit. The most consistent effect was left-lateralization of P_{100}. Hazard produced higher left P_{100} amplitude in the analyses of F_3 vs. F_4 ($F(1,118) = 8.573$, $p = 0.004$, $\eta^2{}_p = 0.068$, Figure 4, upper) and of F_7 vs. F_8 ($F(1,118) = 7.919$, $p = 0.006$, $\eta^2{}_p = 0.063$). Benefit induced higher left P_{100} amplitude in the central C_3 vs. C_4 ($F(1,118) = 6.968$, $p = 0.009$, $\eta^2{}_p = 0.056$, Figure 4, lower) analysis. Contrary to these trends, right dominance of P_{100} amplitude was observed to Benefit in parietal electrodes (P_3 vs. P_4: $F(1,118) = 3.991$, $p = 0.048$, $\eta^2{}_p = 0.033$.

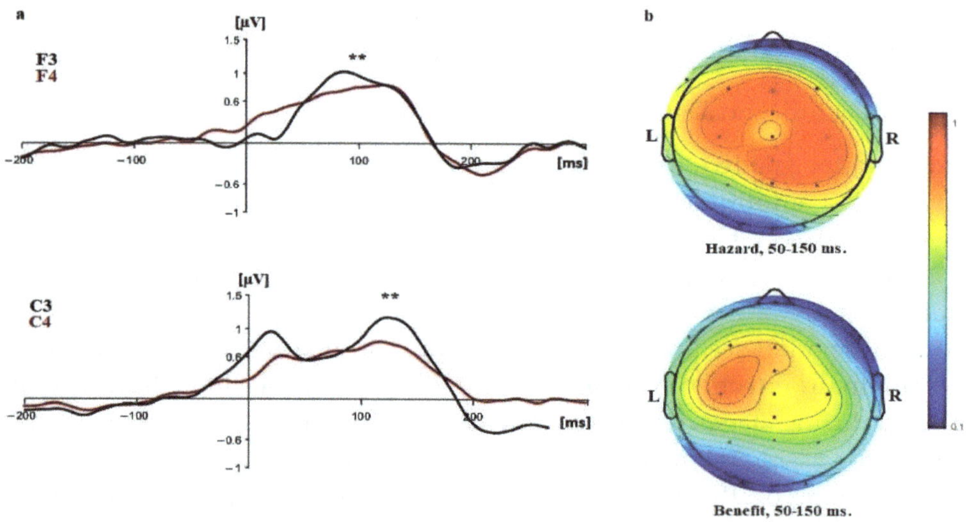

Figure 4. (**a**) ERPs for P_{100} to Hazard (F_3 black line and F_4 red line), upper) and Benefit (C_3 black line and C_4 red line, lower). (**b**) 2-d maps of the mean P_{100} amplitude between 50–150 ms. ** $p < 0.01$.

The Choice stage was characterized by larger P_{100} and P_{300} amplitudes in the left frontal (F_3 vs. F_4: P_{100}, $F(1,118) = 5.054$, $p = 0.026$, $\eta^2{}_p = 0.041$, P_{300}, $F(1,118) = 4.829$, $p = 0.030$, $\eta^2{}_p = 0.039$, F_7 vs. F_8: P_{100}, $F(1,118) = 4.448$, $p = 0.037$, $\eta^2{}_p = 0.036$) and in the right central and parietal electrodes (C_3 vs. C_4: P_{300}, $F(1,118) = 4.503$, $p = 0.036$, $\eta^2{}_p = 0.037$; P_3 vs. P_4: P_{100}, $F(1,118) = 7.327$, $p = 0.008$, $\eta^2{}_p = 0.058$) (see Figure 5).

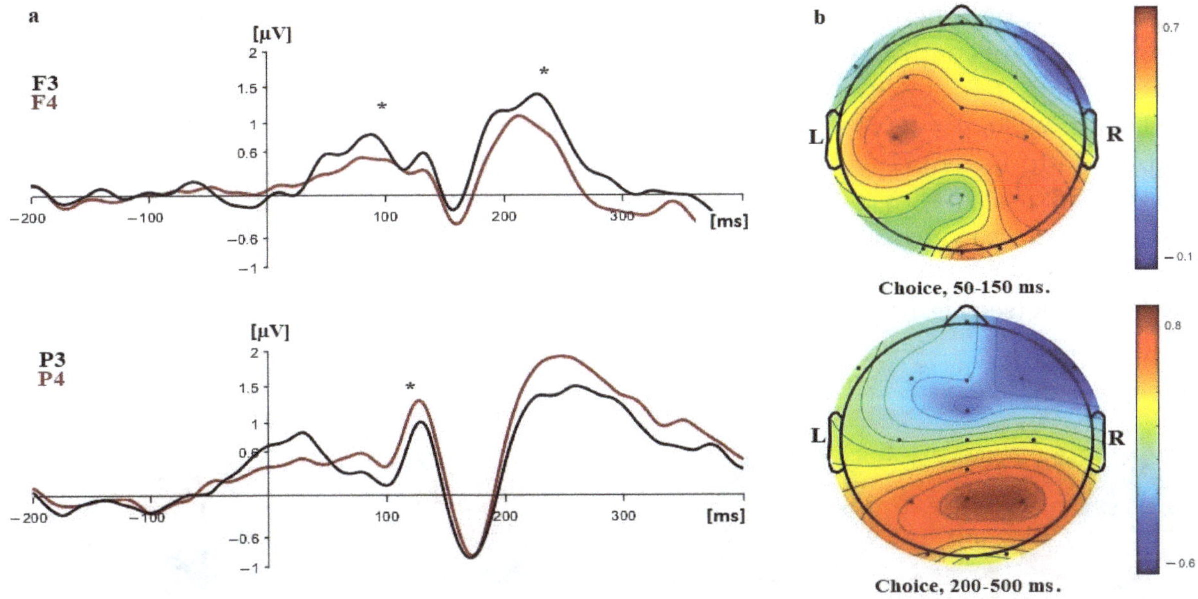

Figure 5. (**a**) ERPs for P_{100} and P_{300} to Choice on F_3 (black line) and F_4 (red line) electrodes (left dominance) and for P_{100} to Choice on P_3 (black line) and P_4 (red line) electrodes (right dominance), * $p < 0.05$. Right upper: 2-d map of mean P_{100} amplitude. (**b**) lower: 2-d map of mean P_{300} amplitude.

In response to Feedback, P_{100} and P_{300} amplitudes in the right central (C3 vs. C4: P100 ($F(1,118) = 5.336$, $p = 0.023$, $\eta^2_p = 0.043$); P_{300} ($F(1,118) = 10.835$, $p = 0.001$, $\eta^2_p = 0.084$) and right parietal (P3 vs. P4: P_{100} ($F(1,118) = 16.849$, $p < 0.0001$, $\eta^2_p = 0.125$); P_{300} ($F(1,118) = 7.843$, $p = 0.006$, $\eta^2_p = 0.062$) electrodes showed lateralization effects. Elevated right parietal response is shown in Figure 6. By contrast, left frontal dominance was observed in F7 vs. F8 P_{300} amplitude ($F(1,118) = 4.378$, $p = 0.039$, $\eta^2_p = 0.036$).

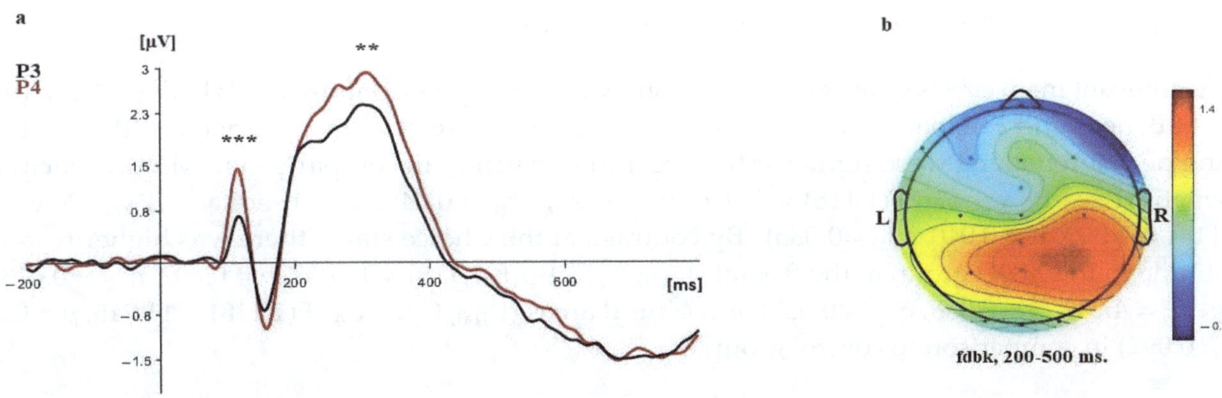

Figure 6. (**a**) ERPs for P_{300} on feedback on P_3 (black line) and P_4 (red line) electrodes. (**b**) 2-d map of mean P_{300} amplitude, ** $p < 0.01$, *** $p < 0.001$.

ERP Amplitudes and Brain Asymmetry in Positive and Negative Feedback Conditions

Significant main effects of feedback condition revealed larger ERP amplitudes in the negative condition at the Benefit (F_3/F_4: P_{100}, $F(1,118) = 4.695$, $p = 0.032$, $\eta^2_p = 0.038$; P_3/P_4: P_{300}, $F(1,118) = 5.985$, $p = 0.016$, $\eta^2_p = 0.048$); Choice (F_3/F_4: P_{100}, $F(1,118) = 5.133$, $p = 0.025$, $\eta^2_p = 0.042$); and Feedback stages (F_3/F_4: P_{100}, $F(1,118) = 6.616$, $p = 0.011$, $\eta^2_p = 0.053$).

There were a few significant feedback condition × side effects in ERPs amplitudes during task performance supporting the hypothesis about hemisphere emotional valence to some extent. The negative feedback condition was characterized by a tendency towards a later hyperactivity in the right central areas, whereas the positive condition induced an earlier stronger left frontal dominance.

However, the left/right hemisphere prevalence was dependent on the task stage, as shown in the following significant condition × side effects. Stronger right dominance in negative condition was observed to Start (P_{300}, C_3 vs. C_4: $F(1,118) = 4.651$, $p = 0.033$, $\eta^2_p = 0.038$) and Hazard (C_3 vs. C_4: $F(1,118) = 3.930$, $p = 0.050$, $\eta^2_p = 0.032$). Left dominance in positive condition was found in P_{100} amplitude to Benefit ($F_{3\ vs.}$ F_4: $F(1,118) = 6.452$, $p = 0.012$, $\eta^2_p = 0.052$) and Choice ($F_{7\ vs.}$ F_8: $F(1,118) = 4.125$, $p = 0.044$, $\eta^2_p = 0.034$). The significant main effects of feedback condition implied a general tendency towards lower early frontal activity in the positive condition. The interactions suggest that this effect was driven primarily by reduced activity in the right hemisphere following positive feedback (see Figure 7).

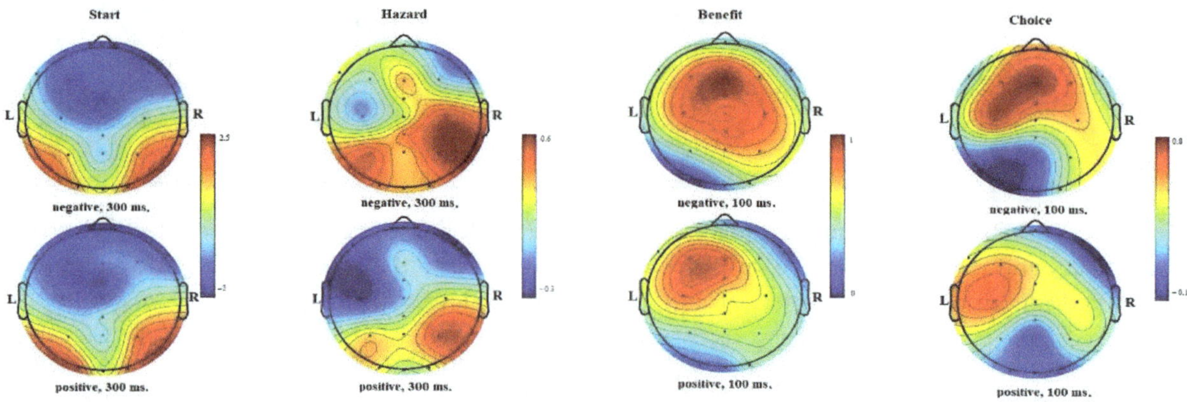

Figure 7. 2-d maps of for P_{300} amplitude to Start and Hazard 300 ms after stimulus onset; and P_{100} to Benefit and Choice in 100 ms after stimulus onset in both feedback conditions: negative and positive.

ERP Amplitudes and Brain Asymmetry Differences in MDD and Hth Groups

Significant main effects of the group factor showed that depressed individuals had weaker parietal P_{300}s at Benefit and Feedback stages, but stronger P_{100} response at Choice. Parietal ERP amplitudes during decision making were significantly larger in Hth group in comparison to MDD participants to Benefit (P_{300}, P_3 vs. P_4: $F(1,118) = 4.926$, $p = 0.028$, $\eta^2_p = 0.040$) and Feedback (P_{300}, P_3 vs. P_4: $F(1,118) = 4.293$, $p = 0.040$, $\eta^2_p = 0.035$). By contrast, at the Choice stage, there was higher response amplitude in the MDD group in the frontal (P_{100}, $F_{3\ vs.}$ F_4: $F(1,118) = 10.052$, $p = 0.002$, $\eta^2_p = 0.078$; F_7 vs. F_8: $F = 4.517$, $p = 0.036$, $\eta^2_p = 0.037$) and central areas ($P_{100,}$ $C_{3\ vs.}$ C_4: $F(1,118) = 11.945$, $p = 0.001$, $\eta^2_p = 0.092$) in comparison to control group.

Significant group × side effects were found to Start in the central electrodes (P_{300}, C_3 vs. C_4: $F(1,118) = 9.138$, $p = 0.003$, $\eta^2_p = 0.072$) with larger right dominance in the MDD group, supporting the hypothesis of the left hypoactivity in depression. There was a significant main effect of the side factor for this ERP with stronger right response; this lateralization was more pronounced in depressed individuals, as shown in Figure 8. Parietal asymmetry to Hazard in the MDD group was characterized by left dominance and Hth group by right dominance (P_3 vs. P_4: P_{100}, $F(1,118) = 6.261$, $p = 0.014$, $\eta^2_p = 0.050$, P_{300}, $F(1,118) = 5.282$, $p = 0.023$, $\eta^2_p = 0.043$), probably, as result of an overreaction to hazards in the MDD group. There was a significant main effect of side on P_{300} parietal response to Hazard, associated with right dominance; the interaction suggests this effect was driven by the healthy group.

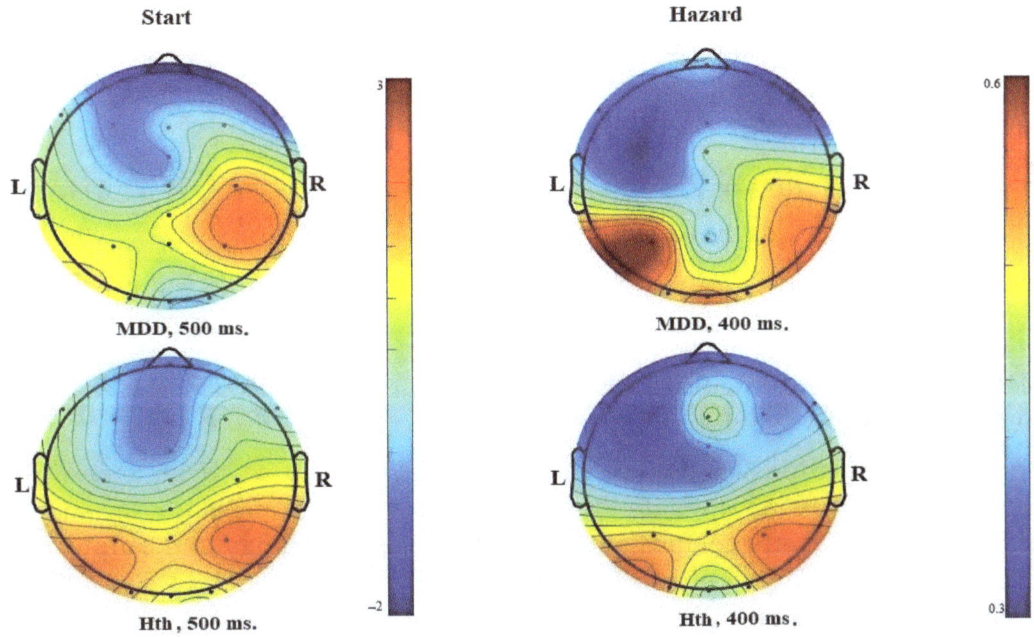

Figure 8. ERPs 2-d maps of the amplitude for P_{300} to Start (500 ms) and Hazard (400 ms) in MDD and Healthy groups.

3.4.3. Effects of Task Factors and Depression on the Task-Induced Alpha Asymmetry Coefficient

The alpha asymmetry coefficient was calculated for each stage at frontal and parietal sites. There was a trend towards dominance of the right hemisphere at the feedback stage. However, none of the means for the whole sample differed significantly from zero on Bonferroni-corrected 1-sample *t*-tests, indicating that task-induced alpha was not lateralized overall.

Effects of independent variables on the task-induced alpha asymmetry coefficient were analyzed with a series of 2 × 2 (feedback condition × group) mixed-model ANOVAs. Several significant main effects of group showed that the coefficient was significantly lower in the MDD group in frontal area to Start ($F(1,118) = 4.95$, $p = 0.028$, $\eta^2_p = 0.040$) and Feedback ($F(1,118) = 4.183$, $p = 0.043$, $\eta^2_p = 0.034$) and in parietal area to Start ($F(1,118) = 14.633$, $p < 0.0001$, $\eta^2_p = 0.110$), Hazard ($F(1,118) = 4.306$, $p = 0.040$, $\eta^2_p = 0.035$), and Choice ($F(1,118) = 8.392$, $p = 0.004$, $\eta^2_p = 0.066$). Means for the coefficient in the two groups are shown in Table 3. The healthy group showed a general trend towards left lateralization (i.e., higher alpha power in the right hemisphere) whereas the depressed participants tended to show the opposite tendency or minimal lateralization). Figure 9 shows topographic maps for the two groups and the difference between them at the feedback stage. No significant main or interactive effects of feedback condition were found.

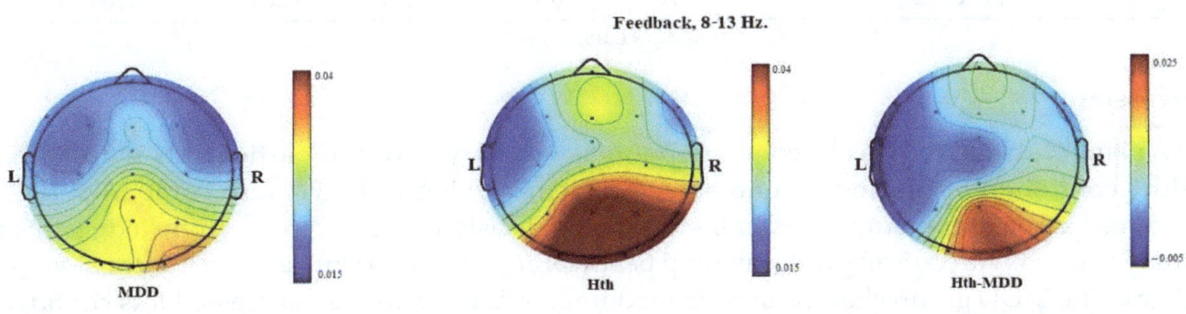

Figure 9. Alpha power spectrum to 'feedback' between 8–13 Hz in MDD and Healthy groups and difference between groups (Hth-MDD).

Table 3. Mean (and SE) values for alpha asymmetry coefficient at multiple task stages in frontal and parietal areas, in healthy and depressed groups.

	Frontal		Parietal	
	Hth	**MDD**	**Hth**	**MDD**
Start	0.091 (0.069)	−0.127 (0.069)	0.484 (0.106)	−0.086 (0.106)
Hazard	0.038 (0.082)	0.002 (0.082)	0.234 (0.103)	−0.067 (0.103)
Benefit	0.075 (0.093)	−0.164 (0.093)	0.114 (0.123)	0.149 (0.123)
Choice	0.104 (0.071)	−0.035 (0.071)	0.320 (0.102)	−0.097 (0.102)
Feedback	0.175 (0.077)	−0.050 (0.077)	0.336 (0.115)	0.181 (0.115)

3.4.4. Correlations between Resting State Alpha Coefficient, Task-Induced Alpha Asymmetry Coefficient, and Task-Induced Amplitude Coefficient

To investigate the relationship between the alpha asymmetry coefficients and asymmetry in P_{300} response, correlations were calculated between the two sets of measures, as shown in Table 4. For this analysis, P_{300} asymmetry coefficients were calculated by analogy to the alpha coefficient, i.e., ln[Right]-ln[Left] [77]. There was only one significant positive correlation between the resting state alpha asymmetry coefficients and the ERP measures: for the parietal response at the Choice stage. However, the task-induced alpha coefficients tended to correlate positively with P_{300} amplitudes, more strongly for the parietal response (range of *r*s: 0.129–0.454) than for the frontal response (range of *r*s: 0.069–0.297). Thus, during task performance, asymmetry in alpha was related to asymmetry in ERP amplitude, although correlation magnitudes were typically small to moderate (Table 4).

Table 4. Correlations between Alpha and P_{300} amplitude asymmetry coefficients.

Alpha Asymmetry Coefficient	P_{300} Amplitude Asymmetry Coefficient				
	Start	**Benefit**	**Hazard**	**Choice**	**Feedback**
Frontal					
Resting State	0.030	0.017	0.028	−0.037	0.082
Start	0.213 *	0.091	0.220 *	0.110	0.091
Benefit	0.165	0.146	0.116	0.289 **	0.147
Hazard	0.213 *	0.133	0.089	0.287 **	0.207*
Choice	0.157	0.178	0.148	0.297 **	0.281 **
Feedback	0.069	0.140	0.182*	0.111	0.124
Parietal					
Resting State	0.135	0.053	0.144	0.185 *	0.109
Start	0.364 **	0.193 *	0.331 **	0.244 **	0.137
Benefit	0.242 **	0.216 *	0.257 **	0.341 **	0.129
Hazard	0.317 **	0.313 **	0.452 **	0.454 **	0.198 *
Choice	0.248 **	0.276 **	0.429 **	0.379 **	0.220 *
Feedback	0.373 **	0.144	0.201 *	0.281 **	0.184 *

Note * $p < 0.05$, ** $p < 0.01$

4. Discussion

The aim of the study was to compare brain asymmetry between participants with MDD and a healthy control group during a multi-stage decision-making task. We also compared ERPs and task-induced alpha as measures of asymmetry during decision-making; to our knowledge, this is the first study to do so. We confirmed affective and behavioral impacts of depression in the decision-making paradigm. The MDD group showed initial mood impairments, and they expressed less confidence in their ability to perform the task. They also took more time to inspect information on costs and benefits of decisional choices. Thus, the task seemed suitable as a test bed for investigating neurocognitive characteristics of depression.

To accomplish the overall study aim we investigated five specific issues as listed previously, with the following broad outcomes. First, analyses of resting alpha provided some limited evidence for left dominance of frontal response in healthy but not depressed participants, as hypothesized. Second, there was strong evidence for lateralization of ERP response during decision-making, depending on task stage, electrode site, and ERP wave. Third, we found support for the hypothesis that persistent negative feedback and processing negative information would increase right-lateralization of ERPs, although the relevant effects on asymmetry were highly specific to stages. Fourth, we confirmed that depression influenced asymmetry in ERP response, although effects were stage-specific and there was no general right dominance in the MDD group. Fifth, task-induced alpha was moderately correlated with ERP amplitude, but only ERPs showed overall lateralization effects. However, healthy participants showed a general trend towards left dominance of alpha response, as predicted. The remainder of this section discusses key issues in more depth and acknowledges some study limitations.

4.1. Asymmetry in ERP Response during Decision-Making

Table 5 summarizes significant ERP lateralization effects. Overall, asymmetry in response was quite prevalent, but lateralization varied with task stage, recording site and ERP component. Both P_{100} and P_{300} responses tended to show right parietal and central lateralization. There was also a tendency for frontal ERPs to be left lateralized, with P_{100} effects reaching significance for Hazard, Benefit, and Choice stages, and P_{300} response showing left lateralization at Choice and Feedback stages. The table also illustrates significant moderator effects, specifying factors that tended to accentuate main effects of side. Positive feedback tended to increase left frontal lateralization of P_{100} response at Benefit and Choice stages, whereas negative feedback increased right lateralization of P_{300} response at the Start stage. We discuss these effects in more detail in this section.

Table 5. Summary of significant lateralization effects on EPR amplitudes

Stage	P_{100}		P_{300}	
	Lateralization	**Moderator Factors**	**Lateralization**	**Moderator Factors**
Start	Right: C, P		Right: F, C, P	C: Neg. Feedback C: MDD
Hazard	Left: F			P: Healthy
Benefit	Left: F, C Right: P	F: Pos. Feedback		
Choice	Left: F Right: P	F: Pos. Feedback	Left: F Right: C	
Feedback	Right: C, P		Left: F Right: C, P	

Note: Effects significant at $p < 0.01$ are bolded. Entries for moderator factors indicate factor that enhanced main effect; e.g., right central lateralization of central P_{300} at Start was stronger in the negative feedback condition (and weaker in the positive condition).

Based on previous lateralization studies [47,48] we tentatively hypothesized an initial right lateralization at Start, followed by a shift to left dominance as the person processes verbal material at the Hazard through Choice stages. Data confirmed the initial right lateralization for both ERP components. Parietal and central right lateralization tended to persist into the later stages. As expected, we also found left lateralization of frontal P_{100} as the person attended to hazard and benefit information and processed this information to arrive at a decision (Choice). A weaker trend towards asymmetry in these stages in P_{300} was significant only at Choice. Right dominance at the start of the trial may reflect the right-hemisphere frontoparietal network for alertness [48]. The influence of this network on ERPs becomes diminished as left-hemisphere language areas are engaged to process the statements of hazard and benefit information. Such dynamic changes in lateralization are consistent with a "state" perspective on asymmetry [18].

Generally, P_{100} reflects early attentive processes controlled by stimulus features [82], sensory selection [83], "cost of attention" [84,85], and "gain control" [86]. It is mostly topographically mapped to visual posterior areas contralaterally to visual stimulus. Anterior P_{100} component originates from frontal generators [87], whereas posterior P_{100} is generated in extrastriate cortex [88], and fusiform gyrus [84]. The current data suggest lateralization of early attention depending on the extent to which attention reflects visuospatial or language-based processes. Lateralization of P_{300} at Start, Choice, and Feedback stages was similar to that for P_{100}, suggesting that it may be sensitive to common attentional networks. P_{300} amplitude asymmetry in the frontal areas may reflect attention engagement, whereas central and parietal P_{300} may indicate executive control and cognitive workload [89,90]. We also expected P_{300} to be sensitive to the cognitive demands of decision-making, given its sensitivity to attention allocation and memory updating [91]. Working memory for verbal or symbolic material tends to be left-lateralized [92] implying stronger left hemisphere response during processing of the hazard and benefit text. However, P_{300} was not lateralized during this stage of the task.

We anticipated that experimental conditions likely to provoke negative emotion such as receiving frequent negative feedback and processing hazard information would tend to elicit hyperactivity in right central areas, whereas positive condition would induce stronger left frontal dominance to benefits, in line with theories of the emotional valence of brain hemispheres [93,94]. Several main effects of feedback condition were associated primarily with stronger frontal P_{100} response in the negative condition at multiple stages. These effects are generally consistent with previous studies suggesting that negative emotion tends to enhance ERP amplitude [95,96], reflecting the high priority of attending to stimuli associated with negative arousal [96]. Feedback condition effects on frontal P_{100} response at Benefit and Choice stages varied with side: reduced frontal activity in the positive condition was especially evident in the right hemisphere. Results also showed a stronger P_{300} right hemisphere response in the negative feedback condition at central sites in Start and Hazard stages. Taken together, these results are consistent with a positive emotional context promoting early left dominance and a negative context leading to later right dominance, as anticipated. However, effect sizes were relatively small, and the effects were significant only at certain stages.

4.2. Decision Making in Depression and Brain Asymmetry

Our literature review suggested two types of effect of major depression on brain functioning. First, depressed patients tend to be over-sensitive to threat [60,61], especially when the task requires inhibition of negative stimuli [62], and under-sensitive to reward [67,68]. Second, the alpha asymmetry literature [2,9,97] implies that avoidance predominates over approach in depression, leading to left frontal hypoactivity. Both characteristics of depression may influence ERPs.

Evidence for greater threat sensitivity and lower reward sensitivity in depressed participants was limited. Depressed patients were expected to show (1) reduced ERP response to benefits relative to hazards, and (2) reduced responsiveness in the positive feedback condition relative to the negative feedback condition, especially at the Feedback stage. Consistent with expectation, depressed participants showed a smaller P_{300} response at the Benefits stage. However, we did not confirm an overall elevated response to hazard information. In fact, there was a lateralized response to Hazard for both P_{100} and P_{300}, with the depressed group showing a stronger left parietal response, and the healthy group showing right lateralization. There were also no significant group × feedback condition effects; depressed patients did not show any general sensitivity to progressive failure at the task. Evidence for expected lateralization effects was limited to the Start stage, at which the depressed group showed a stronger central P_{300} lateralization effect.

4.3. Alpha Asymmetry: Comparison with ERP Data

Previous studies have more often focused on alpha power than ERPs. The present study provided the opportunity to compare two types of EEG measure directly. In accordance with previous studies, we tested for the resting state FAA that was reported as a biological marker of depression [2,7–9,97,98].

We expected that left hyperactivity, associated with approach behavior, would predominate in healthy persons and right hyperactivity, associated with withdrawal behavior, would feature in depressed individuals [24]. Our results confirmed this assumption to a limited extent. There was a general trend towards initial left lateralization at both frontal and parietal sites. There were no significant depression effects in the omnibus ANOVAs, but planned comparisons showed that left dominance in alpha was significant only for healthy individuals, consistent with expectation. The limited evidence for group differences is consistent with data questioning the reliability of depression effects on the FAA [8].

The ERP data suggested early right-lateralization at the start, followed by a more complex pattern of lateralization varying with wave and electrode site in intermediate stages, and a more general central-parietal right lateralization at the final, feedback stage. We did not observe any asymmetry in task-induced alpha at any stage, suggesting that the ERP data are more sensitive to lateralization. For example, there was no counterpart in the alpha data to the significant left frontal lateralization of P100 response evident in the intermediate stages at which the person performs verbal processing. Alpha may be insensitive to specific decision-making processes such as left-lateralized attention to language-based stimuli that are better captured by ERP measures.

The analyses of alpha also showed evidence for depression effects on lateralization of parietal response during Start, Hazard, and Choice stages, and of frontal response at Start and Feedback stages. In each case, the asymmetry coefficient was positive but close to zero in the MDD group. That is, the healthy group showed left dominance (right frontal or parietal hypoactivity, depending on stage), but the depressed individuals showed a more symmetrical response. The relative dominance of the right hemisphere activity in the MDD group compared to healthy controls is consistent with the interrelation of brain asymmetry and depression previously reported [2,9,97].

Previous studies have typically focused on resting FAA, although, similar to our findings, depressed patients had lower left asymmetry during a task requiring processing of facial expression [98]. The present data showed a trend towards a depression effect on resting alpha asymmetry, but it did not reach significance in the analysis of the asymmetry coefficient. Lateralization was stronger during decision-making than at rest, consistent with previous suggestions that frontal asymmetry during affective tasks is a more powerful marker of depression than at rest [19,98,99]. Some studies report that emotion induction is accompanied by alpha desynchronization [100,101]. The strongest effects were observed at the Start stage at which the participant is preparing for task processing. As discussed in the previous section, the anticipated right lateralization of P_{300} response in the MDD group was found only at this stage. Task-induced alpha appears to be a more sensitive indicator of depression effects on lateralization than the ERPs. By contrast, we found that ERP amplitudes were more informative indicators of the dynamical changes in brain asymmetry across task stages then the alpha response, in the whole sample.

The correlational analysis suggested that P_{300} and task-induced alpha provide overlapping but distinct indices of brain activity, consistent with a "trait" model for individual differences in symmetry [2,21]. Positive correlations between alpha power asymmetry and ERP amplitude coefficients, especially in the parietal areas, confirm the consistency of individual differences in lateralization based on two different measurement approaches. However, significant correlations were small to medium in magnitude, implying that the measures are not interchangeable. Resting state alpha asymmetry was only minimally related to P_{300} amplitude, confirming that the resting state may be of limited functional significance for decision-making. However, we might expect that changes in ERP alpha power and ERP amplitude will have opposite directions since alpha oscillations are reverse indicators of brain activity [102,103]. On the other hand, different cognitive tasks such as working memory and Go-NoGo may elicit event-related alpha at parietal sites [104,105].

4.4. Clinical Implications

The present study was designed as basic rather than applied research, but we can suggest some tentative clinical implications. Previous authors have suggested several clinical applications for assessment of FAA, including enhancement of diagnosis, identifying at-risk individuals, and anticipating the outcomes of pharmacological and psychological therapies [6,106]. However, while some studies show promising results, others are more equivocal, and the clinical value of measuring FAA in clients remains to be substantiated [6,8,106,107]. Methodological improvements are necessary to capitalize on the promise of FAA for enhancing diagnosis and anticipating treatment outcomes [3,8].

Consistent with [19], the present findings suggest that task-induced FAA is more strongly linked to depression than resting FAA. Thus, assessment of FAA for diagnostic purposes should be conducted during performance of tasks designed to elicit maximally the abnormal lateralized neurocognitive processes characteristic of depression. The challenge is to define the tasks that are most effective for this purpose. The current study suggests that asymmetry in alpha is not a fixed attribute of depressed patients throughout decision-making. In fact, parietal task-induced alpha asymmetry tended to be the strongest marker for depression, especially early in task processing (Start); the language-based processing at intermediate task stages tended to suppress depression effects. Further research might identify the brain network activated as the person initiates the information search supporting decision-making, such as the frontoparietal network supporting alertness [48], and develop a task version optimized for discrimination of depressed individuals.

The present findings also suggest that resting FAA and ERP measures linked to specific task stages may have diagnostic value over and above task-induced alpha asymmetry, given the modest intercorrelations of the different measures. In the present data, these measures appeared to have only limited diagnostic value. However, further work might develop task paradigms that enhance their ability to discriminate depressed and healthy individuals, such as those using emotionally evocative tasks [3,108]. Such work might support a multivariate diagnostic model, including multiple metrics derived from different tasks or task components. A toolbox for clinical diagnostic purposes could then be defined, using a complex of EEG markers (including ERP and alpha asymmetry metrics) for diagnosis, although further validation work would be needed.

4.5. Limitations

Several study limitations should be noted. First, depression effects on ERPs may vary with severity of illness, depression subtype [53], gender, and age differences. We did not attempt to test these factors as possible moderators of relationships between depression and symmetry of response to keep the number of analyses manageable. However, future research should further address the role of these personal characteristics. Other conditions associated with negative affect such as anxiety may also influence outcomes. Second, identification of asymmetries associated with depression may be enhanced by using more refined measures. For example, individual alpha peak frequency (IAPF), the maximum power value in the individual's EEG frequency spectrum between 7.5 and 12.5 Hz [109], may be used to index FAA [110]. Also, EEG may be combined with other physiological measurements, including brain-imaging [6]. Investigations of stress and emotional factors may be enhanced by assessment of forehead muscle activity and stress hormones, including progesterone in studies of gender [111]. Resting FAA varies with phase of the menstrual cycle [112] and with the presence of PMS [113]. Third, we confirmed that the feedback manipulation we used influenced mood and confidence appropriately. However, an artificial laboratory task may not elicit emotional states representative of real-life depression, such as despair and hopelessness. The effects of the affective variables in this study were fairly modest, although broadly consistent with expectation. Stronger effects might be found with more realistic stressors. Fourth, the effects of depression were quite variable across the different stages of the decision-making task, consistent with other studies demonstrating variability across different information-processing tasks [53,62]. However, given the complexity of decision-making, a more comprehensive framework for decomposing decision-making into different processing components is needed.

5. Conclusions

Impacts of depression on decision-making may have important real-world consequences but the neurocognitive bases for such effects are poorly understood. The present ERP study confirmed that brain response to different stages of a decision-making task is asymmetrical. An initial right lateralization developed into a more complex spatial pattern of asymmetry as the person processed text-based messages on potential benefits and hazards. The effects of depression on lateralization were limited, but we found some evidence for the expected hyperactivity of the right hemisphere in the MDD group, especially in task-induced alpha data. MDD and healthy groups were most strongly discriminated by asymmetry in parietal alpha early in decision-making.

These findings can inform further investigations of asymmetry in depression and its functional significance in decision-making. The results indicate the need for a more nuanced understanding of neurocognitive features of MDD than the conventional linkage between depression and FAA suggests. Depression is not uniformly linked to right lateralization of processing throughout decision-making. The clinician may expect to find abnormalities linked to asymmetry only in specific circumstances. Future applied research should aim to develop tasks that strongly elicit these asymmetrical processes in support of clinical diagnosis and prediction of treatment outcomes.

Author Contributions: Conceptualization, A.K. (Almira Kustubayeva) and G.M.; methodology, A.K. (Almira Kustubayeva) and G.M.; software, A.K. (Almira Kustubayeva) and G.M.; validation, A.K. (Almira Kustubayeva), G.M. and A.K. (Altyngul Kamzanova); formal analysis, A.K. (Almira Kustubayeva) and A.K. (Altyngul Kamzanova); investigation, A.K. (Almira Kustubayeva), A.K. (Altyngul Kamzanova), S.K. and V.P.; resources, A.K. (Almira Kustubayeva), A.K. (Altyngul Kamzanova) and V.P.; data curation, A.K. (Almira Kustubayeva), A.K. (Altyngul Kamzanova), S.K. and V.P.; writing—original draft preparation, A.K. (Almira Kustubayeva) and A.K. (Altyngul Kamzanova); writing—review and editing, G.M.; visualization, A.K. (Almira Kustubayeva) and A.K. (Altyngul Kamzanova); supervision, A.K. (Almira Kustubayeva), G.M.; project administration, A.K. (Almira Kustubayeva); funding acquisition, A.K. (Almira Kustubayeva). All authors have read and agreed to the published version of the manuscript.

References

1. De Aguiar Neto, F.S.; Rosa, J.L.G. Depression biomarkers using non-invasive EEG: A review. *Neurosci. Biobehav. Rev.* **2019**, *105*, 83–93. [CrossRef]
2. Davidson, R.J. Anterior electrophysiological asymmetries, emotion, and depression: Conceptual and methodological conundrums. *Psychophysiology* **1998**, *35*, 607–614. [CrossRef]
3. Allen, J.J.; Reznik, S.J. Frontal EEG Asymmetry as a promising marker of depression vulnerability: Summary and methodological considerations. *Curr. Opin. Psychol.* **2015**, *1*, 93–97. [CrossRef]
4. American Psychiatric Association. *Diagnostic and Statistical Manual of Mental Disorders*, 5th ed.; (DSM-5); American Psychiatric Publishing: Arlington, VA, USA, 2013; 992p, ISBN 978-0-89042-554-1.
5. Nestler, S.; Sander, M.; Egloff, B. Depression and sequential decision-making revisited. *Front. Psychol.* **2019**, *10*, 1492. [CrossRef]
6. Bruder, G.E.; Stewart, J.W.; McGrath, P.J. Right brain, left brain in depressive disorders: Clinical and theoretical implications of behavioral, electrophysiological and neuroimaging findings. *Neurosci. Biobehav. Rev.* **2017**, *78*, 178–191. [CrossRef]

7. Kayser, J.; Bruder, G.E.; Tenke, C.E.; Stewart, J.E.; Quitkin, F.M. Event-related potentials (ERPs) to hemifield presentations of emotional stimuli: Differences between depressed patients and healthy adults in P3 amplitude and asymmetry. *Int. J. Psychophysiol.* **2000**, *3*, 211–236. [CrossRef]
8. Van der Vinne, N.; Vollebregt, M.A.; van Putten, M.J.A.M.; Arns, M. Frontal α asymmetry as a diagnostic marker in depression: Fact or fiction? A meta-analysis. *Neuroimage Clin.* **2017**, *16*, 79–87. [CrossRef]
9. Mumtaz, W.; Malik, A.S.; Yasin, M.A.M.; Xia, L. Review on EEG and ERP predictive biomarkers for major depressive disorder. *Biomed. Signal Proces.* **2015**, *22*, 85–98. [CrossRef]
10. Henriques, J.B.; Davidson, R.J. Left frontal hypoactivity in depression. *J. Abnorm. Psychol.* **1991**, *100*, 535–545. [CrossRef]
11. Davidson, R.J.; Irwin, W. The functional neuroanatomy of emotion and affective style. *Trends Cogn. Sci.* **1999**, *3*, 11–21. [CrossRef]
12. Allen, J.J.B.; Urry, H.L.; Hitt, S.K.; Coan, J.A. The stability of resting frontal electroencephalographic asymmetry in depression. *Psychophysiology* **2004**, *41*, 269–280. [CrossRef] [PubMed]
13. Bruder, G.E.; Fong, R.; Tenke, C.E.; Leite, P.; Towey, J.P.; Stewart, J.E.; McGrath, P.J.; Quitkin, F.M. Regional brain asymmetries in major depression with or without an anxiety disorder: A quantitative electroencephalographic study. *Biol. Psychiatry* **1997**, *41*, 939–948. [CrossRef] [PubMed]
14. Bruder, G.E.; Tenke, C.E.; Warner, V.; Nomura, Y.; Grillon, C.; Hille, J.; Leite, P.; Weissman, M.M. Electroencephalographic measures of regional hemispheric activity in offspring at risk for depressive disorders. *Biol. Psychiatry* **2005**, *57*, 328–335. [CrossRef] [PubMed]
15. Ulrich, G.; Haug, H.J.; Stieglitz, R.D.; Fahndrich, E. EEG characteristics of clinically defined on-drug-responders and non-responders—A comparison clomipramine vs. maprotiline. *Pharmacopsychiatry* **1988**, *21*, 367–368. [CrossRef] [PubMed]
16. Olbrich, S.; van Dinteren, R.; Arns, M. Personalized Medicine: Review and Perspectives of Promising Baseline EEG Biomarkers in Major Depressive Disorder and Attention Deficit Hyperactivity Disorder. *Neuropsychobiology* **2016**, *72*, 229–240. [CrossRef]
17. Adolph, D.; von Glischinski, M.; Wannemüller, A.; Margraf, J. The influence of frontal alpha-asymmetry on the processing of approach and withdrawal-related stimuli—A multichannel psychophysiology study. *Psychophysiology* **2017**, *54*, 1295–1310. [CrossRef]
18. Coan, J.A.; Allen, J.J.B. Frontal EEG asymmetry and behavioral activity and inhibition systems. *Psychophysiology* **2003**, *40*, 106–114. [CrossRef]
19. Stewart, J.L.; Coan, J.A.; Towers, D.N.; Allen, J.J. Resting and task-elicited prefrontal EEG alpha asymmetry in depression: Support for the capability model: Resting and task-elicited asymmetry. *Psychophysiology* **2014**, *51*, 446–455. [CrossRef]
20. Van der Vinne, N.; Vollebregt, M.A.; van Putten, M.J.A.M.; Arns, M. Stability of frontal alpha asymmetry in depressed patients during antidepressant treatment. *NeuroImage Clin.* **2019**, *24*, 102056. [CrossRef]
21. Carver, C.; White, T. Behavioral Inhibition, Behavioral Activity, and Affective Responses to Impending Reward and Punishment: The BIS/BAS Scales. *J. Pers. Soc. Psychol.* **1994**, *67*, 319–333. [CrossRef]
22. Beevers, C.; Meyer, B. Lack of positive experiences and positive expectancies mediate the relationship between BAS responsiveness and depression. *Cogn. Emot.* **2002**, *16*, 549–564. [CrossRef]
23. Kasch, K.L.; Rottenberg, J.; Arnow, B.A.; Gotlib, I.H. Behavioral activity and inhibition systems and the severity and course of depression. *J. Abnorm. Psychol.* **2002**, *111*, 589–597. [CrossRef]
24. Sutton, S.K.; Davidson, R.J. Prefrontal Brain Asymmetry: A Biological Substrate of the Behavioral Approach and Inhibition Systems. *Psychol. Sci.* **1997**, *8*, 204–210. [CrossRef]
25. Santesso, D.L.; Segalowitz, S.J.; Ashbaugh, A.R.; Antony, M.M.; McCabe, R.E.; Schmidt, L.A. Frontal EEG asymmetry and sensation seeking in young adults. *Biol. Psychol.* **2008**, *78*, 164–172. [CrossRef]
26. Jackson, D.C.; Mueller, C.J.; Dolski, I.; Dalton, K.M.; Nitschke, J.B.; Urry, H.L.; Rosenkranz, M.A.; Ryff, C.D.; Singer, B.H.; Davidson, R.J. Now you feel it, now you don't frontal brain electrical asymmetry and individual differences in emotion regulation. *Psychol. Sci.* **2003**, *14*, 612–617. [CrossRef]
27. Grimshaw, G.; Carmel, D. An Asymmetric Inhibition Model of Hemispheric Differences in Emotional Processing. *Front. Psychol.* **2014**, *5*, 489. [CrossRef]
28. Smith, E.E.; Reznik, S.J.; Stewart, J.L.; Allen, J.J. Assessing and conceptualizing frontal EEG asymmetry: An updated primer on recording, processing, analyzing, and interpreting frontal alpha asymmetry. *Int. J. Psychol.* **2017**, *111*, 98–114. [CrossRef]

29. Coan, J.A.; Allen, J.J.; McKnight, P.E. A capability model of individual differences in frontal EEG asymmetry. *Biol. Psychol.* **2006**, *72*, 198–207. [CrossRef]
30. Harmon-Jones, E.; Harmon-Jones, C. Testing the action-based model of cognitive dissonance: The effect of action orientation on postdecisional attitudes. *Pers. Soc. Psychol. Bull.* **2002**, *28*, 711–723. [CrossRef]
31. Nitschke, J.; Nelson, E.; Rusch, B.; Fox, A.; Oakes, T.; Davidson, R. Orbitofrontal cortex tracks positive mood in others viewing pictures of their newborn infants. *NeuroImage* **2004**, *21*, 583–592. [CrossRef]
32. Shankman, S.; Klein, D.; Tenke, C.; Bruder, G. Reward sensitivity in depression: A biobehavioral study. *J. Abnorm. Psychol.* **2007**, *116*, 95–104. [CrossRef] [PubMed]
33. De Freitas, S.B.; Marques, A.A.; Bevilaqua, M.C.; de Carvalho, M.R.; Ribeiro, P.; Palmer, S.; Nardi, A.E.; Dias, G.P. Electroencephalographic findings in patients with major depressive disorder during cognitive or emotional tasks: A systematic review. *Rev. Bras. Psiquiatr.* **2016**, *38*, 338–346. [CrossRef] [PubMed]
34. Proudfit, G.H.; Bress, J.N.; Foti, D.; Kujawa, A.; Klein, D.N. Depression and event-related potentials: Emotional disengagement and reward insensitivity. *Curr. Opin. Psychol.* **2015**, *4*, 110–113. [CrossRef] [PubMed]
35. Bishop, S.J.; Gagne, C. Anxiety, Depression, and Decision Making: A Computational Perspective. *Annu. Rev. Neurosci.* **2018**, *41*, 371–388. [CrossRef]
36. Huys, Q.J.; Daw, N.D.; Dayan, P. Depression: A decision-theoretic analysis. *Annu. Rev. Neurosci.* **2015**, *8*, 1–23. [CrossRef]
37. Kaplan, J.S.; Erickson, K.; Luckenbaugh, D.A.; Weiland-Fiedler, P.; Geraci, M.; Sahakian, B.J.; Charney, D.; Drevets, W.C.; Neumeister, A. Differential performance on tasks of affective processing and decision-making in patients with panic disorder and panic disorder with comorbid major depressive disorder. *J. Affect. Disord.* **2006**, *95*, 165–171. [CrossRef]
38. Wells, A.; Matthews, G. *Attention and Emotion*; Classic Edition; Psychology Press: London, UK, 2015; ISBN 978-131-574-718-7.
39. Treadway, M.T.; Buckholtz, J.W.; Cowan, R.L.; Woodward, N.D.; Li, R.; Ansari, M.S.; Zald, D.H. Dopaminergic mechanisms of individual differences in human effort-based decision-making. *J. Neurosci.* **2012**, *32*, 6170–6176. [CrossRef]
40. Yang, X.H.; Huang, J.; Zhu, C.Y.; Wang, Y.F.; Cheung, E.F.; Chan, R.C.; Xie, G.R. Motivational deficits in effort-based decision making in individuals with subsyndromal depression, first-episode and remitted depression patients. *Psychiatry Res.* **2014**, *220*, 874–882. [CrossRef]
41. Li, Y.; Kang, C.; Qu, X.; Zhou, Y.; Wang, W.; Hu, Y. Depression-related brain connectivity analyzed by eeg event-related phase synchrony measure. *Front. Hum. Neurosci.* **2016**, *10*. [CrossRef]
42. Corwin, J.; Peselow, E.; Feenan, K.; Rotrosen, J.; Fieve, R. Disorders of decision in affective disease: An effect of beta-adrenergic dysfunction? *Biol. Psychiatry.* **1990**, *27*, 813–833. [CrossRef]
43. Muris, P.; van der Heiden, S. Anxiety, depression, and judgments about the probability of future negative and positive events in children. *J. Anxiety Disord.* **2006**, *20*, 252–261. [CrossRef] [PubMed]
44. Mukherjee, M.; Forero, D.F.; Tran, S.; Boulay, M.E.; Bertrand, M.; Bhalla, A.; Cherukat, J.; Al-Hayyan, H.; Ayoub, A.; Revill, S.D.; et al. Suboptimal treatment response to anti-IL-5 monoclonal antibodies in severe eosinophilic asthmatics with airway autoimmune phenomena. *Eur. Respir. J.* **2020**, *56*, 2000117. [CrossRef] [PubMed]
45. Cella, D.; Riley, W.; Stone, A.; Rothrock, N.; Reeve, B.; Yount, S.; Amtmann, D.; Bode, R.; Buysse, D.; Choi, S.; et al. The Patient-Reported Outcomes Measurement Information System (PROMIS) developed and tested its first wave of adult self-reported health outcome item banks: 2005–2008. *J. Clin. Epidemiol.* **2010**, *63*, 1179–1194. [CrossRef] [PubMed]
46. Harmon-Jones, E.; Gable, P.; Price, T. Does negative affect always narrow and positive affect always broaden the mind? Considering the influence of motivational intensity on cognitive scope. *Curr. Dir. Psychol. Sci.* **2013**, *22*, 301–307. [CrossRef]
47. Karolis, V.; Corbetta, M.; Thiebaut de Schotten, M. The architecture of functional lateralisation and its relationship to callosal connectivity in the human brain. *Nat. Commun.* **2019**, *10*. [CrossRef]
48. Clemens, B.; Zvyagintsev, M.; Sack, A.T.; Heinecke, A.; Willmes, K.; Sturm, W. Revealing the functional neuroanatomy of intrinsic alertness using fMRI: Methodological peculiarities. *PLoS ONE* **2011**, *6*, e25453. [CrossRef]

49. Fan, J.; Byrne, J.; Worden, M.S.; Guise, K.G.; McCandliss, B.D.; Fossella, J.; Posner, M.L. The relation of brain oscillations to attentional networks. *J. Neurosci.* **2007**, *27*, 6197–6206. [CrossRef]
50. Petersen, S.; Posner, M. The Attention System of the Human Brain: 20 Years After. *Annu. Rev. Neurosci.* **2012**, *35*, 73–89. [CrossRef]
51. Giustiniani, J.; Gabriel, D.; Nicolier, M.; Monnin, J.; Haffen, E. Neural Correlates of Successful and Unsuccessful Strategical Mechanisms Involved in Uncertain Decision-Making. *PLoS ONE.* **2015**, *10*, e0130871. [CrossRef]
52. Duke, É.; Schnuerch, R.; Heeren, G.; Reuter, M.; Montag, C.; Markett, S. Cortical alpha asymmetry at central and posterior–but not anterior–sites is associated with individual differences in behavioural loss aversion. *Pers. Individ. Differ.* **2018**, *121*, 206–212. [CrossRef]
53. Balconi, M.; Finocchiaro, R.; Canavesio, Y.; Messina, R. Reward bias and lateralization in gambling behavior: Behavioral activity system and alpha band analysis. *Psychiatry Res.* **2014**, *219*, 570–576. [CrossRef]
54. Tenke, C.; Kayser, J.; Stewart, J.; Bruder, G. Novelty P3 reductions in depression: Characterization using principal components analysis (PCA) of current source density (CSD) waveforms. *Psychophysiology* **2009**, *47*, 133–146. [CrossRef]
55. Knott, V.J.; Lapierre, Y.D. Computerized EEG correlates of depression and antidepressant treatment. *Prog. Neuro Psychopharmacol. Biol. Psychiatry* **1987**, *11*, 213–221. [CrossRef]
56. Pierson, A.; Ragot, R.; Van Hooff, J.; Partiot, A.; Renault, B.; Jouvent, R. Heterogeneity of information-processing alterations according to dimensions of depression: An event-related potentials study. *Biol. Psychiatry* **1996**, *40*, 98–115. [CrossRef]
57. Khanna, S.; Mukundan, C.R.; Channabasavanna, S.M. Middle latency evoked potentials in melancholic depression. *Biol. Psychiatry* **1989**, *25*, 494–498. [CrossRef]
58. Elliot, A.J.; Thrash, T.M. Approach-avoidance motivation in personality: Approach and avoidance temperaments and goals. *J. Pers. Soc. Psychol.* **2002**, *82*, 804–818. [CrossRef]
59. Davidson, R.; Pizzagalli, D.; Nitschke, J.; Putnam, K. Depression: Perspectives from Affective Neuroscience. *Annu. Rev. Psychol.* **2002**, *53*, 545–574. [CrossRef]
60. Ilardi, S.S.; Atchley, R.A.; Enloe, A.; Kwasny, K.; Garratt, G. Disentangling attentional biases and attentional deficits in depression: An event-related potential P300 analysis. *Cognit. Ther. Res.* **2007**, *31*, 175–187. [CrossRef]
61. Li, X.; Li, J.; Hu, B.; Zhu, J.; Zhang, X.; Wei, L.; Zhang, L. Attentional bias in MDD: ERP components analysis and classification using a dot-probe task. *Comput. Methods Programs Biomed.* **2018**, *164*, 169–179. [CrossRef]
62. Monnart, A.; Kornreich, C.; Verbanck, P.; Campanella, S. Just swap out of negative vibes? Rumination and inhibition deficits in major depressive disorder: Data from event-related potentials studies. *Front. Psychol.* **2016**, *7*, 1019. [CrossRef]
63. Yang, W.; Zhu, X.; Wang, X.; Wu, D.; Yao, S. Time course of affective processing bias in major depression: An ERP study. *Neurosci. Lett.* **2011**, *487*, 372–377. [CrossRef]
64. Pechtel, P.; Pizzagalli, D.A. Disrupted Reinforcement Learning and Maladaptive Behavior in Women with a History of Childhood Sexual Abuse: A High-Density Event-Related Potential Study. *JAMA Psychiatry* **2013**, *70*, 499. [CrossRef] [PubMed]
65. Moran, T.P.; Schroder, H.S.; Kneip, C.; Moser, J.S. Meta-analysis and psychophysiology: A tutorial using depression and action-monitoring event-related potentials. *Int. J. Psychophysiol.* **2017**, *111*, 17–32. [CrossRef] [PubMed]
66. Clayson, P.E.; Carbine, K.A.; Larson, M.J. A registered report of error-related negativity and reward positivity as biomarkers of depression: P-Curving the evidence. *Int. J. Psychophysiol.* **2020**, *150*, 50–72. [CrossRef] [PubMed]
67. Proudfit, G.H. The reward positivity: From basic research on reward to a biomarker for depression: The reward positivity. *Psychophysiology* **2015**, *52*, 449–459. [CrossRef] [PubMed]
68. Landes, I.; Bakos, S.; Kohls, G.; Bartling, J.; Schulte-Körne, G.; Greimel, E. Altered neural processing of reward and punishment in adolescents with Major Depressive Disorder. *J. Affect.* **2018**, *232*, 23–33. [CrossRef]
69. Ellis, A.J.; Salgari, G.; Miklowitz, D.J.; Loo, S.K. The role of avoidance motivation in the relationship between reward sensitivity and depression symptoms in adolescents: An ERP study. *Psychiatry Res.* **2019**, *279*, 345–349. [CrossRef]
70. Zhou, L.; Wang, G.; Nan, C.; Wang, H.; Liu, Z.; Bai, H. Abnormalities in P300 components in depression: An ERP-sLORETA study. *Nord. J. Psychiatry* **2019**, *73*, 1–8. [CrossRef]

71. Kawasaki, T.; Tanaka, S.; Wang, J.; Hokama, H.; Hiramatsu, K. Abnormalities of P300 cortical current density in unmedicated depressed patients revealed by LORETA analysis of event-related potentials. *Psychiatry Clin. Neurosci.* **2004**, *58*, 68–75. [CrossRef]
72. Salamone, J.D.; Correa, M.; Yohn, S.E.; Yang, J.H.; Somerville, M.; Rotolo, R.A.; Presby, R.E. Behavioral activity, effort-based choice, and elasticity of demand for motivational stimuli: Basic and translational neuroscience approaches. *Motiv. Sci.* **2017**, *3*, 208. [CrossRef]
73. Matthews, G.; Panganiban, A.R.; Hudlicka, E. Anxiety and selective attention to threat in tactical decision-making. *Pers. Individ. Differ.* **2011**, *50*, 949–954. [CrossRef]
74. Matthews, G.; Fallon, C.; Panganiban, A.R.; Wohleber, R.; Roberts, R. Emotional intelligence, information search and decision-making under stress. *Pers. Individ. Differ.* **2014**, *60*, S22. [CrossRef]
75. Kustubayeva, A.; Matthews, G.; Panganiban, A.R. Emotion and information search in tactical decision-making: Moderator effects of feedback. *Motiv. Emotion.* **2012**, *36*, 529–543. [CrossRef]
76. Matthews, G.; Falconer, S. Personality, Coping and Task-Induced Stress in Customer Service Personnel. *Proc. Hum. Factors Ergon. Soc. Annu. Meet.* **2002**, *46*, 963–967. [CrossRef]
77. Coan, J.A.; Allen, J.J.B. Frontal EEG asymmetry as a moderator and mediator of emotion. *Biol. Psychol.* **2004**, *67*, 7–50. [CrossRef] [PubMed]
78. Delorme, A.; Makeig, S. EEGLAB: An open source toolbox for analysis of single-trial EEG dynamics including independent component analysis. *J. Neurosci. Methods* **2004**, *134*, 9–21. [CrossRef] [PubMed]
79. Lopez-Calderon, J.; Luck, S.J. ERPLAB: An open-source toolbox for the analysis of event-related potentials. *Front. Hum. Neurosci.* **2014**, *8*, 213. [CrossRef]
80. The MathWorks Inc. *MATLAB R2019b*; Version 7.10.0 (R2010a); The MathWorks Inc.: Natick, MA, USA, 2019.
81. IBM Corp. *IBM SPSS Statistics for Windows*; Version 25.0; IBM Corp.: Armonk, NY, USA, 2017.
82. Luck, S.J.; Kappenman, E.S. *The Oxford Handbook of Event-Related Potential Components*; Oxford University Press: New York, NY, USA, 2012; ISBN 978-0199328048.
83. Luck, S.J.; Heinze, H.J.; Mangun, G.R.; Hillyard, S.A. Visual event-related potentials index focused attention within bilateral stimulus arrays. II. Functional dissociation of P1 and N1 components. *Clin. Neurophysiol.* **1990**, *75*, 528–542. [CrossRef]
84. Luck, S.J.; Hillyard, S.A.; Mouloua, M.; Woldorff, M.G.; Clark, V.P.; Hawkins, H.L. Effect of spatial cueing on luminance detectability: Psychophysical and electrophysiological evidence for early selection. *Psychol. Hum. Percept. Perform.* **1994**, *20*, 887–904. [CrossRef]
85. Mangun, G.R. Neural mechanisms of visual selective attention. *Psychophysiology* **1995**, *32*, 4–18. [CrossRef]
86. Hillyard, S.A.; Vogel, E.K.; Luck, S.J. Sensory gain control (amplification) as a mechanism of selective attention: Electrophysiological and neuroimaging evidence. *Philos. Trans. R. Soc. B.* **1998**, *353*, 1257–1270. [CrossRef] [PubMed]
87. Clark, V.P.; Fan, S.; Hillyard, S.A. Identification of early visual evoked potential generators by retinotopic and topographic analyses. *Hum. Brain Mapp.* **1994**, *2*, 170–187. [CrossRef]
88. Herrmann, C.S.; Knight, R.T. Mechanisms of human attention: Event-related potentials and oscillations. *Neurosci. Biobehav. Rev.* **2001**, *25*, 465–476. [CrossRef]
89. Posner, M.I. Attention as a cognitive neural system. *Curr. Dir. Psychol. Sci.* **1992**, *1*, 11–14. [CrossRef]
90. Posner, M.I.; Petersen, S. The attention system of the human brain. *Ann. Rev. Psychol.* **1990**, *13*, 25–42. [CrossRef]
91. Polich, J. Updating P300: An integrative theory of P3a and P3b. *Clin. Neurophysiol.* **2007**, *118*, 2128–2148. [CrossRef]
92. Ungerleider, L.G.; Courtney, S.M.; Haxby, J.V. A neural system for human visual working memory. *Proc. Natl. Acad. Sci. USA* **1998**, *95*, 883–890. [CrossRef]
93. Berntson, G.G.; Norman, G.J.; Cacioppo, J.T. Comments: Literality and Evaluative Bivalence: A Neuroevolutionary Perspective. *Emot. Rev.* **2011**, *3*, 344–346. [CrossRef]
94. Heller, W.; Nitschke, J.B. The puzzle of regional brain activity in emotion: A framework for understanding cognition in depression. *Cognit. Emot.* **1998**, *12*, 421–447. [CrossRef]
95. De Pascalis, V.; Strippoli, E.; Riccardi, P.; Vergari, F. Personality, event-related potential (ERP) and heart rate (HR) in emotional word processing. *Pers. Individ. Differ.* **2004**, *36*, 873–891. [CrossRef]
96. Sass, S.M.; Heller, W.; Stewart, J.L.; Silton, R.L.; Edgar, C.; Fisher, J.; Miller, G. Time course of attentional bias to threat in anxiety: Emotion and gender specificity. *Psychophysiology* **2010**, *47*, 247–259. [CrossRef] [PubMed]

97. Nusslock, R.; Walden, K.; Harmon-Jones, E. Asymmetrical frontal cortical activity associated with differential risk for mood and anxiety disorder symptoms: An RDoC perspective. *Int. J. Psychophysiol.* **2015**, *98*, 249–261. [CrossRef] [PubMed]
98. Jesulola, E.; Sharpley, C.F.; Bitsika, V.; Agnew, L.L.; Wilson, P. Frontal alpha asymmetry as a pathway to behavioural withdrawal in depression: Research findings and issues. *Behav. Brain Res.* **2015**, *292*, 56–67. [CrossRef] [PubMed]
99. Jones, N.A.; Field, T.; Davalos, M. Right frontal EEG asymmetry and lack of empathy in preschool children of depressed mothers. *Child Psychiatry Hum. Dev.* **2000**, *30*, 189–204. [CrossRef] [PubMed]
100. Kustubayeva, A.M.; Tolegenova, A.; Matthews, G. EEG-brain activity in different strategies of emotions' self-regulation: Suppression and reappraisal. *Psychol. J.* **2013**, *34*, 51–61.
101. Dennis, T.A.; Solomon, B. Frontal EEG and emotion regulation: Electrocortical activity in response to emotional film clips is associated with reduced mood induction and attention interference effects. *Biol. Psychol.* **2010**, *85*, 456–464. [CrossRef]
102. Pfurtscheller, G.; Stancák, A.; Neuper, C. Post-movement beta synchronization. A correlate of an idling motor area? *Clin. Neurophysiol.* **1996**, *98*, 281–293. [CrossRef]
103. Klimesch, W. EEG-alpha rhythms and memory processes. *Int. J. Psychophysiol.* **1997**, *26*, 319–340. [CrossRef]
104. Klimesch, W. Evoked alpha and early access to the knowledge system: The P1 inhibition timing hypothesis. *Brain Res.* **2011**, *1408*, 52–71. [CrossRef]
105. Jensen, O.; Mazaheri, A. Shaping functional architecture by oscillatory alpha activity: Gating by inhibition. *Front Hum. Neurosci.* **2010**, *4*, 186. [CrossRef]
106. Briesemeister, B.B.; Tamm, S.; Heine, A.; Jacobs, A.M. Approach the good, withdraw from the bad—A review on frontal alpha asymmetry measures in applied psychological research. *Psychology* **2013**, *4*, 261–267. [CrossRef]
107. Gollan, J.K.; Hoxha, D.; Chihade, D.; Pflieger, M.E.; Rosebrock, L.; Cacioppo, J. Frontal alpha EEG asymmetry before and after behavioral activation treatment for depression. *Biol. Psychol.* **2014**, *99*, 198–208. [CrossRef] [PubMed]
108. Meyer, T.; Quaedflieg, C.W.E.M.; Giesbrecht, T.; Meijer, E.H.; Abiad, S.; Smeets, T. Frontal EEG asymmetry as predictor of physiological responses to aversive memories. *Psychophysiology* **2014**, *51*, 853–865. [CrossRef] [PubMed]
109. Klimesch, W. EEG alpha and theta oscillations reflect cognitive and memory performance: A review and analysis. *Brain Res. Rev.* **1999**, *29*, 169–195. [CrossRef]
110. Quaedflieg, C.W.E.M.; Meyer, T.; Smulders, F.T.Y.; Smeets, T. (2015). The functional role of individual-alpha based frontal asymmetry in stress responding. *Biol. Psychol.* **2015**, *104*, 75–81. [CrossRef]
111. Bazanova, O.M.; Nikolenko, E.D.; Barry, R.J. Reactivity of alpha rhythms to eyes opening (the Berger effect) during menstrual cycle phases. *Int. J. Psychophysiol.* **2017**, *1*, 56–64. [CrossRef]
112. Huang, Y.; Zhou, R.; Cui, H.; Wu, M.; Wang, Q.; Zhao, Y.; Liu, Y. Variations in resting frontal alpha asymmetry between high-and low-neuroticism females across the menstrual cycle. *Psychophysiology* **2015**, *52*, 182–191. [CrossRef]
113. Deng, Y.; Jiang, Y.; Li, S.; Zhou, R. Differential trait and state frontal alpha asymmetry in women with premenstrual syndrome. *Motivat. Emot.* **2019**, *43*, 883–893. [CrossRef]

3

Asymmetry of Cerebellar Lobular Development in Ferrets

Kazuhiko Sawada [1,*], Shiori Kamiya [1] and Ichio Aoki [2,3]

1 Department of Nutrition, Faculty of Medical and Health Sciences, Tsukuba International University, Tsuchiura, Ibaraki 300-0051, Japan; s-kamiya@tius.ac.jp
2 Department of Molecular Imaging and Theranostics, National Institute of Radiological Sciences, National Institutes for Quantum and Radiological Science and Technology (QST), Chiba 263-8555, Japan; aoki.ichio@qst.go.jp
3 Institute for Quantum Life Science (iQLS), QST, Chiba 263-8555, Japan
* Correspondence: k-sawada@tius.ac.jp

Abstract: The ferret cerebellum is anteriorly right-lateralized and posteriorly left-lateralized. This study characterized the left/right difference in ferret cerebellar lobular morphology using 3D-rendered magnetic resonance images of fixed brains from seven male and seven female ferrets on postnatal day 90. Asymmetrical lobular morphology showed asymmetrical sublobular development in the anterior vermis, lobulus simplex, and ansiform lobules and additional grooves asymmetrically appearing in the paramedian lobule, lobule VI, and ansiform lobules. Although we observed these asymmetric hallmarks in four cerebellar transverse domains in both sexes, there was no left/right difference in their incidence in each domain. Males showed a significantly higher incidence of the additional grooves in the left side of the ansiform lobules than in females. Data were combined and classified as per the asymmetry quotient (AQ) into left- (AQ < 0) and right-dominant (AQ > 0) groups. There were significantly higher incidences of poor sublobular development of ansiform lobules and additional groove appearing in lobule VI on the right than on the left in the left-dominant group. Asymmetric hallmarks visible on the cerebellar surface of ferrets are relevant to the left-biased volume asymmetry of the central zone of cerebellar transversus domains containing lobule VI and ansiform lobules.

Keywords: asymmetry; sex difference; MRI; volumetry; cerebellum; ferret

---

1. Introduction

Studies have reported cerebellar volume laterality in humans [1], nonhuman primates [2,3], and carnivores [4], including ferrets [5,6]. Interestingly, regional differences in cerebellar volume laterality revealed distinctive torque morphology formed clockwise (anteriorly left-biased and posteriorly right-biased) in humans [2,7] and counterclockwise (anteriorly right-biased and posteriorly left-biased) in ferrets [5,6]. The posterior cerebellum, including lobule VI and ansiform lobules, is functionally lateralized, that is, the right-side controls language and working memory [8,9], while the left side controls cognition [10,11]. Such functional asymmetry is involved in characteristic functional cerebellar organization via cerebrum–cerebellum connections linked contralaterally with the association cortex, not the motor cortex [9]. Thus, cerebellar asymmetry is evaluated volumetrically and functionally but is not examined on the basis of detailed cerebellar morphology. This study characterized the left/right difference in the cerebellar lobular morphology in male and female ferrets using 3D-rendered images obtained from *ex vivo* magnetic resonance (MR) images.

2. Materials and Methods

2.1. Samples

Anatomical MR images of fixed brains from seven male and seven female ferrets on postnatal day 90 obtained in our previous studies [5,6] were used in this study. A preclinical 7.0 T magnetic resonance imaging (MRI) system with a 400 mm inner-diameter-bore magnet (Kobelco and Jastec, Kobe, Japan) and an AVANCE-I console (Bruker BioSpin, Ettlingen, Germany) acquired 3D MR images covering the entire fixed brains using the rapid acquisition with relaxation enhancement (RARE) sequence with the following parameters: Repetition time (TR) = 300 ms; echo time (TE) = 9.6 ms (effective TE = 19.2 ms); RARE factor = 4; field of view (FOV) = 32 × 32 × 40 mm^3; acquisition matrix = 256 × 256 × 256; voxel size = 125 × 125 × 156 μm^3; number of acquisitions (NEX) = 2; and total scan time = 2 h 43 min 50 s.

2.2. Volumetry

Volumetric analysis was conducted using 3D MR images of the cerebellum. The left and right cerebellar sides were divided at the midline, which was defined by the position of the cerebral longitudinal fissure. Cerebellar transverse domains were segmented semi-automatically into four zones: Anterior zone (AZ; lobules I–V of the vermis), central zone anterior (CZa; lobules VI and the lobules simplex), central zone posterior (CZp; lobules VII of the vermis and ansiform lobules), and posterior zone (PZ; lobules VIII–IXa of the vermis and paramedian lobule) [5]. Segmented areas of each domain were measured using the SliceOmatic software version 4.3 (TomoVision, Montreal, Canada), and the volume of each domain was calculated by multiplying the combined areas by the slice thickness (156.25 μm). The asymmetry quotient (AQ) was calculated using the formula $((R - L)/\{(R + L) \times 0.5\})$ and was used to assess the volume laterality of each domain. The direction of asymmetry was indicated by the AQ values: Positive value = rightward bias and negative value = leftward bias [12].

2.3. 3D-Rendered Images

The cerebellar cortex was segmented semi-automatically on MR images using Amira ver. 5.2 (Visage Imaging, Inc., San Diego, CA, USA) on the basis of image contrast. The images were rendered in 3D using the surface projection algorithm, which best visualizes the surface. Then, the 3D-rendered images were rotated and manipulated to best visualize the cerebellar morphology by linear registration using SliceOmatic software. Finally, asymmetric morphological changes (i.e., poor sublobular development and additional grooves) were noted in the left and right sides of each cerebellar transverse domain on the 3D-rendered images. The cerebellar lobules/sublobules were identified with reference to the textbook of Lawes and Andrews (1998) [13].

2.4. Statistical Analysis

The incidence of asymmetry in sublobular development and additional grooves was estimated in each cerebellar transverse domain segmented with reference to expression patterns of zebrin II/aldolase C in other mammals [14,15]. Left-/right-side or sexual differences were evaluated using the chi-square test. In addition, the relationship between morphological asymmetry and volume laterality in each cerebellar transverse domain was evaluated. Then, data from males and females were combined and classified on the basis of AQ values into left-dominant (AQ < 0) and right-dominant (AQ > 0) groups. The incidence of asymmetry in sublobular development and additional grooves was estimated in left- and right-dominant groups of all transverse domains, and left-/right-side or intergroup differences were evaluated using the chi-square test.

2.5. Ethics

All experiments were conducted in accordance with the Guide for the Care and Use of Laboratory Animals by the National Institutes of Health (NIH, Bethesda, MD, USA). The study, and all its procedures, was approved by the Institutional Animal Care and Use Committee of Tsukuba International University, Japan. All efforts were made to minimize the number of animals used and their suffering.

3. Results

3.1. Types of Cerebellar Gross Anatomical Asymmetry

The cerebellar morphological asymmetry was roughly classified into two types: Asymmetrical lobular/sublobular development and asymmetrical appearance of additional grooves. Figure 1 illustrates the types of morphological asymmetry of the ferret cerebellum.

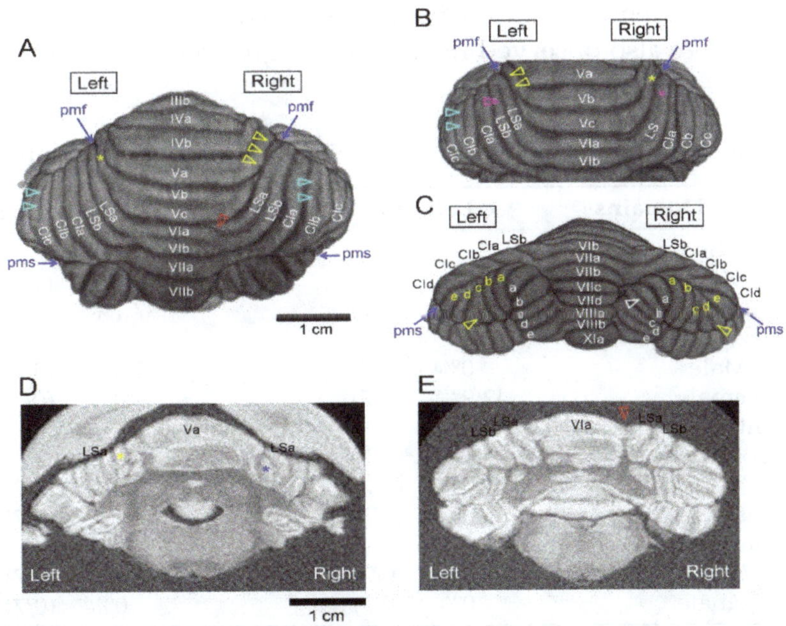

Figure 1. Typical asymmetric morphology in the ferret cerebellum. (**A**) Dorsal view of 3D-rendered cerebellar image showing asymmetrically poor development of the sublobule in the anterior vermis and additional grooves emerging asymmetrically in the lobulus simplex (LS) and ansiform lobules. Sublobule Vb/c was visible at the left end on the cerebellar surface (yellow asterisk) but not at the right end, which was covered by adjacent sublobules (yarrow arrowheads). Additional grooves were found asymmetrically in sublobule VIa of the right paravermis (red arrowhead) and crus I sublobules (right CIb and left CIc) (light-blue arrowheads). (**B**) Dorsal view of 3D-rendered cerebellar image showing asymmetrically poor development of the LS. The sulcus demarcating LS sublobules was present on the left (purple arrowhead) but not on the right (purple asterisk). Sublobule Vc was visible at the right end on the cerebellar surface (yellow asterisk) but not at the left end, which was covered by adjacent sublobules (yarrow arrowheads). Additional grooves emerging asymmetrically were seen in the left CIb (light-blue arrowheads). (**C**) Posterior view of 3D-rendered cerebellar image showing additional grooves emerging asymmetrically in crus II (CII) sublobules (left CIIc and right CIId) (yellow arrowheads) and the paramedian sublobule (right PMb) (white arrowhead). Yellow a–e letters indicate CII sublobules; white a–e letters indicate PM sublobules. (**D**) Coronal (transaxial) MR image showing asymmetrically poor sublobular development in the anterior vermis. The blue asterisk indicates the poorly developed right Vc sublobule, which was covered by the adjacent sublobules Va and LSa on the cerebellar surface. The yellow asterisk indicates contralateral Vc sublobules, which were visible on the cerebellar surface. (**E**) Coronal (transaxial) MR image showing an additional groove appearing in sublobule VI of the right paravermis (red arrowhead). CI, crus I of ansiform lobule; CII, crus II of ansiform lobule; LS, lobulus simplex; PM, paramedian lobule; MR, magnetic resonance.

Sublobules were poorly developed on the left or right, which was covered by adjacent lobules/sublobules (Figure 1A,D). Such asymmetry was seen primarily in the anterior vermis and secondarily in the lobulus simplex and ansiform lobules. The asymmetrical lobular development was also characterized by underdeveloped sulci demarcating the sublobules on the left or right (Figure 1B). This asymmetry was found primarily in lobule VI and the lobulus simplex. Additional grooves appeared asymmetrically in sublobules of paravermian lobule VI, ansiform lobules, and the paramedian lobule (Figure 1A,C). Particularly, the additional groove appearing in the right paravermian lobule VI was distinct from those appearing in other lobules; it infolded loosely and made a distinctive asymmetric profile in lobule VI on coronal MR images (Figure 1E).

3.2. *Incidence of Cerebellar Asymmetrical Morphology*

The highest incidence of asymmetrically poor development of sublobules was observed in the AZ (corresponding to the anterior vermis) on both left and right sides in 57.1% of males and on the right in 57.1% of females. The incidence did not differ between left and right sides and at ipsilateral sides between sexes (Table 1). We also observed no additional grooves asymmetrically appearing in AZ sublobules (Table 2).

Table 1. Incidences of asymmetrically poor sublobule development in male and female ferrets.

Transverse Domains	Left Side		-	Right Side	
Anterior zone					
Male	57.1%	(4/7)		57.1%	(4/7)
Female	14.3%	(1/7)		57.1%	(4/7)
Central zone anterior					
Male	0%	(0/7)		42.9%	(3/7)
Female	42.9%	(3/7)		0%	(0/7)
Central zone posterior					
Male	0%	(0/7)		28.6%	(2/7)
Female	0%	(0/7)		42.9%	(3/7)
Posterior zone					
Male	0%	(0/7)		0%	(0/7)
Female	0%	(0/7)		0%	(0/7)

The number of individuals exhibiting the poor sublobular development at each side is shown in parentheses.

Table 2. Incidences of asymmetrically appearing additional cerebellum indentations in male and female ferrets.

Transverse Domains	Left Side		-	Right Side	
Anterior zone					
Male	0%	(0/7)		0%	(0/7)
Female	0%	(0/7)		0%	(0/7)
Central zone anterior					
Male	0%	(0/7)		42.9%	(3/7)
Female	0%	(0/7)		42.9%	(3/7)
Central zone posterior					
Male	57.1%	(4/7) *		28.6%	(2/7)
Female	0%	(0/7)		0%	(0/7)
Posterior zone					
Male	42.9%	(3/7)		57.1%	(4/7)
Female	28.6%	(2/7)		28.6%	(2/7)

The number of individuals showing the additional grooves at each side is shown in parentheses. * $p < 0.05$ male vs. female (chi-square test).

In the CZa, the lobulus simplex was poorly developed on the right in 42.9% of males and on the left in 42.9% of females (Table 1). Additional grooves appeared in paravermian lobule VI on the right in 42.9% of males and 28.6% of females but not on the left in both sexes (Table 2).

In the CZp, sublobules in ansiform lobules were poorly developed on the right in 28.6% of males and 42.9% of females. Although ansiform sublobules on the left were well developed in both males and females, we did not detect a statistical left/right difference in the incidence of asymmetrically poor development of ansiform sublobules in both sexes (Table 1). Additional grooves were found in ansiform lobules on the left in 57.1% of males and on the right in 28.6% of males (Table 2). However, there were no additional grooves in either the left or the right of ansiform lobules in females (Table 2). We observed a significant sexual difference in the incidence of additional grooves only in the left CZp, which was significantly higher in males compared to females (Table 2).

There were no asymmetrically poorly developed sublobules in the PZ in both males and females (Table 1). Additional grooves appeared asymmetrically on the left and right of the paramedian sublobules in both males and females without a significant sexual difference and a left/right difference (Table 2).

3.3. *Relationship with Regional Cerebellar Volume Laterality*

Volumes of left and right sides and mean AQ values of each transverse domain are shown in Table S1 in the Supplementary Materials.

We observed significant differences in the incidence of asymmetry in sublobular development and additional grooves appearing in the left-dominant group between the left and right sides of the CZa and CZp. Poor sublobular development appeared more frequently in the right CZp compared to the left CZp in the left-dominant group (Table 3). There was a significantly greater incidence of additional grooves in the right CZa compared to the left CZa in the left-dominant group (Table 4). Therefore, the right-dominant appearance of the poor development of CZp sublobules and additional grooves in the CZa might be associated with left-lateralized volumes of these cerebellar domains.

Table 3. Incidence of asymmetrically poor development of cerebellar sublobules in ferrets with left- or right-dominant volume laterality in cerebellar transverse domains.

Transverse Domains	Left-Dominant (AQ < 0)		Right-Dominant (AQ > 0)	
Anterior zone				
Left side	66.7%	(2/3)	27.3%	(3/11)
Right side	33.3%	(1/3)	63.6%	(7/11)
Central zone anterior				
Left side	30.0%	(3/10)	50.0%	(2/4)
Right side	20.0%	(2/10)	25.0%	(1/4)
Central zone posterior				
Left side	0%	(0/10)	0%	(0/4)
Right side	40.0%	(4/10) *	25.0%	(1/4)
Posterior zone				
Left side	0%	(3/8)	0%	(0/6)
Right side	0%	(4/8)	0%	(0/6)

The number of individuals exhibiting the poor sublobular development at each side is shown in parentheses. * $p < 0.05$ left side vs. right side in left-dominant group (chi-square test).

Table 4. Incidence of asymmetrically appearing additional grooves in ferrets with left- or right-dominant volume laterality in cerebellar transverse domains.

Transverse Domains	Left-Dominant (AQ < 0)		Right-Dominant (AQ > 0)	
Anterior zone				
Left side	0%	(0/3)	0%	(0/11)
Right side	0%	(0/3)	0%	(0/11)
Central zone anterior				
Left side	0%	(0/10)	0%	(0/4)
Right side	40.0%	(4/10) *	50.0%	(2/4)
Central zone posterior				
Left side	30.0%	(3/10)	25.0%	(1/4)
Right side	20.0%	(2/10)	0%	(0/4)
Posterior zone				
Left side	37.5%	(3/8)	33.3%	(2/6)
Right side	50.0%	(4/8)	33.3%	(2/6)

The number of individuals showing the additional grooves at each side is shown in parentheses. * $p < 0.05$ left side vs. right side in left-dominant group (chi-square test).

4. Discussion

The cerebellum is functionally lateralized by making cerebrum–cerebellum connections linked contralaterally with the association cortex, not the motor cortex [9,16]. Right-handed humans showed mirror linkage of the torque asymmetry between the cerebrum and cerebellum, i.e., counterclockwise versus clockwise [7]. The left-lateralized volume of the CZp in the ferret cerebellum plays a role in poor sublobular development in right ansiform lobules. Such left-lateralized development might be involved in left CZp function, such as place-based navigation [10].

Another asymmetric profile appearing in relation to the cerebellar volume laterality is the additional groove in the right paravermian lobule VI, especially in ferrets with the left-biased volume of the CZa. A meta-analysis of task-based neuroimaging studies has shown that the left lobule VI is involved in spatial processing, while the right lobule VI is involved in language and working memory processing [8]. As cerebellar morphological lateralization is related to cerebrum–cerebellum connections [9], the right lobule VI might infold by an enchantment of connectivity to the left cerebral hemisphere.

There is a significant male-over-female incidence in additional grooves appearing in the left CZp, which mainly emerge in left ansiform lobules, indicating sexual differences in CZp function. Sex-related paw preferences have a significant correlation with cerebellar volume asymmetry in dogs [4]. However, ansiform lobules might not be related to paw preferences. In humans, handedness is not related to the superior posterior cerebellar lobule volume, including crura I and II, in terms of interhemispheric connectivity in cortical systems [17]. In contrast, the emergence of additional indentations, called secondary and tertiary sulci, in the cerebral cortex might be associated with regional cortical growth [18]. A preliminary study revealed the possibility of adult cerebellar neurogenesis in ferrets [19], as reported in humans and mice [20]. As volumetric asymmetry of the ferret cerebellum is evident during puberty to adolescence [6], regional cerebellar growth by adult neurogenesis might be involved in the appearance of additional sex-related grooves. Further studies are needed to elucidate this.

5. Conclusions

A distinctive cerebellar morphological asymmetry has been documented in humans [7], nonhuman primates [2], and carnivores [4,5], although the direction and degree of asymmetry are altered by species and/or sexes [2–7] but not by genetic factors [7]. As the rodent cerebellum developed symmetrically [21], ferrets would be useful models for investigating the pathogenesis underlying human neurodevelopmental disorders with disturbances in morphological cerebellar asymmetry, such as autistic spectrum disorder [22], schizophrenia [23,24], dyslexia [25], and attention-deficit hyperactivity disorder [26]. Asymmetric hallmarks of the cortical surface morphology visible on the cerebellar surface of ferrets are relevant to the left-biased volume asymmetry of the CZ of cerebellar transversus domains containing lobule VI and ansiform lobules in ferrets. The findings provide a new insight into assessments of cerebellar asymmetry on the basis of cerebellar surface morphology.

Author Contributions: K.S. designed the study; K.S. and S.K. performed the experiments and analyzed the data; K.S. and I.A. wrote the manuscript; the final version of the manuscript was approved by all authors. All authors have read and agreed to the published version of the manuscript.

Acknowledgments: The authors wish to thank Nobuhiro Nitta (Molecular Imaging Center, National Institute of Radiological Sciences, Chiba, Japan) for the MRI measurements. The authors would like to thank Enago (www.enago.jp) for the English language review.

References

1. Synder, P.J.; Bilder, R.M.; Wu, H.; Bogerts, B.; Lieberman, J.A. Cerebellar volume asymmetries are related to handedness: A quantitative MRI study. *Neuropsychologia* **1995**, *33*, 407–419. [CrossRef]
2. Phillips, K.; Hopkins, W.D. Exploring the relationship between cerebellar asymmetry and handedness in chimpanzees (*Pan troglodytes*) and capuchins (*Cebus apella*). *Neuropsychologia* **2007**, *45*, 2333–2339. [CrossRef] [PubMed]
3. Cantalupo, C.; Freeman, H.; Rodes, W.; Hopkins, W. Handedness for tool use correlates with cerebellar asymmetries in chimpanzees (*Pan troglodytes*). *Behav. Neurosci.* **2008**, *122*, 191–198. [CrossRef] [PubMed]
4. Koyun, N.; Aydinlioğlu, A.; Aslan, K. A morphometric study on dog cerebellum. *Neurol. Res.* **2011**, *33*, 220–224. [CrossRef]
5. Sawada, K.; Horiuchi-Hirose, M.; Saito, S.; Aoki, I. Male prevalent enhancement of leftward asymmetric development of the cerebellar cortex in ferrets (*Mustela putorius*). *Laterality* **2015**, *20*, 723–737. [CrossRef]
6. Sawada, K.; Aoki, I. Age-dependent sexually-dimorphic asymmetric development of the ferret cerebellar cortex. *Symmetry* **2017**, *9*, 40. [CrossRef]
7. Rosch, R.E.; Ronan, L.; Cherkas, L.; Gurd, J.M. Cerebellar asymmetry in a pair of monozygotic handedness-discordant twins. *J. Anat.* **2010**, *217*, 38–47. [CrossRef]
8. Valera, E.M.; Faraone, S.V.; Biederman, J.; Poldrack, R.A.; Seidman, L.J. Functional neuroanatomy of working memory in adults with attention-deficit/hyperactivity disorder. *Biol. Psychiatry* **2005**, *57*, 439–447. [CrossRef]
9. Wang, D.; Buckner, R.L.; Liu, H. Cerebellar asymmetry and its relation to cerebral asymmetry estimated by intrinsic functional connectivity. *J. Neurophysiol.* **2013**, *109*, 46–57. [CrossRef]
10. Iglói, K.; Doeller, C.F.; Paradis, A.L.; Benchenane, K.; Berthoz, A.; Burgess, N.; Rondi-Reig, L. Interaction between hippocampus and cerebellum crus I in sequence-based but not place-based navigation. *Cereb. Cortex* **2015**, *25*, 4146–4154. [CrossRef]
11. Sokolov, A.A. The cerebellum in social cognition. *Front. Cell Neurosci.* **2018**, *12*, 145. [CrossRef]
12. Hopkins, W.D.; Marino, L. Asymmetries in cerebral width in nonhuman primate brains as revealed by magnetic resonance imaging (MRI). *Neuropsychologia* **2000**, *38*, 493–499. [CrossRef]
13. Lawes, I.N.C.; Andrews, P.L.R. Neuroanatomy of the ferret brain. In *Biology and Diseases of the Ferret*, 2nd ed.; Fox, Ed.; Lippincott Williams and Wilkins: Baltimore, MD, USA, 1998; pp. 71–102.
14. Ozol, K.; Hayden, J.M.; Oberdick, J.; Hawkes, R. Transverse zones in the vermis of the mouse cerebellum. *J. Comp. Neurol.* **1999**, *412*, 95–111. [CrossRef]
15. Sillitoe, R.V.; Hawkes, R. Whole-mount immunohistochemistry: A high-throughput screen for patterning defects in the mouse cerebellum. *J. Histochem. Cytochem.* **2002**, *50*, 235–244. [CrossRef]
16. Siniscalchi, M.; Franchini, D.; Pepe, A.M.; Sasso, R.; Dimatteo, S.; Vallortigara, G.; Quaranta, A. Volumetric assessment of cerebral asymmetries in dogs. *Laterality* **2011**, *16*, 528–536. [CrossRef]
17. Rosch, R.E.; Cowell, P.E.; Gurd, J.M. Cerebellar asymmetry and cortical connectivity in monozygotic twins with discordant handedness. *Cerebellum* **2018**, *17*, 191–203. [CrossRef]

18. Sawada, K.; Fukunishi, K.; Kashima, M.; Imai, N.; Saito, S.; Aoki, I.; Fukui, Y. Regional difference in sulcal infolding progression correlated with cerebral cortical expansion in cynomolgus monkey fetuses. *Congenit. Anom. (Kyoto)* **2017**, *57*, 114–117. [CrossRef]
19. Kamiya, S.; Sawada, K. Immunohistochemical characterization of postnatal changes in cerebellar cortical cytoarchitectures in ferrets. *Anat. Rec. (Hoboken)*, in press.
20. Ahlfeld, J.; Filser, S.; Schmidt, F.; Wefers, A.K.; Merk, D.J.; Glaß, R.; Herms, J.; Schüller, U. Neurogenesis from Sox2 expressing cells in the adult cerebellar cortex. *Sci. Rep.* **2017**, *7*, 6137. [CrossRef]
21. Dorr, A.E.; Lerch, J.P.; Spring, S.; Kabani, N.; Henkelman, R.M. High resolution three-dimensional brain atlas using an average magnetic resonance image of 40 adult C57Bl/6J mice. *Neuroimage* **2008**, *42*, 60–69. [CrossRef]
22. Hodge, S.M.; Makris, N.; Kennedy, D.N.; Caviness, V.S., Jr.; Howard, J.; McGrath, L.; Steele, S.; Frazier, J.A.; Tager-Flusberg, H.; Harris, G.J. Cerebellum, language, and cognition in autism and specific language impairment. *J. Autism Dev. Disord.* **2010**, *40*, 300–316. [CrossRef] [PubMed]
23. Levitt, J.J.; McCarley, R.W.; Nestor, P.G.; Petrescu, C.; Donnino, R.; Hirayasu, Y.; Kikinis, R.; Jolesz, F.A.; Shenton, M.E. Quantitative volumetric MRI study of the cerebellum and vermis in schizophrenia: Clinical and cognitive correlates. *Am. J. Psychiatry* **1999**, *156*, 1105–1107. [PubMed]
24. Sheng, J.; Zhu, Y.; Lu, Z.; Liu, N.; Huang, N.; Zhang, Z.; Tan, L.; Li, C.; Yu, X. Altered volume and lateralization of language-related regions in first-episode schizophrenia. *Schizophr. Res.* **2013**, *148*, 168–174. [CrossRef] [PubMed]
25. Kibby, M.Y.; Fancher, J.B.; Markanen, R.; Hynd, G.W. A quantitative magnetic resonance imaging analysis of the cerebellar deficit hypothesis of dyslexia. *J. Child Neurol.* **2008**, *23*, 368–380. [CrossRef] [PubMed]
26. Castellanos, F.X.; Giedd, J.N.; Marsh, W.L.; Hamburger, S.D.; Vaituzis, A.C.; Dickstein, D.P.; Sarfatti, S.E.; Vauss, Y.C.; Snell, J.W.; Lange, N.; et al. Quantitative brain magnetic resonance imaging in attention-deficit hyperactivity disorder. *Arch. Gen. Psychiatry* **1996**, *53*, 607–616. [CrossRef] [PubMed]

4

How Ecology Could Affect Cerebral Lateralization for Explorative Behaviour in Lizards

Beatrice Bonati [1,*], Caterina Quaresmini [2], Gionata Stancher [3,4] and Valeria Anna Sovrano [2,4]

1 Department of Chemistry, Life Sciences and Environmental Sustainability, University of Parma, Parco Area delle Scienze 11/A, 43124 Parma, Italy
2 Department of Psychology and Cognitive Sciences, University of Trento, 38068 Rovereto (Trento), Italy; caterina.quaresmini@gmail.com (C.Q.); valeriaanna.sovrano@unitn.it (V.A.S.)
3 Rovereto Civic Museum Foundation, 38068 Rovereto (Trento), Italy; gionata.stancher@unitn.it
4 Center for Mind/Brain Sciences, University of Trento, 38068 Rovereto (Trento), Italy
* Correspondence: beatrice.bonati@unipr.it

Academic Editor: Lesley Rogers

Abstract: As recent studies have shown a left-eye preference during exploration in *Podarcis muralis*, which could be strictly related to its territoriality, we tested the same behaviour in a similar species, but one living in different habitats and showing a different ecology. In particular, we assessed the preferential turning direction in adults of a non-territorial lizard, *Zootoca vivipara*, during the exploration of an unknown maze. At the population level, no significant preference emerged, possibly for the lack of the territorial habit and the characteristics of the natural environment. Nevertheless, females turned to the left more frequently than males did. We hypothesize this as a motor bias, possibly due to a necessity for females to be coordinated and fast in moving in the environment, because of their viviparous condition and the resultant reduction of physical performance during pregnant periods, which are likely to increase vulnerability to predators.

Keywords: brain asymmetry; eye preference; lateralization; lizard; motor bias; territoriality

1. Introduction

Scientists have collected a large amount of evidence supporting behavioural bias spread across vertebrates, and even invertebrates [1–3]. This is even clearer if we consider that being lateralized could bring benefits, hence, affecting the fitness of individuals that present it [4–6].

Brain asymmetries can be manifested and studied as behavioural visual asymmetries, or the preferential use of a specific eye for looking at a type of stimulus, with the latter being especially easily evident in animals with laterally-placed eyes [7,8]. We know that different reactions to right-and left-placed stimuli have been ascertained in several species, verifying the specialization of the brain to perceive information with the left or right eye and in elaborating it with the contralateral hemisphere, according to the nature of the cue (for review, see [1,4,8]).

Being so lateralized could be advantageous by allowing better processing of two tasks at the same time, each one perceived with an eye, and then elaborated by the contralateral hemisphere [4,8,9]. This can enhance a lateralized individual's cognition to simultaneously attend to multiple cues [4,10,11]. As the behaviours involved, i.e., lateralized, are generally usual and important for survival, such as feeding and vigilance, it could be extremely advantageous that they can be performed simultaneously [12–14].

Recently, the scientific interest about lateralized species has increased for mammals, as well as for birds [15–18]. Lizards are an interesting model for studying visual lateralization because they have almost complete decussation of the optic chiasma and they lack the larger number of interhemispheric connections present in mammals, allowing cues perceived with one eye to be processed almost entirely with the contralateral half of the brain [19,20]. Each visual system could then work largely independently [21]. Some previous works focused on *Podarcis muralis*, a lizard species widespread in Europe, highlighting that this species is lateralized for some crucial daily behaviours [22]. According to the bibliography, this species shows preferences in using the left eye in predatory tasks (detailed observation of stimuli), and the right eye in vigilance and exploratory tasks (global attention and spatial processing of stimuli), also in the wild [23–27]. Speculations hypothesized that the lateralization present in this species could be related to its strong territoriality [28,29] and consequent habit of exploring with a high vigilance level during its activities; hence, laterality in this lizard could be evolved as an adaptive character in response to specific environmental needs [22,30]. In this work, we attempted to investigate an eventual form of lateralization in a non-territorial and elusive lizard species, *Zootoca vivipara*, with different life habits [31], environment, and needs than to *P. muralis*, so as to compare results for both species, and attempt to understand the importance/weight of ecological conditions on the manifestation of behavioural and cerebral biases. Starting from the study conducted by Csermely et al. [32], we focused on exploration, an activity closely related to life in the natural environment and biology.

2. Materials and Methods

2.1. Subjects and Housing

From June to July we collected 10 wild adult *Zootoca vivipara* lizards, five males and five females, from Ampola Lake, a biotope in the southwestern area of Trentino, near the town Tiano di Sopra (TN). We obtained the required administrative permit for capturing the lizards from the wild from Comunità Alto Garda e Ledro (prot. 11083/11.4, 25 May 2012). Captures were made by noosing or hands; the lizards were put in cloth bags immediately after and carried to the terraria. Behavioural observations were carried out in the research and the didactical station SperimentArea, situated in Rovereto (Trento, Italy). Here the lizards were housed in 80 × 50 × 40 cm glass terraria or 40 × 40 × 30 cm plastic cages, under the natural Italian summer photoperiod (16:8 h light/dark cycle) and temperature (25–35 °C) regulated with artificial lighting, if necessary. Each terrarium had a floor covered with a sand substratum with the addition of soil, bark, and musk, other than rocks and bricks for refuge and/or basking. The lizards were fed daily with multivitamin powder-dusted mealworm larvae (*Tenebrio molitor*) and crickets; water was provided *ad libitum*. In order to maintain the correct substratum humidity, the terrain was adjusted daily with water vaporization, if necessary. Once entering the terrarium, the lizards were allowed to accustom themselves to the new environment for seven days before the tests started. At the end of the experiment lizards were released at the same site of capture; none of them was harmed by the experiment, which was carried out under license from Italian authorities.

2.2. Apparatus

In order to compare the explorative behaviour of *Zootoca vivipara* with that of *Podarcis muralis*, we employed the same experimental apparatus previously used in Csermely et al. [32] (Figure 1), modified, consisting of a 54 × 66 cm PVC base maze with 10 cm high sides. Thirteen 12 × 10 × 6 cm blocks were scattered regularly on the base at the distance of 6 cm each other; four additional 6 × 10 × 6 cm blocks were located against two sides of the base; their length was limited to one-half of that of the others so as to maintain the regular reciprocal distance among the blocks. The blocks' presence had to induce the exploring lizard to continuously change direction when it arrived at the T-crossroads, then forcing it to decide to go either to the left or to the right. The blocks were attached to the base with adhesive tape. They were made of a series of commercial Duplo® bricks (Lego A/S, Billund, Denmark) and covered with plastic adhesive paper with marble coloration to prevent the lizards from climbing them. Experiments were conducted without transparent cover, for possible interferences of the reflectance of neon light placed on the top of the maze. The apparatus was located in a circular tub

(110 cm of diameter, 50 cm high), necessary to contain animals in case of escape and to avoid possible surrounding influences on the individual behaviour. In addition, four black corrugated honeycomb panels were collocated all around the apparatus, working as screens for the operator.

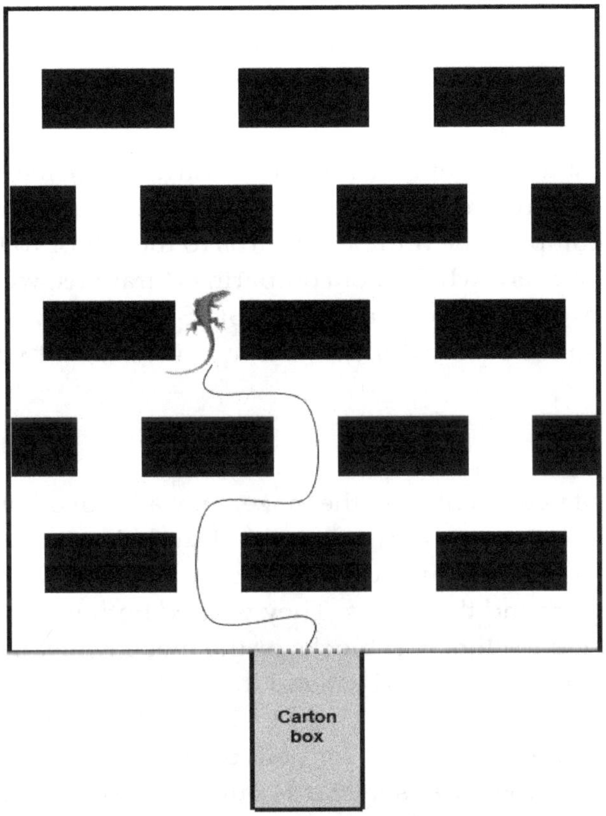

Figure 1. Schematic 2D representation of the experimental apparatus (adapted from [32]).

2.3. Procedure

Before the beginning of the tests, we allowed lizards to thermoregulate at least 30 min under the light of a 50-W halogen lamp, allowing them to reach the temperature for maximal locomotor performance, necessary to express correct exploring behaviour. Experiments were conducted in the same place as the lizard housing, hence, with the same light and temperature conditions. Afterwards, a lizard was gently removed from the terrarium and placed in a 15 × 9 × 6.5 cm carton box external to the maze, but attached to it. The lizard remained in the box for 5 min to acclimatize; thereafter, the operator, located behind a black Poliplak® screen (RÖHM GmbH, Sontheim/Brenz, Germany), using a thin cable, lifted up the PVC gateway that had prevented the lizard from entering the maze through the opening before the beginning of the test. The test started when the lizard entered the maze. After 20 min, if the lizard did not spontaneously enter it, the operator beat, with a small stick, the distal part of the box containing the lizard to encourage it to move out. The lizard could move freely within the maze for 20 min. During the experiment, the gateway remained open; hence, the lizard could come back to the box. At the end, it was returned to its terrarium and the maze floor and walls were cleaned with ethyl alcohol to prevent any possible effect of chemical cues on subsequent individuals.

The tests were carried out when the air temperature was within the 27–35 °C range. Light was homogeneous and both natural and artificial by a neon lamp placed on the experimental apparatus. We considered the following behaviour parameters: when the subject entered the maze, we assessed (1) the rotation of the head to the left or the right, and (2) the frequency of direction of the turn (leftward or rightward). Afterward, while the lizard was exploring the maze, we observed (3) the delay time (duration of hesitation) at each T-crossroads, and (4) the duration of each turning, (5) the total frequency of direction of turning; and (6) when passing a T-crossroad for the first time (excluding any possible olfactory influence).

All tests were recorded with a digital mini DV colour video camera Sony "Handycam" DCR-SR58 (Sony, Tokyo, Japan) 17.0 × 9.0 × 8.0 cm placed above the maze. Frame by frame analysis of the footage was possible by the Windows Live Movie Maker 6.0 video software (Microsoft Corporation, Redmond, WA, USA).

2.4. Statistical Analyses

We used the binomial test to compare the number of turns to the left or to the right performed by each lizard and the individual preference in turning the head. The Wilcoxon matched-pairs signed ranks test (T+) was used to compare the number of turns to the left or to the right and the preference in turning the head in the group as a whole. For comparing durations, we used the Mann–Whitney U test (U). Calculations have been performed using the SPSS 18.0 for Windows software [33]. Means are ± Standard Error (SE) and the probability, set at $\alpha = 0.05$, was two-tailed throughout, unless otherwise stated.

3. Results

Although all lizards hesitated in entering the maze, they all moved out of the box and completed the experiment. Some lizards, before exiting, required a stimulation by gently tapping on the starting box with a stick. During experiments lizards did not appear frightened but explored the environment, walking inside it and turning around the blocks. They walked both in the central and lateral routes of the maze; sometimes they tried to climb the blocks or the maze walls. During the exploration some individuals arrived near the entrance box and entered it, but they shortly moved back out to the maze. During the experiment lizards moved for 619.15 ± 71.45 s and froze for 580.85 ± 57.82 s, without any difference inside the group and between sexes for both the time of movement and immobility.

Immediately after entering the maze six lizards out of 10 (four males and two females) rotated the head to the right (binomial test; $p = 0.289$), two lizards (both females) to the left, and two lizards (one male and one female) did not rotate the head before entering.

Three lizards (one male and two females) out of 10 performed the first turn immediately after entering the maze on the left and seven lizards (four males and three females) out of 10 on the right (binomial test; $p = 0.3438$).

The subsequent movements of the lizards were in various directions, moving progressively further from the entering point. The delay time for turning at each T-crossroad showed similar results for both the left and right directions (2.53 ± 0.90 s and 2.00 ± 0.72 s, respectively; $z = -0.227$; $p = 0.821$), and also between sexes (males left: 3.96 ± 1.12 s; females left: 1.10 ± 0.24 s; $U = -0.522$; $p = 0.690$; males right: 3.23 ± 0.89 s; females right: 0.78 ± 0.09 s; $U = -1.567$; $p = 0.117$). During each T-crossroad turning, lizards kept the head right-turned for 4.62 ± 0.88 s and left-turned for 6.19 ± 0.23 s ($U = -0.076$; $p = 0.940$); no differences emerged between sexes in keeping the head right-turned (males: 4.74 ± 0.97 s; females: 4.51 ± 0.90; $U = -0.522$; $p = 0.6$) and left-turned (males: 8.66 ± 3.26 s; females: 3.73 ± 0.52 s; $U = -0.83$; $p = 0.4$).

The average number of turns per lizard per test was 27.70 ± 3.19, with no significant differences between sexes (males: 25.80 ± 2.75, females: 29.60 ± 4.01; $U = 11.500$; $p = 0.834$). Statistical analyses did not reveal any population-level bias for turning to the left or to the right among the lizards (13.2 ± 2.30 and 14.5 ± 1.68, respectively; $T+ = -0.153$; $p = 0.878$) and between sexes for the right turning ($T+ = -0.674$; $p = 0.500$), but females showed a bias in turning left compared with males ($T+ = -2.032$; $p = 0.042$). Males performed 9.80 ± 1.40 left-turns and 16.0 ± 2.00 right-turns ($T+ = -1.826$, $p = 0.068$) and females performed 16.60 ± 2.67 left-turns vs. 13.0 ± 1.342 right-turns ($T+ = -1.214$, $p = 0.225$). If we consider the average number of turns that lizards performed when encountering a T-crossroad for the first time (i.e., without any olfactory influence) there emerged a preference in turning right (8.5 ± 1.02) compared with the left direction (5.9 ± 0.78; $T+ = -1.963$, $p = 0.050$) in the population.

This result is due to the males' choice (right: 8.5 ± 1.02; left: 4.4 ± 0.52) more than the females' choice (right: 8.0 ± 0.72; left: 7.4 ± 0.72; Table 1). Moreover, females turned more frequently than males to the left (T+ = −2.032; p = 0.042) than to the right (T+ = −0.412; p = 0.680).

Considering the total number of turns per lizard to the left or to the right, 2 individuals of the 10 tested showed a preference for turning right (Binomial test; p = 0.029 and p = 0.035), both males (Table 2).

Table 1. Number of first turns for lizards when encountering a T-crossroad for the first time. p-values refer to binomial test comparisons.

Lizard	Sex	Left	Right	Tot	p
1	M	4	15	19	0.0192
2	M	5	10	15	0.3018
3	M	7	9	16	0.8036
4	M	3	6	9	0.5078
5	M	3	5	8	0.7266
6	F	5	5	10	1.2461
7	F	9	6	15	0.6072
8	F	8	12	20	0.5034
9	F	10	9	19	1.0000
10	F	5	8	13	0.5811

Table 2. Number of turns for lizard for test. p-values refer to binomial test comparisons.

Lizard	Sex	Left	Right	Tot	p
1	M	7	19	26	0.0290
2	M	13	23	36	0.1325
3	M	16	15	31	1.0000
4	M	6	17	23	0.0347
5	M	7	6	13	1.0000
6	F	11	7	18	0.4807
7	F	17	12	29	0.4583
8	F	30	18	48	0.1114
9	F	17	16	33	1.0000
10	F	8	12	20	0.5034

By the number of first turn performed by each lizard it emerged that only one individual (a male) showed a preference, in particular in turning rightward (binomial test; p = 0.0192).

4. Discussion

Overall, our lizards resulted in not showing any evident bias or side preference in exploring a novel environment. Hence, the explorative behaviour of *Zootoca vivipara* lizards does not seem to be controlled by a form of lateralization. This is interesting as this result is in strong contrast with what was found by Csermely et al. [32] in *Podarcis muralis*. In fact, although experiments were conducted in the same way, and with the same experimental apparatus, *P. muralis* evidenced a strong bias in turning left, that the authors associated to a visual guided bias during exploration, i.e., a visual lateralization [32]. As such, these results suggest that differences emerging between these species are probably due to their remarkably different ecology, although, at present, there is no evidence of a clear explanation for the differential lateralization of the two species.

As a first point, we observed that although during the experiment almost all *Z. vivipara* individuals gave good clear signals of exploration, they all showed hesitation in entering the maze and the time they spent in exploring was similar to the time they spent in freezing. This poor activity and the overall low level of confidence in the maze could be related to the secretive behaviour of *Z. vivipara* and, in particular, likened to the thermally-heterogeneous habitats where this species is commonly found, allowing less active movements in general and, at the same time, more time spent in thermoregulation [34,35].

Results on behavioural lateralization highlighted in *P. muralis* have been explained by the authors with its strong territoriality and its consequent natural high predisposition to explore [32]. A support of this is the fact that, in Csermely et al. [32], an evident higher frequency of turning emerged, especially in males, mainly motivated by the need to defend their own area. In contrast, our *Z. vivipara* lived in a wild, cold-climate environment, characterized by the presence of unique ecological factors potentially influencing the explorative behaviour (therefore, the *Z. vivipara* lateralization). For example, the human impact and presence in such areas is generally low, in contrast with the high anthropic level locations, where *P. muralis* was studied by Csermely et al. [32] lived. This could force individuals to maintain a high level of attention and vigilance, pushing towards a stronger lateralization in the explorative behaviour.

Nevertheless, an overall female bias in turning left emerged here, referring also to the first and more spontaneous encounter with a T-crossroad. Whereas the lack of turning preferences in the overall T-maze could be due to the low sample used in these experiments, the turning bias in the first T-crossroad could be explained either as a visual lateralization or a motor lateralization. As a visual lateralization, the direction of choice is consistent with that found in *P. muralis*, and with previous studies, which appointed to the right hemisphere the capability of processing global aspects of the environment [14,32,36]. However, it is in strong contrast with the evidence that, in *P. muralis*, the turning bias is found in males, not in females [32]. As this previous result could be linked with males' territorial attitude, we suggest that *Z. vivipara* females' visual preference could be related to the viviparous nature of several populations of this species, which constrains female individuals in having a longer reproductive period in respect to oviparous females, and a consequently higher level of attention compared with male individuals [34]. During gestation, females must be more vigilant to guarantee the offspring's survival, hence, to increase their fitness. However, gestation incurs some costs, such as a shift in thermoregulatory needs and locomotor impairment [34,35,37–39]. Pregnant individuals are physically limited by their body increase which may affect and reduce their fleetness and speed, thus, with locomotor costs. Being lateralized, in particular for the same direction in the same population, could be advantageous for the possibility of coordination in behaviour between individuals, in particular for anti-predatory tasks [4]. This is especially true for social/gregarious species [4,40,41]. Although there is no evidence of gregarious habits in *Zootoca vivipara*, the absence of territoriality allows tolerance between individuals, and a coordination in moving may become, for these lizards, one of the evolutionary strategies for contrasting costs of viviparity. This could become a hypothesis of explanation of the necessity for female lizards to be specialized in vigilance as a group, especially in moving.

Movement, particularly in exploratory behaviour, is preceded by a high-level observation that probably guides the subsequent choice of direction. There are several indications of left-eye processing in using the environmental layout to guide locomotion to a target site using spatial information [42]. However, we emphasize that the female leftward preference in turning, which emerged at T-crossroads is not supported by the head rotation durations we measured during each T-crossroad turning. These comparisons, easily indicative of visual system involvement, did not show any significance, not sustaining a visual influence in the choice of direction. It is therefore possible to advance the hypothesis in this context, that the left-turning females' bias highlighted by this work may be evidence of footedness, hence, a motor bias more than a visual one.

Very differently to *P. muralis,* closely related to dry and bare environments, *Z. vivipara* is strictly dependent on habitats, as wetlands, where the vegetation cover is prominent and could become a visual impediment between individuals. Thus, it could be difficult for these individuals to maintain a visual link in groups of conspecifics. This is also true during thermoregulatory exposure. In fact, because of their viviparity, female lizards preferentially used the half-basking behaviour (partially hidden), although basking in the open is more efficient [34]. This allowed these lizards to significantly reduce the risk of facing exposure to predators, optimizing the trade-off between predation risks and basking efficiency [34,43,44]. In this context, it could be disadvantageous or simply necessary to visually coordinate the behaviour, but it may help to synchronise a motor response.

All this contributes to explaining the different response *Z. vivipara* provide compared with *P. muralis*, i.e., the main absence of lateralization and the different sex evidence, also underlining the importance and close relationship between the living environment and conditions and the evolution of biases.

In conclusion, our results show, that in general *Z. vivipara* is not lateralized in exploring a new environment. However, females showed a bias for turning left during exploration, possibly more easily explained as a motor bias. As these results are in contrast with what emerged in *P. muralis* individuals in previous studies, which showed a visual lateralization especially in males, we propose it could be related to the different ecology of the species, in particular, with differences of the territorial and viviparous natures. Moreover, this is a confirmation of the crucial role of the real-life environment and habits in the emergence and evolution of cerebral lateralization, supporting its advantageous nature, which contributes in its manifestation in different contexts.

Acknowledgments: This study was supported by a grant obtained from the collaboration between the Department of Cognitive Sciences and the Municipality of Rovereto about the study on the biodiversity of the Trentino's environmental heritage. We wish to thank Tiziana Cumer for her help with the experiments and the Natural History Museum of Parma University for having kindly provided part of the scientific material. B.B. is sincerely grateful to Filippo Merusi, Cristina Menta, and Giorgio Dieci.

Author Contributions: All authors participated in conceiving and designing the experiments; and G.S. and C.Q. performed the experiments and analysed the data.

References

1. Vallortigara, G.; Chiandetti, C.; Sovrano, V.A. Brain asimmetry (animal). *Wires Cogn. Sci.* **2011**, *2*, 146–157. [CrossRef] [PubMed]
2. Rogers, L.J.; Vallortigara, G.; Andrew, R.J. *Divided Brains: The Biology and Behaviour of Brain Asymmetries*; Cambridge University Press: Cambridge, UK, 2013.
3. Frasnelli, E.; Vallortigara, G.; Rogers, L.J. Left–right asymmetries of behaviour and nervous system in invertebrates. *Neurosci. Biobehav. Rev.* **2012**, *36*, 1273–1291. [CrossRef] [PubMed]
4. Vallortigara, G.; Rogers, L.J. Survival with an asymmetrical brain: Advantages and disadvantages of cerebral lateralization. *Behav. Brain Sci.* **2005**, *28*, 102–178. [CrossRef] [PubMed]
5. Güntürkün, O.; Diekamp, B.; Manns, M.; Nottelmann, F.; Prior, H.; Schwarz, A.; Skiba, M. Asymmetry pays: Visual lateralization improves discrimination success in pigeons. *Curr. Biol.* **2000**, *10*, 1079–1081. [CrossRef]
6. Rogers, L.J. A Matter of Degree: Strength of Brain Asymmetry and Behaviour. *Symmetry* **2017**, *9*, 57. [CrossRef]
7. Vallortigara, G.; Rogers, J.L.; Bisazza, A. Possible evolutionary origins of cognitive brain lateralization. *Brain Res. Rev.* **1999**, *30*, 164–175. [CrossRef]
8. Sovrano, V.A.; Bisazza, A.; Vallortigara, G. Lateralization of response to social stimuli in fishes: A comparison between methods and species. *Physiol. Behav.* **2001**, *74*, 237–244. [CrossRef]
9. Rogers, L.J.; Zucca, P.; Vallortigara, G. Advantages of having a lateralized brain. *Proc. R. Soc. B* **2004**, *271*, S420–S422. [CrossRef] [PubMed]

10. Rogers, L.J. Advantages and disadvantages of lateralization. In *Comparative Vertebrate Lateralization*; Rogers, L.J., Andrew, R.J., Eds.; Cambridge University Press: Cambridge, UK, 2002.
11. Reddon, A.R.; Gutiérrez-Ibáñez, C.; Wylie, D.R.; Hurd, P.L. The relationship between growth, brain asymmetry and behavioural lateralization in a cichlid fish. *Behav. Brain Res.* **2009**, *201*, 223–228. [CrossRef] [PubMed]
12. Casper, L.M.; Dunbar, R.I.M. Asymmetries in the visual processing of emotional cues during agonistic interactions by gelada baboons. *Behav. Process.* **1996**, *37*, 57–65. [CrossRef]
13. Bisazza, A.; Pignatti, R.; Vallortigara, G. Detour tests reveal task and stimulus-specific behavioural lateralisation in mosquitofish (*Gambusia holbrooki*). *Behav. Brain Res.* **1997**, *89*, 237–242. [CrossRef]
14. MacNeilage, P.F.; Rogers, L.J.; Vallortigara, G. Origins of the left & right brain. *Sci. Am.* **2009**, *301*, 60–67. [PubMed]
15. Malaschichev, Y. Asymmetry of righting reflexes in sea turtles and its behavioral correlates. *Physiol. Behav.* **2016**, *157*, 1–8. [CrossRef] [PubMed]
16. Stancher, G. Cold blooded minds: Cognition in reptiles. In *Animal Flatmates: In the Mind of Our Closest Animal Friends*; Malavasi, M., Ed.; Smashwords Edition: Los Gatos, CA, USA, 2016.
17. Robins, A. Lateralized visual processing in anurans: New vistas though ancient eyes. In *Behavioral and Morphological Asymmetries in Vertebrates*; Malashichev, Y.B., Deckel, A.W., Eds.; Landes Bioscience: Georgetown, TX, USA, 2006.
18. Robins, A.; Chen, P.; Beazley, L.D.; Dunlop, S.A. Lateralized predatory responses in the ornate dragon lizard (*Ctenophorus ornatus*). *NeuroReport* **2005**, *16*, 849–852. [CrossRef] [PubMed]
19. Deckel, A.W. Laterality of aggressive response in Anolis. *J. Exp. Zool.* **1995**, *272*, 194–200. [CrossRef]
20. Butler, A.B.; Northcutt, G. Ascending tectal efferent projections in the lizard *Iguana iguana*. *Brain Res.* **1971**, *35*, 597–601. [CrossRef]
21. Schaeffel, F.; Howland, H.C.; Farkas, L. Natural accommodation in the growing chicken. *Vision Res.* **1986**, *26*, 1977–1993. [CrossRef]
22. Bonati, B.; Csermely, D. Lateralization in lizards: Evidence of presence in several contexts. In *Behavioral Lateralization in Vertebrates*; Csermely, D., Regolin, L., Eds.; Springer: Berlin/Heidelberg, Germany, 2013.
23. Bonati, B.; Csermely, D.; Sovrano, V.A. Advantages in exploring a new environment with the left eye in lizards. *Beahv. Process.* **2013**, *97*, 80–83. [CrossRef] [PubMed]
24. Csermely, D.; Bonati, B.; Romani, R. Lateralisation in a detour test in the common wall lizard (*Podarcis muralis*). *Laterality* **2010**, *15*, 535–547. [CrossRef] [PubMed]
25. Bonati, B.; Csermely, D.; López, P.; Martín, J. Lateralization in the escape behaviour of the common wall lizard (*Podarcis muralis*). *Behav. Brain Res.* **2010**, *207*, 1–6. [CrossRef] [PubMed]
26. Bonati, B.; Csermely, D. Complementary lateralization in the exploratory and predatory behaviour of the common wall lizard (*Podarcis muralis*). *Laterality* **2011**, *16*, 462–470. [CrossRef] [PubMed]
27. Martín, J.; López, P.; Bonati, B.; Csermely, D. Lateralization when monitoring predators in the wild: A left eye control in the common wall lizard (*Podarcis muralis*). *Ethology* **2010**, *116*, 1226–1233. [CrossRef]
28. Edsman, L. Territoriality and resource defense in wall lizards (*Podarcis muralis*). In *Studies in Herpetology: Proceedings of the European Herpetological Meeting (3rd Ordinary General Meeting of the Societas Europaea Herpetologica)*; Rocek, Z., Ed.; Charles University: Prague, Czech Republic, 1985.
29. Edsman, L. Territoriality and Competition in wall Lizards. Ph.D. Thesis, University of Stockholm, Stockholm, Sweden, 1990.
30. Bonati, B.; Csermely, D.; Sovrano, V.A. Looking at a predator with the left or right eye: asymmetry of response in lizards. *Laterality* **2013**, *18*, 329–339. [CrossRef] [PubMed]
31. Gvozdík, L.; Van Damme, R. Evolutionary maintenance of sexual dimorphism in head size in the lizard *Zootoca vivipara*: A test of two hypotheses. *J. Zool.* **2003**, *259*, 7–13. [CrossRef]
32. Csermely, D.; Bonati, B.; López, P.; Martín, J. Is the *Podarcis muralis* lizard left-eye lateralised when exploring a new environment? *Laterality* **2011**, *16*, 240–255. [CrossRef] [PubMed]
33. IBM SPSS, Corp. *PASW Statistic 18.0 for Windows: Base, Professional Statistics and Advanced Statistics*; IBM Corp.: Chicago, IL, USA, 2011.
34. Bleu, J.; Heulin, B.; Haussy, C.; Meylan, S.; Massot, M. Experimental evidence of early costs of reproduction in conspecific viviparous and oviparous lizards. *J. Evol. Biol.* **2012**, *25*, 1264–1274. [CrossRef] [PubMed]

35. Gvoždík, L. To heat or to save time? Thermoregulation in the lizard *Zootoca vivipara* (Squamata: Lacertidae) in different thermal environments along an altitudinal gradient. *Can. J. Zool.* **2002**, *80*, 479–492. [CrossRef]
36. Posner, M.J.; Petersen, S.E. The attention system of the human brain. *Annu. Rev. Neurosci.* **1990**, *13*, 25–42. [CrossRef] [PubMed]
37. De Marco, V.; Guillette, L.J. Physiological cost of pregnancy in a viviparous lizard (*Sceloporus jarrovi*). *J. Exp. Zool.* **1992**, *262*, 383–390. [CrossRef]
38. Olsson, M.; Shine, R.; Bak-Olsson, E. Locomotor impairment of gravid lizards: is the burden physical or physiological? *J. Evol. Biol.* **2000**, *13*, 263–268. [CrossRef]
39. Lin, C.-X.; Zhang, L.; Ji, X. Influence of pregnancy on locomotor and feeding performances of the skink, *Mabuya multifasciata*: Why do females shift thermal preferences when pregnant? *Zoology* **2008**, *111*, 188–195. [CrossRef] [PubMed]
40. Ghirlanda, S.; Vallortigara, G. The evolution of brain lateralization: A game-theoretical analysis of population structure. *Proc. Biol. Sci.* **2014**, *271*, 853–857. [CrossRef] [PubMed]
41. Ghirlanda, S.; Frasnelli, E.; Vallortigara, G. Intraspecific competition and coordination in the evolution of lateralization. *Philos. Trans. R. Soc. Lond. B* **2009**, *364*, 861–866. [CrossRef] [PubMed]
42. Andrew, R.J.; Rogers, L.J. The nature of lateralisation in tetrapods. In *Comparative Vertebrate Lateralisation*; Rogers, L.J., Andrew, R.J., Eds.; Cambridge University Press: Cambridge, UK, 2002.
43. Christian, K.A.; Tracy, C.R. The effect of the thermal environment on the ability of hatchling Galapagos land iguanas to avoid predation during dispersal. *Oecologia* **1981**, *49*, 218–223. [CrossRef] [PubMed]
44. Clobert, J.; Oppliger, A.; Sorci, G.; Ernande, B.; Swallow, J.G.; Garland, T., Jr. Trade-offs in phenotypic traits: Endurance at birth, growth, survival, predation and susceptibility to parasitism in a lizard, *Lacerta vivipara*. *Funct. Ecol.* **2000**, *14*, 675–684. [CrossRef]

5

Asymmetry for Symmetry: Right-Hemispheric Superiority in Bi-Dimensional Symmetry Perception

Giulia Prete [1,*], Mara Fabri [2], Nicoletta Foschi [3] and Luca Tommasi [1]

[1] Department of Psychology, Health and Territory, G. d'Annunzio University of Chieti-Pescara, Chieti 66013, Italy; luca.tommasi@unich.it

[2] Department of Clinical and Experimental Medicine, Neuroscience and Cell Biology Section, Polytechnic University of Marche, Ancona 60121, Italy; m.fabri@univpm.it

[3] Regional Epilepsy Centre, Neurological Clinic, Ospedali Riuniti, Ancona 60126, Italy; n.foschi@ospedaliriuniti.marche.it

* Correspondence: giulia.prete@unich.it

Academic Editor: Lesley Rogers

Abstract: A right-hemispheric superiority has been shown for spatial symmetry perception with mono-dimensional stimuli (e.g., bisected lines). Nevertheless, the cerebral imbalance for bi-dimensional stimuli is still controversial, and the aim of the present study is to investigate this issue. Healthy participants and a split-brain patient (D.D.C.) were tested in a divided visual field paradigm, in which a square shape was presented either in the left or right visual field and they were asked to judge whether a dot was placed exactly in the center of the square or off-center, by using the left/right hand in two separate sessions. The performance of healthy participants was better when the stimuli presented in the left visual field (LVF) were on-center rather than off-center. The performance of D.D.C. was higher than chance only when on-center stimuli were presented in the LVF in the left hand session. Only in this condition did his accuracy not differ with respect to that of the control group, whereas in all of the other conditions, it was lower than the controls' accuracy. We conclude that the right-hemispheric advantage already shown for mono-dimensional stimuli can be extended also to bi-dimensional configurations, confirming the right-hemispheric superiority for spatial symmetry perception.

Keywords: perceptual symmetry; cerebral hemispheres; split-brain patient; spatial processing; bi-dimensional stimuli

---

1. Introduction

Symmetry is easily detected by the visual system, and the way in which humans and other animals process visual symmetry is a central issue both in psychology and neuroscience. In fact, several models have been proposed in the attempt to explain how symmetry is detected and analyzed by the brain (e.g., [1–7]). Among the most acknowledged models, the perceptual rules proposed by Gestalt psychologists suggested that our preference for symmetric configurations ("symmetry bias") could be considered as a consequence of the perceptual preference for regularity and balance, compared to randomness and imbalance, by the human visual system. A debated point in this context concerns the possibility that such a regularity is extracted automatically, or it calls attentional processes into play (see [3] for a review). In support of the first point of view, it has been shown that patients with hemispatial neglect ("blind" for the left visual field as a consequence of a right-hemispheric lesion) show a preference for symmetrical arrangements in both visual fields, confirming that preattentive processes are responsible for figure-ground organization [8–10]. Other important results in this context come from those patients who have undergone surgical resection of callosal fibers, in the attempt to avoid the spread of epileptic foci between the two cerebral hemispheres, the so called "split-brain patients" [11]. In a series of experiments carried out with a split-brain patient, Funnell, Corballis, and Gazzaniga [12] showed that the right disconnected hemisphere is superior to the left hemisphere in perceptual matching tasks with mirror-reversed stimuli. By presenting stimuli consisting of either color pictures of nameable objects, black-and-white line drawings, or abstract geometrical forms, the authors concluded that the left hemisphere is specialized in pattern recognition, whereas the right hemisphere is specialized in spatial processing (see also [13]). The split-brain patients' literature is strongly linked to that of perceptual symmetry, because a number of authors suggested that at least when talking about vertical symmetry perception, this mechanism is due to the symmetrical morphology of our brain. In other words, it has been suggested that the preferential activation of two homologue areas in the left and right hemispheres is the basis for the automatic detection of symmetry in the physical world. In this "callosal hypothesis", the detection of symmetry may be favored by the activity of two specular areas in the left and right halves of the brain, which are connected by means of the fibers constituting the corpus callosum [1,2,14–16]. In this frame, it has been suggested that both the left and the right hemispheres are capable of low-level perceptual processing, and that hemispheric asymmetries arise at later stages of visual processing, in associative areas representing the two sides of visual space [17]. It has to be highlighted, however, that contrasting models have been recently suggested [18,19]. The fact that higher order cortical areas are involved in the detection of symmetrical patterns was confirmed in a functional magnetic resonance imaging (fMRI) study [20]: it was shown that independently of the size and the geometrical configuration of the stimuli, as well as independently of the recruitment of attentional control, symmetrical arrangements activated associative visual areas, in particular V3, V4, V7, and lateral occipital areas (for similar results see also [21,22], for a review see [23]).

A right-hemispheric superiority for symmetry detection has been found in healthy participants by means of the divided visual field paradigm. Wilkinson and Halligan [24] presented lines which could be either perfectly divided into two halves (bisected lines) or divided into two asymmetrical segments (misbisected lines), either in the left visual field (LVF) or in the right visual field (RVF), and participants were asked to judge whether each stimulus was symmetrical or asymmetrical. The performance of participants was better in terms of both accuracy and response times when bisected lines, but not misbisected lines, were presented in the LVF, concluding in favor of a right-hemispheric preference for symmetry. Besides the advantage of the right hemisphere in geometrical processing, the authors explained their results also by referring to the differential hemispheric specialization for low and high spatial frequencies. In particular, they concluded that the cerebral asymmetry they found could also be due to the fact that the right hemisphere is more strictly linked than the left hemisphere to the magnocellular visual pathway. This pathway is more sensitive to the low spatial frequencies of the stimuli, which are processed faster than the high spatial frequencies [25], and this could be intended as a further reason for the faster detection of symmetry by the right hemisphere. According to the authors, the short stimulus exposure used in the divided visual field paradigm (tachistoscopic presentation), together with the lateralized presentation of the stimuli (eccentricity), may facilitate the low spatial frequency analysis and thus the right-hemispheric processing. The same right-hemispheric superiority for low spatial frequencies has been confirmed also by means of complex visual stimuli, both in healthy participants and in split-brain patients (e.g., [26–28]). Nevertheless, in the same study Wilkinson and Halligan [24] failed to find a cerebral imbalance in the detection of symmetry when "double axes stimuli" (squares in which a circle could be placed on-center or off-center) were presented, explaining this finding as possibly attributable to the fact that square bisection activates bilateral networks. In a following fMRI study, Wilkinson and Halligan [29] found that the cerebral substrate of the LVF advantage for detecting the presence/absence of symmetry in lines is the right anterior cingulate gyrus. Bertamini and Makin [30] found that symmetry processing induced occipital alpha Event Related Desynchronization (ERD) in the right hemisphere, confirming at the electrophysiological level the stronger right- than left-hemispheric involvement in symmetry detection (see also [31,32]). In another electroencephalographic (EEG) study, Makin and colleagues [33] also showed that the

Sustained Posterior Negativity is stronger for reflection than for rotation and translation, and that this is true when participants were explicitly required to detect the presence of regularity in the stimuli.

The right-hemispheric causal involvement in symmetry detection has been demonstrated by means of transcranial magnetic stimulation (TMS) studies: Bona and colleagues [34] applied TMS over the left or right lateral occipital cortex while participants were asked to distinguish symmetrical from asymmetrical random dot patterns. The authors found that both hemispheres are involved in the task, but that the right-hemispheric stimulation leads to a stronger disruption of symmetry detection with respect to the left-hemispheric stimulation (see also [35]). TMS was also exploited together with an adaptation paradigm, revealing that when applied between adaptation and test stimuli, TMS applied over the dorsolateral extrastriate cortex, but not over V1/V2, reduced adaptation effects to dot patterns [36].

Only in one study among those reviewed above, has the cerebral asymmetry for double axes figures been investigated [24], and the authors failed to find significant differences in the ability to detect symmetry between the left and right hemispheres. Starting from this evidence, the main aim of the present study is to further assess this issue both in healthy participants and in a split-brain patient. In particular, in a divided visual field paradigm, participants were presented with stimuli consisting of a square containing a dot placed either in its exact center or slightly off-center. They were asked to judge whether the circle was/was not placed exactly in the center of the square. We hypothesized that, as found in previous works with single axis stimuli, a LVF superiority may be observed also for double axes stimuli, starting from the several studies of a right-hemispheric superiority for symmetry detection. To this aim, we almost quadrupled the number of healthy participants with respect to the study of Wilkinson and Halligan (from 12 to 44 participants), we further shortened the tachistoscopic presentation time (from 170 ms to 150 ms), and we also tested a complete callosotomy patient in order to obtain data from each surgically disconnected hemisphere. Additionally, in contrast to Wilkinson and Halligan, we asked participants to take part in two separate sessions, differing from one another in the hand used to respond, in order to consider the hand of the response as a further within-subject factor in the statistical design. Specifically, we did not expect to find differences in healthy participants according to the hand used to respond (the use of one hand does not allow us to test the unilateral responses in the intact brain), but we expected that the use of one hand in the split-brain patient would ensure the contralateral hemispheric involvement (due to the contralateral organization of the motor pathways; e.g., [37–39]). By using these changes, we expected to confirm that the performance is better when symmetrical (on-center) stimuli were presented in the LVF, both in healthy participants and—importantly—in the patient. The right-hemispheric superiority for spatial processing in split-brain patients has already been shown [12,13], but it has not been investigated for symmetry detection. In a study involving two split-brain patients, including the patient tested here, Corballis et al. [40] found a right-hemispheric superiority when patients were asked to distinguish between canonical and mirror-reversed letters (F and R), concluding that this task depends on matching to an exemplar (the canonical oriented letter), for which the right-hemisphere is dominant (as opposed to the left-hemispheric superiority in letter naming). In contrast to that study, in the present study we presented geometrical shapes, for which no comparison with a "model" is required, and thus we aimed at investigating the pure hemispheric imbalance in symmetry detection.

2. Materials and Methods

2.1. Participants

D.D.C. is an Italian male patient suffering from medically intractable epilepsy, who has had the corpus callosum (CC) surgically sectioned in the attempt to avoid the spread of epileptic foci between the cerebral hemispheres. He underwent the first partial section of CC in 1994, when he was 18-year old, and the complete section in 1995; the anterior commissure was also resected (see Figure 1). D.D.C. was 38 years old at the time of the test, his postoperative IQ was 83, and his laterality quotient was +40 (for more details, see [41]). The patient declared that he wrote with his left hand until he was 10, and then he was forced to use the right hand. D.D.C. is free from perceptual or motor impairments, and he has intact linguistic skills in both hemispheres [41]. He was tested at the Epilepsy Center of the Polytechnic University of Marche (Torrette of Ancona), during a pause between routine neurological examinations.

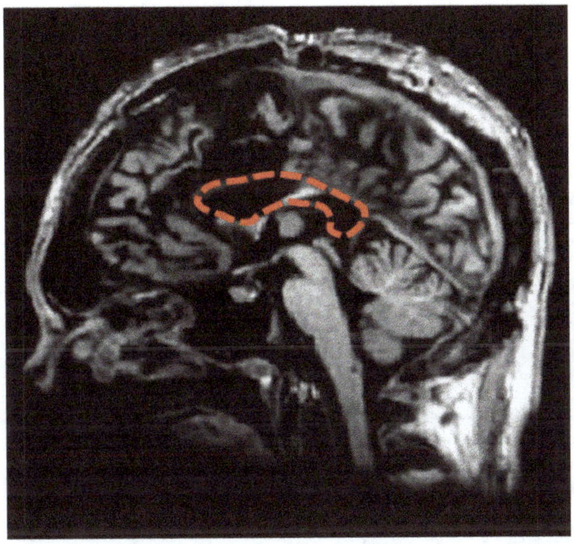

Figure 1. Midsagittal MRI of patients: the figure shows D.D.C.'s brain, showing the complete absence of callosal fibers (in the area delimited by the red-dashed line).

The control group was composed of 44 healthy volunteers (22 female; age: M = 25.5 ± 0.89). All were right-handed as assessed by the Edinburgh Handedness Inventory ([42]; M = 67.31 ± 2.28), had normal or corrected-to-normal vision, and none of them had any neurological or psychiatric history. These participants were tested at the Psychobiology Laboratory of the University of Chieti.

Informed consent was obtained from all participants prior to the experiment and the experimental procedures were conducted in accordance with the guidelines of the Declaration of Helsinki.

2.2. Stimuli

Stimuli consisted of a square designed by means of the software Microsoft PowerPoint 2007 (Microsoft Corp., Redmond, WA, USA). The square shape had black contours and it encompassed a white area measuring 7.6 × 7.6 cm (width × height; 4.2 × 4.2 degrees of visual angle, seen at a distance of 72 cm, on a screen with a resolution of 1280 × 768 pixels). The perimeter of the figure measured 0.3 mm in thickness. A black circular dot with a diameter measuring 0.9 cm was placed within the square. The dot was placed perfectly in the center of the square in half of the stimuli (On-Center condition), whereas in the other half it was placed 3 mm (0.18° of the visual angle) away from the center (Off-Center condition: 25% above, 25% below, 25% left, and 25% right, with respect to the center of the square).

2.3. Procedure

Each trial started with a vertical red line, measuring 2 mm in thickness and 16 cm in height, presented in the center of a white screen for 1000 ms. In the following 150 ms the red line remained visible, and a stimulus was presented in the center of the left or right half of the screen (the center of the square was placed at 3.7° of the visual angle from the center of the screen, with the innermost edge placed at 1.6° of the visual angle). Finally, a white screen was presented until the participant gave the response, and then the next trial started.

Each participant took part into two sessions, each composed of 96 trials. In each session, the stimulus was presented 48 times in the left visual field (LVF) and 48 times in the right visual field (RVF). For each visual field, 24 trials consisted of the square containing the dot in the center (On-Center condition), and 24 trials consisted in the square containing the dot moved away from the center (Off-Center condition, with 6 trials for each position: up, down, left, right; see Figure 2). The presentation order of the trials was randomized within and among participants.

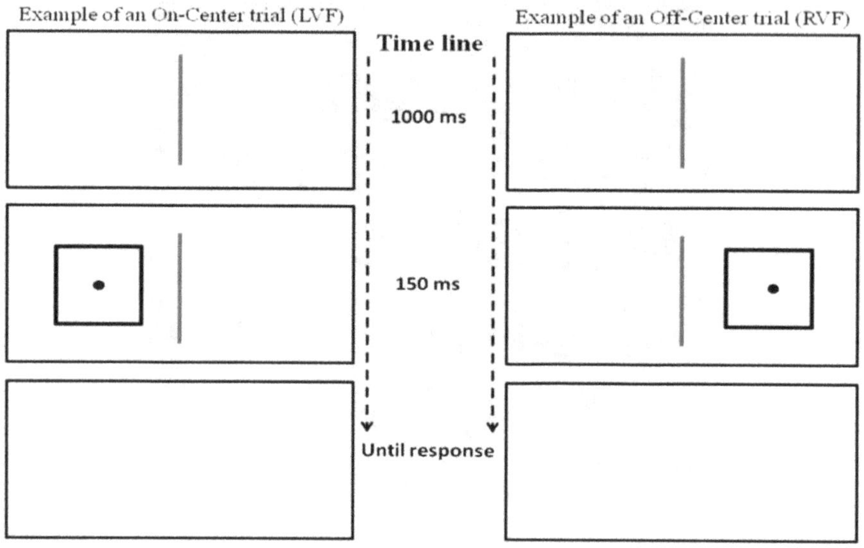

Figure 2. An example of (1) an On-Center trial, in which a symmetrical stimulus is presented in the Left Visual Field (LVF, **left panel**) and (2) an Off-Center trial, in which an asymmetrical stimulus is presented in the Right Visual Field (RVF, **right panel**).

Participants were tested in isolation. Before the beginning of the experiment, 4 trials were presented to allow the participants to become familiar with the task. They were asked to maintain their gaze in the center of the screen for the whole task, on the red line (a red line was used instead of the most conventional central fixation cross, in order to avoid possible cues concerning the exact center of the screen on the horizontal plane), and to evaluate in each trial the position of the dot inside the square. Specifically, they were asked to press one key when the dot was perfectly placed in the center of the square, and a different key when the dot was not in the center. They were also informed that the dot position could be a few millimeters away from the exact center of the square, in any direction (up, down, left, right). In the two experimental sessions, participants were required to carry out the task using either the left hand or the right hand, and the order of the two sessions was balanced among the participants. D.D.C. started with the right hand session.

The paradigm was controlled by means of E-Prime software (Psychology Software Tools Inc., Pittsburgh, PA, USA), and lasted about 15 min.

3. Results

3.1. Control Group

Data were analyzed by means of an analysis of variance (ANOVA), in which the Inverse Efficiency Score (IES) was the dependent variable. The IES was calculated by dividing the response times obtained in the correct responses by the proportion of correct responses in each condition. Reaction times were excluded when they were lower than 150 ms and higher than 1500 ms (3.11% of the trials). In a first ANOVA, Order of sessions (first session: Left hand, Right hand) and Sex of participants (Female, Male) were considered as between-subjects factors, and Hand of response (Left, Right), Visual field of presentation (Left, Right), and Condition (On-Center, Off-Center) were considered as within-subjects factors. Neither Order of sessions, nor Sex of participants were significant, nor did they interact with the other factors, thus they were excluded from the main analysis.

The ANOVA was carried out considering three within-subject factors: Hand of response (Left, Right), Visual field of presentation (Left, Right), and Condition (On-Center, Off-Center), and the IES was considered as the dependent variable. When required, the Duncan test was used for post-hoc comparisons. The main effect of Condition was significant ($F_{(1,43)} = 4.060$, $p = 0.050$, $\eta_p^2 = 0.09$), showing that the performance of participants was better in the On-Center condition (922.76 ± 101.46), than in the Off-Center condition (1423.06 ± 132.46). Importantly, the interaction between Condition and Visual field was significant ($F_{(1,43)} = 6.196$, $p = 0.017$, $\eta_p^2 = 0.13$). Post-hoc comparisons revealed that when stimuli were presented in the LVF, the performance of participants was better in the On-Center condition than in the Off-Center condition ($p < 0.001$). Moreover, in the On-Center condition, the performance was better when stimuli were presented in the LVF than in the RVF, and the opposite was true for the Off-Center condition, even if both comparisons failed to reach statistical significance (On-Center: $p = 0.088$; Off-Center: $p = 0.083$; Figure 3). Other main effects and interactions were not significant.

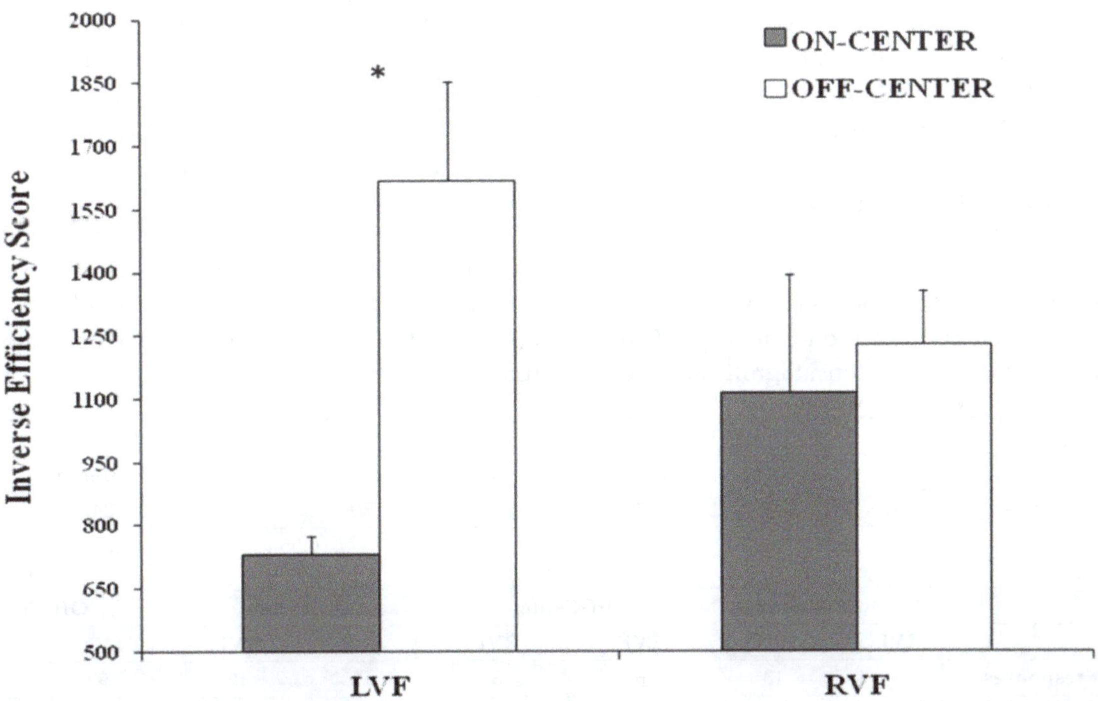

Figure 3. Interaction between the Visual field of presentation (Left, Right) and Condition (On-Center, Off-Center) on the Inverse Efficiency Score (response times of the correct responses divided by the proportion of correct responses) in healthy participants. Bars represent standard errors and the asterisk shows the significant comparison.

3.2. D.D.C.

The results of D.D.C. were analyzed by using a binomial distribution analysis and chi-square tests (as in [39]). The binomial distribution was computed considering the frequency of correct responses in each condition (Hand of response × Visual field × Condition). The results showed that the patient's responses were given at the chance level (50%) in any condition in the Right hand session, and in the On-Center condition-RVF in the Left hand session. In the Left hand session, his performance was significantly below the chance level for the Off-Center condition in both LVF and RVF, whereas it was significantly above the chance level only in the On-Center condition-LVF (Table 1).

Table 1. The frequencies of correct responses of patient D.D.C., and respective probabilities in the binomial distribution, in the Left hand session (upper panel) and in the Right hand session (lower panel), for stimuli presented in the Left Visual Field (LVF) and in the Right Visual Field (RVF), in the On-Center and Off-Center condition. Significant results are represented in bold.

Session	Results	LVF		RVF	
		On-Center	Off-Center	On-Center	Off-Center
Left hand	Correct responses	20	6	13	3
	Binomial: *p*	**<0.001**	**0.008**	0.149	**<0.001**
Right hand	Correct responses	11	9	13	12
	Binomial: *p*	0.149	0.078	0.149	0.161

Chi-square tests were used to compare the frequency of correct responses in the LVF vs RVF, as well as in the On-Center vs Off-Center conditions, in each session (Left hand, Right hand). Only the comparison between the On-Center and Off-Center conditions in the Left hand session was significant, showing that the patient correctly categorized the stimuli more frequently in the On-Center condition (Table 2). Thus, in order to better investigate this effect, chi-square tests were also computed for all of the interactions between VF and Condition. In the Right hand session, the comparisons were not significant. In the Left hand session, the comparisons between LVF and RVF were not significant either for the On-Center or for the Off-Center conditions, but D.D.C. categorized stimuli better in the On-Center condition than in the Off-Center condition, when presented with both in the LVF ($\chi^2 = 7.54$, $p = 0.006$) and in the RVF ($\chi^2 = 6.25$, $p = 0.012$; see Table 2).

Table 2. The frequencies of correct responses of patient D.D.C., Chi-square values and respective significance levels in the Left hand session and in the Right hand session, for stimuli presented in the Left Visual Field (LVF) and in the Right Visual Field (RVF), in the On-Center and Off-Center condition, as well as their interactions. Significant results are represented in bold.

Results	LEFT HAND				RIGHT HAND			
	LVF	**RVF**	**On-Center**	**Off-Center**	**LVF**	**RVF**	**On-Center**	**Off-Center**
Correct responses	26	16	33	9	20	25	24	21
Chi²	2.38		13.71		0.55		0.2	
p	0.122		**<0.001**		0.456		0.655	
	On-Center		**Off-Center**		**On-Center**		**Off-Center**	
	LVF	**RVF**	**LVF**	**RVF**	**LVF**	**RVF**	**LVF**	**RVF**
Correct responses	20	13	6	3	11	13	9	12
Chi²	1.485		1		0.167		0.428	
p	0.223		0.317		0.683		0.513	
	LVF		**RVF**		**LVF**		**RVF**	
	On-Center	**Off-Center**	**On-Center**	**Off-Center**	**On-Center**	**Off-Center**	**On-Center**	**Off-Center**
Correct responses	20	6	13	3	11	9	13	12
Chi²	7.54		6.25		0.2		0.04	
p	**0.006**		**0.012**		0.655		0.841	

3.3. Control Group vs. D.D.C.

The mean percentage of correct responses for each condition obtained in the control group was compared with the percentage of D.D.C.'s correct responses, by means of exact *t*-tests, using the percentage of responses by the patient as a reference value for each session (Left hand and Right hand), separately (as in [39,43]).

The results showed that healthy participants gave more correct responses than D.D.C. in all conditions and in both sessions (for all comparisons: $3.39 < t_{(43)} < 18.21$, $p \leq 0.001$), with the exception of the On-Center condition-LVF in the Left hand session, where no difference between the patient's performance and the control group's performance was observed ($t_{(43)} = -1.23$, $p = 0.225$; Figure 4).

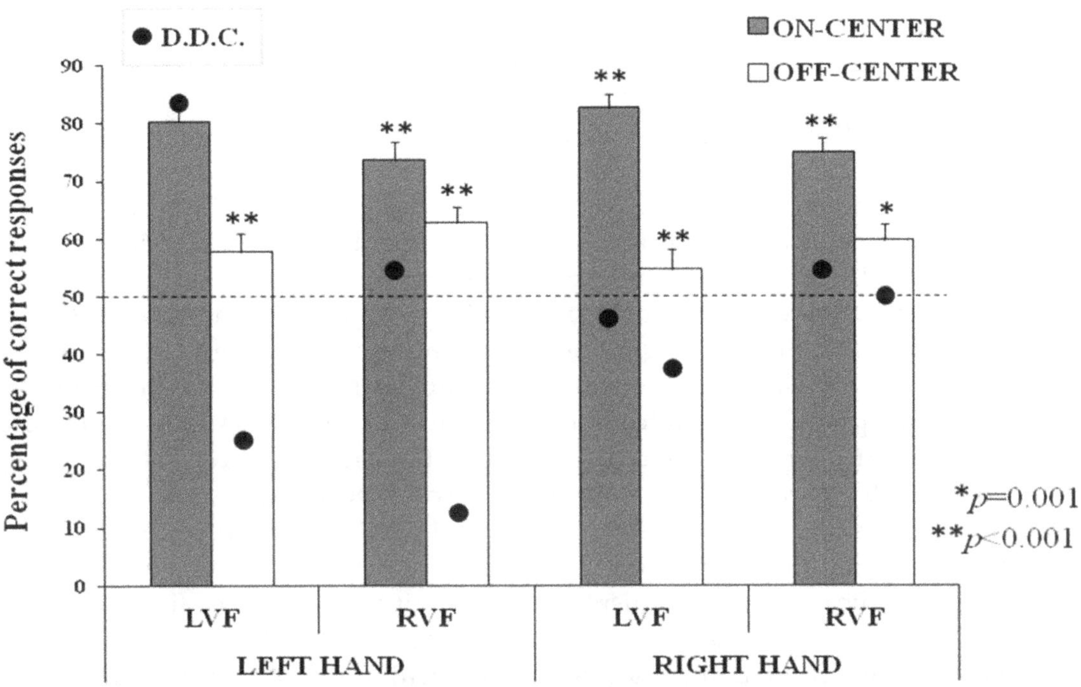

Figure 4. The percentage of correct responses in the left hand session (on the left) and in the right hand session (on the right), for On-Center stimuli (gray columns) and Off-Center stimuli (white columns) presented in the Left Visual Field (LVF) and in the Right Visual Field (RVF). The columns represent the results of healthy participants (bars represent standard errors), and black circles represent the results of D.D.C. Dashed lines represent chance levels (50%). Asterisks show the significant comparisons between the performance of D.D.C. and healthy controls.

4. Discussion

The main aim of the present study was to investigate the possible hemispheric imbalance in the processing of visual symmetry for double-axes stimuli. As reviewed in the Introduction, a right-hemispheric superiority has been found in symmetry detection when mono-dimensional stimuli are presented, but no asymmetries have been found using bi-dimensional stimuli [24]. Nevertheless, we found that the right hemisphere is superior compared to the left hemisphere in the detection of bi-dimensional symmetry, both in healthy participants and in a callosotomized patient.

It has to be highlighted that in the sample of healthy participants, we did not find significant differences depending on the hand used to respond. Although, we did not hypothesize that the use of one hand would lead to statistical differences in the healthy sample, we did expect that in the patient with complete callosal section, the use of one hand would highlight the effects of the activity of the contralateral hemisphere. Indeed, in the split-brain literature the collection of responses given with one hand has been repeatedly exploited as a tool to test the contralateral hemispheric activity (e.g., [37–39]). We found that D.D.C.'s performance was at the chance level in all of the conditions when he provided the responses using his right hand, suggesting that the left disconnected hemisphere is not capable of discerning symmetry from asymmetry. Moreover, in the left hand session, the performance of the patient was below the chance level when off-center stimuli were presented, suggesting that the right disconnected hemisphere cannot correctly judge asymmetry or, alternatively, that a right-hemispheric bias for symmetry influences this result. A possible alternative explanation could be that the patient shows a simple response bias for on-center stimuli, but the fact that the percentage of correct responses for on-center stimuli presented in the LVF is 54% (random level), together with the fact that such a bias is present only when the left hand is used, makes this possibility less likely. Moreover, in the left hand session a main effect of symmetry confirmed that a "symmetry bias" is present in the right hemisphere (on-center stimuli were better categorized than off-center stimuli), for stimuli presented both in the LVF and in the RVF. Finally, the comparison between the performance of D.D.C. and the control group confirmed that only when the left hand was used and symmetric (on-center) stimuli were presented in the LVF was the comparison not significant, meaning that D.D.C. had the same accuracy level as the controls, whereas in all of the other conditions his performance was largely below that of the control group. Considered together, these results show that the right disconnected hemisphere of the split-brain patient can correctly process symmetry in bi-dimensional stimuli. The fact that the right (disconnected) hemisphere is superior to the left hemisphere in a number of tasks requiring spatial processing [12,13] is not a possible explanation for the present results. In fact, if it were the case, we should find a better performance in D.D.C. with both symmetrical and asymmetrical stimuli presented in the LVF. Similarly, a possible hemispheric difference in visual processing has to be discarded: by using the binocular rivalry paradigm, it has been shown, in two split-brain patients, that both hemispheres are able to process simple and complex stimuli (colored disks and faces), revealing a typical degree of binocular rivalry in both hemispheres [44–46]. Moreover, by means of binocular rivalry paradigms there is evidence of a redundancy effect [47], meaning that both hemispheres processed visual stimuli similarly and a callosal dysfunction can constitute an advantage in response times only when stimuli presented in both visual fields must be compared to each other [48]. The evidence of a right-hemispheric superiority which is specific for symmetry allows us to conclude that the symmetry bias is lateralized in the right hemisphere.

Regarding the healthy participants, the first crucial result found here is that they were better at categorizing symmetrical (on-center) rather than asymmetrical (off-center) stimuli, independently of the visual field of presentation. This evidence confirms the "symmetry bias" [23], that is the preference for symmetrical over asymmetrical configurations already proposed by the Gestalt theory. Some evidence has been collected concerning such a bias, showing that the human visual system detects symmetry more easily than asymmetry. First of all, symmetry detection is faster than asymmetry detection [49] and it affects the performance of observers even when it is not crucial for the task [50], as well as when the symmetrical arrangement constitutes the distracters during a visual search task [51]. Finally, it has been shown that symmetry is detected before eye movements are made towards a symmetric object, meaning that symmetry detection occurs also in the absence of overt attention [52]. This bias can have evolutionary roots, since symmetry is a relevant cue in the biological and physical world, so much so that it has been verified that it is innate and it is present in human infants (e.g., [53]), as well as in other species (e.g., [54]). The callosal hypothesis suggests that the symmetry bias could be due to the activity of two homologous areas in the two hemispheres, connected by means of the callosal fibers [1,2,14–16]. Starting from this view, it is predicted that when two patterns are presented in the two visual fields, they should be detected faster when they are symmetrical than when they are asymmetrical. Similarly, concerning split-brain patients, it can be expected that the absence of callosal connections should reveal no difference between the bilateral presentation of symmetrical or asymmetrical configurations. This prediction has been confirmed in split-brain and acallosal patients [55]. In the present study, we did not present stimuli bilaterally, and thus we did not aim at further exploring this issue, but we decided to present bi-dimensional stimuli in each visual field separately, in order to assess the specific propensity of each disconnected hemisphere at detecting bi-dimensional symmetry. To our knowledge, this is the first time a right-hemispheric superiority for bi-dimensional symmetry detection has been shown in a callosotomized patient. Moreover, the right-hemispheric bias for symmetry found in D.D.C. has been also confirmed in our control group: the results showed that when stimuli were presented in the LVF, the performance was better in the on-center than in the off-center condition, suggesting that the right hemisphere "prefers" symmetrical patterns also in healthy participants. The same conclusion might be suggested by the almost significant result showing a better discrimination of the on-center condition in the LVF than in the RVF. Moreover, a slightly better discrimination of the off-center condition in the RVF than in the LVF seems to suggest a complementary superiority in the two hemispheres in healthy brains, with a right-hemispheric preference for symmetry processing and an opposite left-hemispheric preference for asymmetry processing. Nevertheless, further investigations are needed in order to verify this hypothesis.

The right-hemispheric superiority in bi-dimensional symmetry detection are in accordance with the results by Verma et al. [56]. By presenting symmetric and asymmetric geometric figures in the periphery of each visual field, the authors found that both right-handed and left-handed participants with left-hemispheric speech dominance were more accurate when symmetrical stimuli were presented in the LVF (whereas contrasting cerebral asymmetries were found in participants with right-hemispheric dominance for speech). Differently from the results of the present study and from the results by Verma and colleagues [56], Wilkinson and Halligan [24] did not find a hemispheric imbalance in healthy participants, by using a divided visual field paradigm and double-axes stimuli. As reviewed above, however, we manipulated a number of parameters which could explain the difference in the results between the two studies, e.g., we lowered the presentation time of the stimuli. Also the eccentricity of the stimuli differed between the two studies, although it has been shown that this parameter did not influence symmetry detection [57]. Moreover, we tested a number of participants: Wilkinson and Halligan, in fact, divided their whole sample into different subgroups, each carrying out a different task. Thus, in that study 12 participants carried out the task with the double-axes stimuli (for more details on their study see the Introduction). Nevertheless, the results of the present study confirm those by Wilkinson and Halligan with single-axis stimuli; in fact, we found that the right hemisphere is superior to the left hemisphere in correctly judging symmetrical patterns. In single axis conditions, Wilkinson and Halligan exploited the "classical" bisection paradigm to assess symmetry perception, in which participants are asked to divide a line into two equal segments or to evaluate a pre-bisected line as composed of two symmetrical or asymmetrical segments. By using this paradigm, a number of studies confirmed the presence of "pseudo-neglect" in healthy participants (i.e., the systematic trend to bisect a line leftward than at its real center), and the opposite bias in patients suffering from neglect, who "ignore" the left hemispace and bisect the line rightmost rather than at the veridical center (for a review see [58]). A central issue in this context is the difference found in the performance of neglect patients according to the mono- or bi-dimensional stimuli they were required to bisect: in fact, if on one hand the rightward bisection is considered a "landmark" of hemispatial neglect, on the other hand, no such bias has been found when neglect patients were asked to find the central point of bi-dimensional stimuli. For instance, this dissociation has been evidenced by Halligan and Marshall [59] with a neglect patient: the patient showed the bias in horizontal and vertical line bisection, but he did not show biases when required to place a dot in the center of a square or of a circle. Conversely, however, MacDonald-Nethercott and colleagues [60] found the same magnitude of pseudoneglect (leftward bias) in healthy participants by using both lines and elliptical shapes.

A possible dissociation has been suggested between vertical and horizontal spatial processing: Churches and colleagues [61] have recently shown that independent of the shape of the bi-dimensional images, a consistent correlation exists between the biases within each dimension (vertical, horizontal) across different shapes, but that there is no correlation between the vertical and horizontal bias when the two dimensions are compared to one another. The authors concluded that the parietal ("where") route is involved in vertical plane processing, and that the occipital ("what") route is responsible for horizontal plane processing. This suggestion is in line with other studies, showing that the parietal cortex is mostly involved in line bisection (mono-dimensional stimuli), whereas the occipital extrastriate cortex is mostly involved in bi-dimensional stimuli activating the object-based route instead of the parietal space-based route (e.g., [62]). This is also a possible explanation for the dissociation found with neglect patients between mono- and bi-dimensional stimuli, in whom the spatial deficit is mainly due to a parietal or temporo-parietal lesion [58], and it is also confirmed by TMS evidence in healthy subjects. As reviewed above, in two different studies Bona and colleagues [34,35] showed that a right-hemispheric stimulation disrupted symmetry detection in a stronger fashion than a left-hemispheric stimulation, when TMS was applied over the lateral occipital cortex. The involvement of the occipital cortex in multi-dimensional symmetrical patterns has been also confirmed in other fMRI and EEG studies [21,22].

We can conclude that the occipital, object-based visual route is responsible for the processing of bi-dimensional stimuli, and that this is also the cerebral substrate for symmetry detection when stimuli are bi-dimensional [36,62]. The present results confirm the "symmetry bias" consisting of the preference for symmetrical rather than asymmetrical configurations [23], and also show that such a bias is right-lateralized in the human brain. These speculations are based on the results we collected with healthy participants, but also—and importantly—with a patient with a complete section of the corpus callosum. This evidence is in line with other results collected before, by using different paradigms [60], and by exploiting both neuroimaging and electrophysiological measurements [21,22], as well as brain stimulation techniques [34,35]. We can also hypothesize that the same cerebral substrate could be the basis for the processing of three-dimensional stimuli, and thus for the detection of symmetry in the real world, but further work is needed in order to assess these hypotheses.

Acknowledgments: We thank very much D.D.C. for his willingness to collaborate in this study. We thank Gabriele Polonara for providing us with the MRI images of D.D.C., and Gabriella Venanzi for scheduling the patient's exams. Finally, we thank Elisabetta Conti and Margherita Davado, who helped us in recruiting and testing healthy participants.

Author Contributions: G.P. and L.T. conceived and designed the experiment; G.P., M.F., and N.F. performed the experiment; G.P. analyzed the data and wrote the paper; M.F. and L.T. revised the paper.

References

1. Tyler, C.W. Empirical aspects of symmetry perception. *Spat. Vis.* **1995**, *9*, 1–7. [CrossRef] [PubMed]
2. Wagemans, J. Detection of visual symmetries. *Spat. Vis.* **1995**, *9*, 9–32. [CrossRef] [PubMed]
3. Wagemans, J. Characteristics and models of human symmetry detection. *Trends Cogn. Sci.* **1997**, *1*, 346–352. [CrossRef]
4. Treder, M.S. Behind the looking glass: A review on human symmetry perception. *Symmetry* **2010**, *2*, 510–543. [CrossRef]
5. Van der Helm, P.A. Symmetry perception. In *The Oxford Handbook of Perceptual Organization*; Wagemans, J., Ed.; Oxford University Press: Oxford, UK, 2014.
6. Beck, D.M.; Pinsk, M.A.; Kastner, S. Symmetry perception in humans and macaques. *Trends Cogn. Sci.* **2005**, *9*, 405–406. [CrossRef] [PubMed]
7. Makin, A.D.; Wright, D.; Rampone, G.; Palumbo, L.; Guest, M.; Sheehan, R.; Cleaver, H.; Bertamini, M. An electrophysiological index of perceptual goodness. *Cereb. Cortex* **2016**, *26*, 4416–4434. [CrossRef] [PubMed]
8. Driver, L.; Baylis, G.C.; Rafal, R. Preserved figure-ground segregation and symmetry detection in visual neglect. *Nature* **1992**, *360*, 73–75. [PubMed]
9. Cattaneo, Z.; Fantino, M.; Silvanto, J.; Tinti, C.; Pascual-Leone, A.; Vecchi, T. Symmetry perception in the blind. *Acta Psychol.* **2010**, *134*, 398–402. [CrossRef] [PubMed]
10. Cattaneo, Z.; Bona, S.; Monegato, M.; Pece, A.; Vecchi, T.; Herbert, A.M.; Merabet, L.B. Visual symmetry perception in early onset monocular blindness. *Visual Cogn.* **2014**, *22*, 963–974. [CrossRef]
11. Prete, G.; Tommasi, L. Split-Brain Patients. In *Encyclopedia of Evolutionary Psychological Science*; Shackelford, T.K., Weekes-Shackelford, V.A., Eds.; Springer International Publishing AG: Cham (ZG), Switzerland, 2017; pp. 1–5.
12. Funnell, M.G.; Corballis, P.M.; Gazzaniga, M.S. A deficit in perceptual matching in the left hemisphere of a callosotomy patient. *Neuropsychologia* **1999**, *37*, 1143–1154. [CrossRef]
13. Corballis, P.M.; Funnell, M.G.; Gazzaniga, M.S. A dissociation between spatial and identity matching in callosotomy patients. *Neuroreport* **1999**, *10*, 2183–2187. [CrossRef] [PubMed]
14. Herbert, A.M.; Humphrey, G.K. Bilateral symmetry detection: Testing a 'callosal' hypothesis. *Perception* **1996**, *25*, 463–480. [CrossRef] [PubMed]
15. Corballis, M.C.; Beale, I.L. *The Psychology of Left and Right*; Lawrence Erlbaum: Oxford, UK, 1976; pp. x–227.

16. Braitenberg, V. Reading the structure of brains. *Netw. Comput. Neural* **1990**, *1*, 1–11. [CrossRef]
17. Corballis, P.M. Visuospatial processing and the right-hemisphere interpreter. *Brain Cogn.* **2003**, *53*, 171–176. [CrossRef]
18. Wright, D.; Makin, A.D.J.; Bertamini, M. Electrophysiological responses to symmetry presented in the left or in the right visual hemifield. *Coretx* **2017**, *86*, 93–108. [CrossRef] [PubMed]
19. Ban, H.; Yamamoto, H.; Fukunaga, M.; Nakagoshi, A.; Umeda, M.; Tanaka, C.; Ejima, Y. Toward a common circle: Interhemispheric contextual modulation in human early visual areas. *J. Neurosci.* **2006**, *26*, 8804–8809. [CrossRef] [PubMed]
20. Sasaki, Y.; Vanduffel, W.; Knutsen, T.; Tyler, C.; Tootell, R. Symmetry activates extrastriate visual cortex in human and nonhuman primates. *Proc. Natl. Acad. Sci. USA* **2005**, *102*, 3159–3163. [CrossRef] [PubMed]
21. Tyler, C.W.; Baseler, H.A.; Kontsevich, L.L.; Likova, L.T.; Wade, A.R.; Wandell, B.A. Predominantly extra-retinotopic cortical response to pattern symmetry. *Neuroimage* **2005**, *24*, 306–314. [CrossRef] [PubMed]
22. Palumbo, L.; Bertamini, M.; Makin, A. Scaling of the extrastriate neural response to symmetry. *Vis. Res.* **2015**, *117*, 1–8. [CrossRef] [PubMed]
23. Sasaki, Y. Processing local signals into global patterns. *Curr. Opin. Neurobiol.* **2007**, *17*, 132–139. [CrossRef] [PubMed]
24. Wilkinson, D.T.; Halligan, P.W. The effects of stimulus symmetry on landmark judgments in left and right visual fields. *Neuropsychologia* **2002**, *40*, 1045–1058. [CrossRef]
25. Breitmeyer, B.G. Simple reaction time as a measure of the temporal response properties of transient and sustained channels. *Vis. Res.* **1975**, *15*, 1411–1412. [CrossRef]
26. Prete, G.; Capotosto, P.; Zappasodi, F.; Laeng, B.; Tommasi, L. The cerebral correlates of subliminal emotions: An eleoencephalographic study with emotional hybrid faces. *Eur. J. Neurosci.* **2015**, *42*, 2952–2962. [CrossRef] [PubMed]
27. Prete, G.; D'ascenzo, S.; Laeng, B.; Fabri, M.; Foschi, N.; Tommasi, L. Conscious and unconscious processing of facial expressions: Evidence from two split-brain patients. *J. Neuropsychol.* **2015**, *9*, 45–63.
28. Prete, G.; Laeng, B.; Fabri, M.; Foschi, N.; Tommasi, L. Right hemisphere or valence hypothesis, or both? The processing of hybrid faces in the intact and callosotomized brain. *Neuropsychologia* **2015**, *68*, 94–106. [CrossRef] [PubMed]
29. Wilkinson, D.T.; Halligan, P.W. Stimulus symmetry affects the bisection of figures but not lines: Evidence from event-related fMRI. *NeuroImage* **2003**, *20*, 1756–1764. [CrossRef] [PubMed]
30. Bertamini, M.; Makin, A.D. Brain activity in response to visual symmetry. *Symmetry* **2014**, *6*, 975–996. [CrossRef]
31. Wright, D.; Makin, A.D.; Bertamini, M. Right-lateralized alpha desynchronization during regularity discrimination: Hemispheric specialization or directed spatial attention? *Psychophysiology* **2015**, *52*, 638–647. [CrossRef] [PubMed]
32. Makin, A.D.; Rampone, G.; Wright, A.; Martinovic, J.; Bertamini, M. Visual symmetry in objects and gaps. *J. Vis.* **2014**, *14*, 1–12. [CrossRef] [PubMed]
33. Makin, A.D.; Rampone, G.; Pecchinenda, A.; Bertamini, M. Electrophysiological responses to visuospatial regularity. *Psychophysiology* **2013**, *50*, 1045–1055. [CrossRef] [PubMed]
34. Bona, S.; Herbert, A.; Toneatto, C.; Silvanto, J.; Cattaneo, Z. The causal role of the lateral occipital complex in visual mirror symmetry detection and grouping: An fMRI-guided TMS study. *Cortex* **2014**, *51*, 46–55. [CrossRef] [PubMed]
35. Bona, S.; Cattaneo, Z.; Silvanto, J. The causal role of the occipital face area (OFA) and lateral occipital (LO) cortex in symmetry perception. *J. Neurosci.* **2015**, *35*, 731–738. [CrossRef] [PubMed]
36. Cattaneo, Z.; Mattavelli, G.; Papagno, C.; Herbert, A.; Silvanto, J. The role of the human extrastriate visual cortex in mirror symmetry discrimination: A TMS-adaptation study. *Brain Cogn.* **2011**, *77*, 120–127. [CrossRef] [PubMed]
37. Gazzaniga, M.S. The split brain in man. *Sci. Am.* **1967**, *217*, 24–29. [CrossRef] [PubMed]
38. Levy, J.; Trevarthen, C.; Sperry, R.W. Perception of bilateral chimeric figures following hemispheric deconnexion. *Brain* **1972**, *95*, 61–78. [CrossRef] [PubMed]
39. Prete, G.; Fabri, M.; Foschi, N.; Tommasi, L. Geometry, landmarks and the cerebral hemispheres: 2D spatial reorientation in split-brain patients. *J. Neuropsychol.* **2016**. [CrossRef] [PubMed]
40. Corballis, M.C.; Birse, K.; Paggi, A.; Manzoni, T.; Pierpaoli, C.; Fabri, M. Mirror-image discrimination and reversal in the disconnected hemispheres. *Neuropsychologia* **2010**, *48*, 1664–1669. [CrossRef] [PubMed]

41. Fabri, M.; Polonara, G.; Mascioli, G.; Paggi, A.; Salvolini, U.; Manzoni, T. Contribution of the corpus callosum to bilateral representation of the trunk midline in the human brain: An fMRI study of callosotomized patients. *Eur. J. Neurosci.* **2006**, *23*, 3139–3148. [CrossRef] [PubMed]
42. Oldfield, R.C. The assessment and analysis of handedness: The Edinburgh Inventory. *Neuropsychologia* **1971**, *9*, 97–114. [CrossRef]
43. Prete, G.; Fabri, M.; Foschi, N.; Brancucci, A.; Tommasi, L. The "consonance effect" and the hemispheres: A study on a split-brain patient. *Laterality* **2015**, *20*, 257–269. [CrossRef] [PubMed]
44. O'shea, R.P.; Corballis, P.M. Binocular rivalry between complex stimuli in split-brain observers. *Brain Mind* **2001**, *2*, 151–160. [CrossRef]
45. O'Shea, R.P.; Corballis, P.M. Binocular rivalry in split-brain observers. *J. Vis.* **2003**, *3*, 610–615. [CrossRef] [PubMed]
46. Miller, J. Exaggerated redundancy gain in the split brain: A hemispheric coactivation account. *Cogn. Psychol.* **2004**, *49*, 118–154. [CrossRef] [PubMed]
47. Ritchie, K.L.; Bannerman, R.L.; Turk, D.J.; Sahraie, A. Eye rivalry and object rivalry in the intact and split-brain. *Vis. Res.* **2013**, *91*, 102–107. [CrossRef] [PubMed]
48. Ritchie, K.L.; Bannerman, R.L.; Sahraie, A. Redundancy gain in binocular rivalry. *Perception* **2014**, *43*, 1316–1328. [CrossRef] [PubMed]
49. Wagemans, J.; Van Gool, L.; D'ydewalle, G. Detection of symmetry in tachistoscopically presented dot patterns: Effects of multiple axes and skewing. *Atten. Percept. Psychophys.* **1991**, *50*, 413–427. [CrossRef]
50. Van der Helm, P.A.; Treder, M.S. Detection of (anti) symmetry and (anti) repetition: Perceptual mechanisms versus cognitive strategies. *Vis. Res.* **2009**, *49*, 2754–2763. [CrossRef] [PubMed]
51. Wolfe, J.M.; Friedman-Hill, S.R. On the role of symmetry in visual search. *Psychol. Sci.* **1992**, *3*, 194–198. [CrossRef]
52. Kootstra, G.; de Boer, B.; Schomaker, L.R. Predicting eye fixations on complex visual stimuli using local symmetry. *Cog. Comp.* **2011**, *3*, 223–240. [CrossRef] [PubMed]
53. Bornstein, M.H.; Ferdinandsen, K.; Gross, C.G. Perception of symmetry in infancy. *Dev. Psychol.* **1981**, *17*, 82. [CrossRef]
54. Mascalzoni, E.; Osorio, D.; Regolin, L.; Vallortigara, G. Symmetry perception by poultry chicks and its implications for three-dimensional object recognition. *Proc. R. Soc. Lond. B Biol. Sci.* **2011**, *279*, 841–846. [CrossRef] [PubMed]
55. Roser, M.; Corballis, M.C. Interhemispheric neural summation in the split brain with symmetrical and asymmetrical displays. *Neuropsychologia* **2002**, *40*, 1300–1312. [CrossRef]
56. Verma, A.; Van der Haegen, L.; Brysbaert, M. Symmetry detection in typically and atypically speech lateralized individuals: A visual half-field study. *Neuropsychologia* **2013**, *51*, 2611–2619. [CrossRef] [PubMed]
57. Rampone, G.; O'Sullivan, N.; Bertamini, M. The Role of Visual Eccentricity on Preference for Abstract Symmetry. *PLoS ONE* **2016**, *11*, e0154428. [CrossRef] [PubMed]
58. Karnath, H.O.; Rorden, C. The anatomy of spatial neglect. *Neuropsychologia* **2012**, *50*, 1010–1017. [CrossRef] [PubMed]
59. Halligan, P.W.; Marshall, J.C. Figural modulation of visuo-spatial neglect: A case study. *Neuropsychologia* **1991**, *29*, 619–628. [CrossRef]
60. Macdonald-Nethercott, E.M.; Kinnear, P.R.; Venneri, A. Bisection of shapes and lines: Analysis of the visual and motor aspects of pseudoneglect. *Percept. Mot. Skills* **2000**, *91*, 217–226. [CrossRef] [PubMed]
61. Churches, O.; Loetscher, T.; Thomas, N.A.; Nicholls, M.E. Perceptual biases in the horizontal and vertical dimensions are driven by separate cognitive mechanisms. *Q. J. Exp. Psychol.* **2017**, *70*, 444–460. [CrossRef] [PubMed]
62. Fink, G.R.; Marshall, J.C.; Weiss, P.H.; Shah, N.J.; Toni, I.; Halligan, P.W.; Zilles, K. 'Where' depends on 'what': A differential functional anatomy for position discrimination in one-versus two-dimensions. *Neuropsychologia* **2000**, *38*, 1741–1748. [CrossRef]

6

Lateralization of the Avian Magnetic Compass: Analysis of its Early Plasticity

Dennis Gehring [1], **Onur Güntürkün** [2,3], **Wolfgang Wiltschko** [1] **and Roswitha Wiltschko** [1,*]

1 FB Biowissenschaften, Goethe-Universität Frankfurt am Main, Max-von-Laue-Str. 13, D-60438 Frankfurt am Main, Germany; d.gehring@ect.de (D.G.); wiltschko@zoology.uni-frankfurt.de (W.W.)
2 Abteilung Biopsychologie, Fakultät für Psychologie, Ruhr-Universität Bochum, D-44780 Bochum, Germany; Onur.Guentuerkuen@rub.de
3 Stellenbosch Institute for Advanced Study (STIAS), Wallenberg Research Centre at Stellenbosch University, Stellenbosch 7600, South Africa
* Correspondence: wiltschko@bio.uni-frankfurt.de

Academic Editor: Lesley J. Rogers

Abstract: In European Robins, *Erithacus rubecula*, the magnetic compass is lateralized in favor of the right eye/left hemisphere of the brain. This lateralization develops during the first winter and initially shows a great plasticity. During the first spring migration, it can be temporarily removed by covering the right eye. In the present paper, we used the migratory orientation of robins to analyze the circumstances under which the lateralization can be undone. Already a period of 1$^1/_2$ h being monocularly left-eyed before tests began proved sufficient to restore the ability to use the left eye for orientation, but this effect was rather short-lived, as lateralization recurred again within the next 1$^1/_2$ h. Interpretable magnetic information mediated by the left eye was necessary for removing the lateralization. In addition, monocularly, the left eye seeing robins could adjust to magnetic intensities outside the normal functional window, but this ability was not transferred to the "right-eye system". Our results make it clear that asymmetry of magnetic compass perception is amenable to short-term changes, depending on lateralized stimulation. This could mean that the left hemispheric dominance for the analysis of magnetic compass information depends on lateralized interhemispheric interactions that in young birds can swiftly be altered by environmental effects.

Keywords: avian magnetic compass; lateralization; right eye/left brain system; plasticity; commissures; Cryptochrome 1a

---

1. Introduction

In most vertebrates studied up to now, several perceptual, cognitive, and motor systems display a left–right difference of neural processing [1,2]. This ubiquity of functional brain asymmetries is probably the result of some fundamental benefits. Indeed, various studies could demonstrate in several species, ranging from fish to humans, that those individuals that are more strongly lateralized in a certain function also display higher performances when this function is tested [3–5]. This is possibly due to three mechanisms. First, asymmetries can selectively increase the perceptual or motor learning effect in one hemisphere. This is the case for, e.g., birds where the eyes are so laterally placed that most of the visual input derives from monocular vision. Thus, increased perceptual training of one eye can result in higher discrimination ability with this side [6]. The second mechanism for an advantage of asymmetry is directly related: increased learning with one perceptual or motor system also decreases reaction times, resulting in a time advantage of the dominant side [7,8]. The third mechanism of an advantage is parallel and complementary processing during task execution. If, for example, lateralized and non-lateralized chicks are tested in a foraging task that requires them to find grains scattered among pebbles and, at the same time, monitor overhead for a flying model predator, the strongly lateralized birds can conduct both tasks efficiently and in parallel [9]. Thus, hemispheric specialization seems to increase parallel processing by enabling separate processing of complementary information into the two hemispheres [10].

An important function that has been found to be lateralized is the avian magnetic compass. Information is obtained in the right eye and processed in the left hemisphere of the brain: with only their right eye open, birds could use their magnetic compass in the normal way, whereas they were disoriented when they had to use their left eye alone [11–15]. The reception of magnetic directional information is associated with the visual system. The Radical Pair Model, proposed by Ritz and colleagues [16], assumes that magnetoreception is based on spin-chemical processes in specialized photopigments; the eye was suggested as the site for magnetoreception, with cryptochromes as molecules forming the crucial radical pairs. Experimental evidence supports this model: radio-frequency fields in the MHz-range, a diagnostic tool for radical pair processes [17] disrupt magnetoreception (e.g., [18–22]). Furthermore, Cryptochrome 1a was found in the retina of birds, located along the disks of the outer segments of the UV/V cones [23], activated by light of the short wavelengths that allows birds magnetic compass orientation [24].

The first behavioral experiments documenting a lateralization of the magnetic compass in favor of the right eye/left hemisphere were performed with migratory birds, European Robins, *Erithacus rubecula* (Turdidae), and Australian Silvereyes, *Zosterops l. lateralis*, making use of their spontaneous directional preferences during the migratory phase [11,12]. Later studies, however, questioned these findings, reporting that migratory birds, among them European Robins, were oriented in their migratory direction even if they had to rely on their left eye alone [25–27]. Yet, there were marked differences between these studies, an important one being a difference in the test season: the tests documenting the lateralization of the magnetic compass had been spring experiments with birds returning to their breeding grounds whereas the tests not finding a lateralization were predominantly autumn experiments with birds mainly following an innate course (see [28]). A follow-up study testing the same robins consecutively during the first three migration seasons indicated that lateralization of the magnetic compass was not present in very young robins, but develops only after the first autumn migration [29]: initially, the magnetic compass was not lateralized and the birds could orient with their right as well as their left eye. During the following spring migration and the second autumn migration, in contrast, the same birds could no longer orient with their left eye alone—the magnetic compass had become lateralized in favor of the right eye/left brain hemisphere. Yet, in the beginning, the lateralization proved to be flexible with considerable plasticity: during spring migration, covering the right eye for 6 h prior to the orientation tests could temporarily restore the ability for magnetic compass orientation to the left eye. During the subsequent autumn migration, however, the same treatment no longer had any effect. These results strongly indicate that the magnetic compass asymmetry requires a developmental period: while it is absent during the first autumn and subsequently susceptible to change during the first spring, it becomes more strongly fixed beginning with the second autumn.

The flexible phase during spring migration is of particular interest because it allows some insights into the processes leading to the lateralization of the avian magnetic compass. Here, we report behavioral experiments during the first spring migration of migratory European Robins, designed to analyze in more detail the time-span required to restore magnetoreception to the left eye, the extent and the duration of this effect and the circumstances under which it takes place.

2. Results

The various test conditions are listed in Table 1. The results are summarized in Table 2, indicating significant differences between various treatments and the respective binocular controls; for the data of the individual birds, see Tables S1–S3a,b in the Supplementary Material.

2.1. The Effect of Monocular Pre-Exposure

Our previous study [29] had shown that, during the first spring migration, covering the right eye for 6 h had temporarily restored the ability for magnetic compass orientation to the left eye. This raised the question of how this treatment affected the right eye. The respective data are given in Figure 1: after having the right eye covered for 6 h, the robins could orient with their right eye (6hpeL-R) as well as with their left eye (6peL-L). Obviously, disrupting the input from the right eye for 6 h had no adverse effect on ability of the right eye/left hemisphere to process magnetic compass orientation; it just seems to remove the lateralization.

Table 1. Definition of the test conditions and their abbreviations.

Abbreviation	Test Condition
Bi	binocularly tested, control
L	monocularly left-eyed
6peL-L	6 h pre-exposed monocularly left-eyed, tested left-eyed
6peL-R	6 h pre-exposed monocularly left-eyed, tested right-eyed
1½peL-L	1½ h pre-exposed monocularly left-eyed, tested left-eyed
1½peL/1½-L	1½ h pre-exposed monocularly left-eyed, then 1½ h without eye cover, tested left-eyed
3peRFBi-Bi	3 h binocularly pre-exposed in an RF field (1.314 MHz, 480 nT), tested binocularly
3peRFL-L	3 h monocularly left-eyed pre-exposed in a RF field(1.314 MHz, 480 nT), tested left-eyed
3pe92R-92R	3 h right-eyed pre-exposed in a 92 μT field, tested right-eyed in the 92 μT field
3pe92L-92L	3 h left-eyed pre-exposed in a 92 μT field, tested left-eyed in the 92 μT field
3pe92L-92R	3 h left-eyed pre-exposed in a 92 μT field, tested right-eyed in the 92 μT field

If not indicated otherwise, the birds were pre-exposed and tested in the geomagnetic field. RF field: radio frequency field.

Table 2. Orientation after various lengths and modes of monocular pre-exposure. Twelve birds were tested in all test conditions (48 birds altogether, see Tables in Supplementary Material).

Year	Condition	Test Magnetic Field	n	Med. r_b	α_N	r_N	ΔBi	ΔX
2011	Bi	geomagnetic field	4	0.79	354°	0.80 ***		
"	6peL-L	"	3	0.81	21°	0.92 ***	+27° *d	X_1
"	6peL-R	"	3	0.91	28°	0.66 **	+32° n.s	+7 *s
2012	Bi	"	3	0.45	15°	0.62 **		
"	L	"	3	0.48	(12°)	0.22 n.s.	(−3°) *s	X_2
"	1½peL-L	"	3	0.77	11°	0.85 ***	−4°n.s.	(−11° *s)
"	1½peL/1½-L	"	3	0.60	(322°)	0.22 n.s.	(−53°) *d	(−50° n.s.)
2013 I	Bi	geomagnetic field	3	0.92	351°	0.65 **		
"	3pe92R-92R	92 nT	3	0.90	22°	0.74 ***	+31°n.s.	
2013 II	Bi	geomagnetic field	3	0.82	10°	0.95 ***		
"	3peRFBi-Bi	"	3	0.44	15°	0.59 *	+5° *s	X_3
"	3peRFL-L	"	3	0.41	(180°)	0.18 n.s.	(+170°) ***s	(−165° *s)
"	3pe92L-92L	92 nT	4	0.50	354°	0.80 ***	−16° n.s.	X_4
"	3pe92L-92R	92 nT	3	0.83	(287°)	0.21 n.s.	(−103°) ***	(−67° **s)

For the definition of the test conditions, see Table 1. n, tests per bird; med-r_b, median vector length per birds; α_N, r_N, direction and length of grand mean vector, with asterisks indicating significant directional preference by the Rayleigh test [30] (α_N in parentheses if not significant). ΔBi, difference to the respective binocular control, and ΔX, difference to the X-sample above, with asterisk indication a significance of the difference by the Mardia Watson Wheeler test (d) and the Mann–Whitney U-test (s). *** $p < 0.001$; ** $p < 0.01$; * $p < 0.05$; n.s.: not significant.

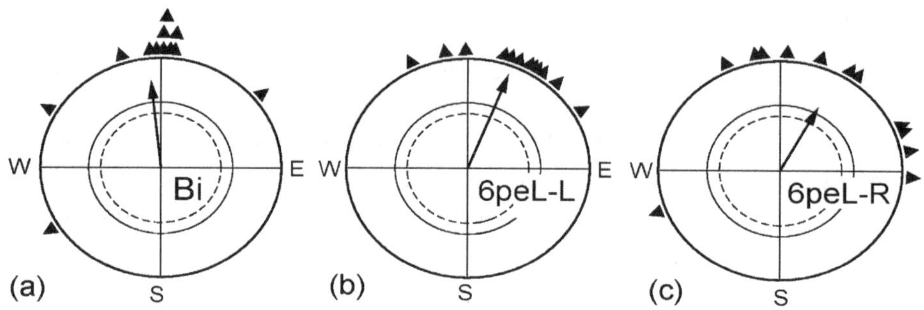

Figure 1. Effect of covering the right eye for 6 h prior to the test. (**a**) Untreated binocular control; (**b**) Birds tested monocularly left-eyed after having the right eye covered for 6 h; (**c**) Birds tested monocularly right-eyed after having the right eye covered for 6 h. The triangles at the periphery of the circle indicate the mean headings of the individual birds; the arrow represents the grand mean vector in relation to the radius of the circle = 1, and the inner circles mark the 5% (dotted) and the 1% significance border of the Rayleigh test [30].

Another question concerned the duration of the interval required to restore the ability to use information from the left eye and how long the effect would last. The data are given in Figure 2. When the right eye was covered immediately before the test (L), the monocularly left-eyed birds were disoriented, documenting lateralization in favor of the right eye. If the birds had been monocularly left-eyed already 1¹/2 h before the tests began (1¹/2peL-L), they showed normal orientation with their left eye, not different from when they were tested as binocular controls (Bi). However, this effect of removing the lateralization proved to be rather short-lived: when the birds had been monocularly left-eyed for 1¹/2 h, followed by a binocular period of another 1¹/2 h and were then tested left-eyed immediately afterwards (1¹/2peL/1¹/2-L), they were disoriented (Figure 2d)—lateralization had set in again.

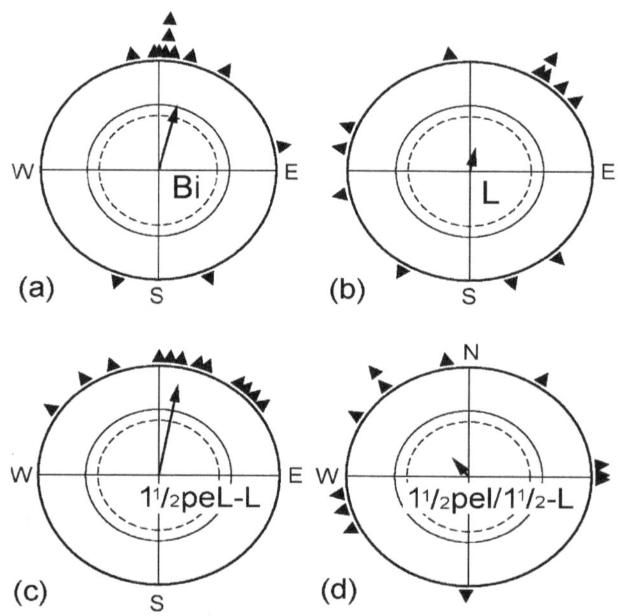

Figure 2. Time required for removing the lateralization in favor of the right eye. (**a**) Untreated binocular control; (**b**) Birds tested monocularly left eyed; their right eye was covered immediately before the tests began, indicating the lateralization in favor of the right eye; (**c**) Birds tested monocularly left eyed after having the right eye covered 1¹/2 h before the beginning of the tests; (**d**) Birds tested monocularly left eyed after having the right eye covered for 1¹/2 h, and then the cover was removed for 1¹/2 h before the beginning of the tests. Symbols as in Figure 1.

2.2. Pre-Exposure in Altered Magnetic Conditions

The previously described tests showing a temporary removal of lateralization as an effect of covering the right eye had been performed in the local geomagnetic field. With the following treatments, we tested for possible effects of the magnetic conditions during monocular deprivation.

First, we pre-exposed birds binocularly to a radio-frequency field that had been shown to disrupt magnetic orientation [19]. This meant that the birds did not receive interpretable magnetic information during a period 3 h immediately before the tests began (3peRFBi-Bi). Immediately after the pre-exposure, these birds were significantly oriented in their migratory direction in the geomagnetic field (see Figure 3b), even if the distribution of their mean headings shows a certain increase in scatter. Birds that were exposed monocularly left-eyed to the radio frequency field for 3 h immediately before they were tested left-eyed (3peRFL-L), in contrast, were disoriented in the geomagnetic field immediately afterwards (Figure 3c). Covering the right eye for a period of 3 h, twice as long as the one used in the previous series, should have been sufficient to enable the birds to use their left eye for obtaining magnetic compass orientation, yet in this case, it did not work. Obviously, receiving only visual information from the left eye could not remove the lateralization. Our data clearly show that interpretable directional information from the magnetic field is essential for allowing the processing of magnetic information by the left eye again.

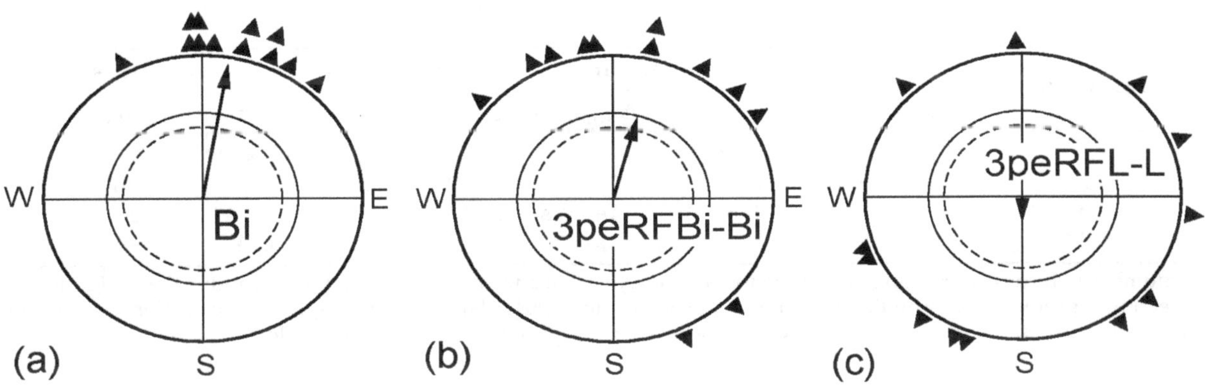

Figure 3. Effect of denying the birds interpretable magnetic information before the tests. (**a**) Untreated binocular control; (**b**) Birds exposed binocularly to a radio frequency for 3 h prior to being tested binocularly in the local geomagnetic field; (**c**) Birds exposed monocularly left-eyed to the radio frequency field for 3 h prior to being tested monocularly left-eyed in the geomagnetic field. Symbols as in Figure 1.

In a next step, we exposed the birds prior to the tests for 3 h to a magnetic field of 92 μT, twice as strong as the local geomagnetic field. Robins cannot spontaneously cope with such field strengths, but become able to orient in it if they had a chance to adjust to this intensity before the tests. In a previous study, 1 h pre-exposure to such a strong field had proven sufficient to allow orientation [31]. We tested two different groups of birds: Group I was pre-exposed with the right eye open and subsequently tested monocularly right-eyed (3pe92R-92R). Group II was pre-exposed and tested monocularly left-eyed (3pe92L-92L). The results are given in Figure 4: both groups of birds were oriented in the strong magnetic field. However, there was a difference between the groups: while the right-eyed birds were oriented in their migratory direction right away, with the headings of the three tests not different from each other, the left eyed birds were first disoriented and oriented only from the third test onward, with only the distribution of the forth headings significantly different from the disoriented first round (see Table 3). When left-eyed, the birds thus required more time to adjust to the stronger field.

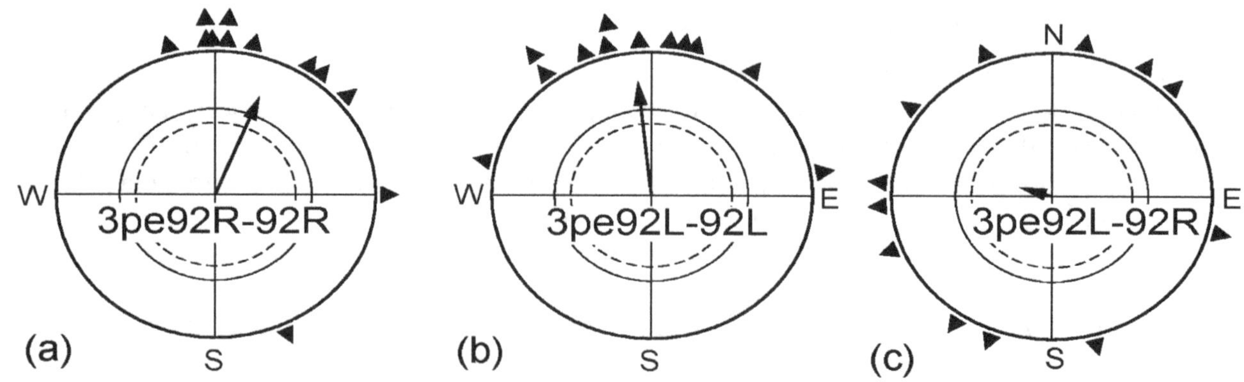

Figure 4. Adjusting to higher magnetic intensities. (**a**) Birds of group I pre-exposed monocularly right-eyed for 3 h in a magnetic field of 92 μT, twice the intensity of the geomagnetic field, and then were tested in that field; (**b**) Birds of group II pre-exposed monocularly left-eyed for 3 h in the strong magnetic field then tested in that field; (**c**) Birds of group II pre-exposed monocularly left-eyed for 3 h in the strong magnetic field and then tested monocularly right-eyed in that field. For the orientation of the untreated control birds, see Figure 3a and Table 2. Symbols as in Figure 1.

Table 3. Orientation of the robins pre-exposed and tested in the 92 μT-field.

Test Round	Monocularly Right-Eyed Birds				Monocularly Left-Eyed Birds			
	N	α	r	Δ Round 1	*N*	α	r	Δ Round 1
1	12	8°	0.87 ***		11	(304°)	0.38 n.s.	
2	11	(20°)	0.46 n.s	+12° n.s.	12	(10°)	0.36 n.s.	+66° n.s.
3	10	22°	0.64 **	+14° n.s.	11	3°	0.54 *	+59° n.s.
4					12	13°	0.74 ***	+69° *

N, number of birds contributing; α, r, direction and length of mean vector, with asterisks at r indicating a significant directional preference by the Rayleigh Test [30] (Batschelet, 1981). The column Δ Round 1 gives differences to the behavior in the first test round, with asterisks indicating significance; symbols as in Table 2.

Birds that had been pre-exposed monocularly left-eyed to the 92 μT field for 3 h were tested monocularly right-eyed in the same 92 μT field; however, they were disoriented (Figure 4c). While covering the left eye per se did not interfere with the ability of the right eye to mediate magnetic directional information (see Figure 1c), the right eye/left hemisphere could not cope with the increased intensity if it had not experienced the respective magnetic condition before. For adjusting to higher field strengths, processing of such input in the respective hemisphere seems to be required—there appears to be no transfer from the right to the left hemisphere where the adjustment to higher magnetic intensities is concerned.

3. Discussion

Our data show that, during the first spring migration, the lateralization of the magnetic compass in favor of the right eye/left hemisphere of the brain can be easily undone by covering the right eye for a short time. However, this activation of the left eye/right hemisphere system does, in turn, not seem to affect the right eye. Interpretable magnetic information mediated by the left eye is essentially required to remove the lateralization. When the left eye system is activated, it can adjust to intensities outside the functional window of the magnetic compass (see [32]), but if it does, this ability is not transferred to the right eye system.

The directional information from the magnetic field originates in the retina and is transmitted by the visual nerve to higher centers in the brain (e.g., [33–35]). There are two main ascending visual systems in the bird brain that reach the telencephalon: one is the tectofugal system that runs from the retina via the optic tectum to the thalamic *nucleus rotundus*, which, in turn, projects to the entopallium. The second is the thalamofugal system that ascends from the retina via a thalamic link to a telencephalic area called wulst [36]. Anatomical and physiological studies in pigeons could demonstrate that both systems display asymmetries with a dominance of the left hemisphere. The tectofugal system is characterized by diverse anatomical and physiological asymmetries along its route [37–41]. Consequently, left-sided tectofugal lesions result in more severe visual deficits than right-sided ones [42,43]. In the thalamofugal system, the left- but not the right-sided wulst is able to importantly modify activity patterns of the tectofugal pathway [44]. Thus, both ascending visual pathways are lateralized with a superiority of the right eye and constitute a leading role of the left hemisphere, e.g., in recognizing and categorizing objects [45,46]. This could also be the reason for the normal dominance of the right eye/left hemisphere system in magnetoreception. At the same time, several commissural fibers that run through the tectal and posterior commissures are asymmetrically organized in birds such that the left tectum is less inhibited by its right counterpart than vice versa [47]. As a consequence, the dominant left hemisphere is able to inhibit the subdominant right. Inhibitory interactions are possibly crucial when only one function for which one hemisphere is dominant has to be executed [48]. Against this background, we will discuss our findings.

3.1. *Fast Re-Activation of the Left Eye/Right Hemisphere System for Sensing Magnetic Directions*

A mere 1½ h of covering the right eye enabled the robins to orient with their left eye. This extends the findings of our previous study [29] and shows that the lateralization of magnetic compass orientation is still amenable to changes during the first spring migration. Ninety minutes is probably too short for major anatomical changes within the visual pathway [49]. It is more likely that the causal mechanisms for re-activation of the left eye system are related to the short-term synaptic plasticity of the strength of commissural synapses. As the dominant left hemisphere is able to inhibit the subdominant right [47,48], the functional asymmetry of the magnetic compass could be constituted via asymmetrically organized inhibitory interactions between the two hemispheres. Both the left and the right hemispheres are obviously able to do the task during the first spring migration, but, under normal conditions, the dominant left hemisphere (right eye) would inhibit the subdominant right half brain (left eye). This asymmetrical inhibition is abolished after forcing the animal to use the left eye alone for 1½ h. However, these birds return to their left hemispheric dominance after just another further 1½ h of binocular vision. Thus, left hemisphere (right eye) dominance seems to be the normal state of the magnetic compass system. In young birds, this condition is subject to plasticity after the accumulation of left eye experience, but it returns to its previous status once the right eye can be used again.

The short time of 1½ h required to enable birds to use their left eye during spring migration could also explain some of the seemingly controversial findings in the literature. Engels and colleagues [27] reported that they did not find lateralization of the magnetic compass in their spring experiments with robins. In their method section, the authors quote previous studies [25,50] that imply that the covering of the right eye occurred at least 2 h before the tests began, often earlier—this would have allowed sufficient time for the neural circuit to process information from the left eye again.

3.2. *Conditions Required for the Re-Activation of the Left Eye/Right Hemisphere System*

The findings of the second part of our study are more difficult to interpret because they touch the still open question of whether the reception of magnetic directions is an integrated part of vision or magnetic information is processed more or less independently as a sense of its own.

Learning visual discrimination tasks takes longer with the left eye/right hemisphere than with the right eye, and in several cases of bilateral learning, the right hemisphere did not share the knowledge, but had to be trained separately (e.g., [51,52]; for review, see [53]). It is unclear whether the longer time required for the left eye/right hemisphere system to adjust to higher magnetic intensities represents a parallel case. We exposed the robins prior to the tests for 3 h to a higher magnetic field of 92 μT. As shown previously [31], robins need about 1 h to orient in this field strength. Robins allowed to use their right eye were oriented right away, but this was not so for the left-eyed birds; they took considerably longer. This appears to be in accordance with the results of discrimination studies mentioned above. The adjustment to higher magnetic intensities means that the birds become able to interpret a slightly different activation pattern on the retina (see [16,31]); it can start only after the ability to process magnetic information has been restored to left eye/right hemispheres. However, this alone can probably not account for the longer delay of the left eye system, as our experiments show that it requires only 1½ h, possibly less. It means that the left eye system is indeed considerably slower in performing the adjustment, requiring much longer than the 1 h observed in binocular birds [31].

Once the left eye system could orient in the stronger magnetic field of 92 μT, this ability was not directly transferred to the right eye system. This is contrary to the results of most visual discriminations tasks, which found a more efficient transfer of visual discrimination from the left eye to the right eye [43,51,52]. This is assumed to be due to the more bilateral left hemispheric visual representation in the tectofugal pathway that enables the right eye system to swiftly access left eye information [38]. The fact that our result pattern runs contrary to these data from visual pattern discrimination studies indicates that magnetic compass information is processed differently from visual patterns. It could also be related to the thalamofugal wulst system where cluster *N* was suggested to be a central hub of magnetic compass processing ([35], but see [54]). At least in pigeons, the wulst is known to modify lateralized activity patterns of the tectofugal pathway [41,44] and to thereby affect interhemispheric exchange of information [43].

An important finding in the experiments with left-eyed birds is that exposure to a radio-frequency field that disrupts magnetic orientation [18,19] did not result in an ability to orient with the left eye, although this eye had had access to visual information. Obviously, the change in asymmetry concerning magnetic compass information is not the result of mere right-eye monocular occlusion. What is required for this kind of change is the ability to sense interpretable magnetic compass information with the left eye during periods of absence of right eye input—if this specific requirement is not met, the normal left hemispheric (right eye) dominance prevails. This, too, seems to indicate that magnetic directional information is processed differently from visual input, with the specific magnetic stimulus necessary to overcome the normal lateralization in favor of the right eye system. However, it is also conceivable that magnetic compass information is just a specific kind of visual input within the visual system and that disruption of this input through a radio-frequency field makes it impossible for the left eye/right hemisphere system to regain the ability to process this specific input class. Details of how magnetic compass information is processed have to be analyzed in further studies.

3.3. Lasting Flexibility in the Avian Magnetic Compass?

Our results clearly show that, during the first spring migration, both hemispheres are in principle able to process magnetic compass information. Indeed, in a histological study [23], Cry1a, the putative receptor molecule, was found in both eyes alike in robins almost a year old, i.e., after spring migration was finished. Older robins were not examined, but at least in Domestic Chickens, *Gallus gallus*, Cry1a was still present in both eyes when they are more than two years old [55]. This suggests that magnetic directional information could still be provided by the left eye and processed in the right hemisphere, but that it is actively suppressed by the left hemisphere—information from the left eye is no longer processed as long as corresponding information from the right eye is transmitted to the brain. However, if this is interrupted, it can be replaced by that from the left eye. The observation that the right eye system is not affected by being temporarily covered and that the re-gained ability to use the information from the left eye is lost rather quickly when the right eye is open again demonstrates the dominance of the right eye/left hemisphere in processing magnetic directional information.

For this study, we used young robins during their first spring migration, i.e., birds less than one year old; older birds roughly 1½ years old had proven less flexible in an earlier study [29]. It seems possible that changes of asymmetry are easier during early ontogeny and less flexible in adult individuals. Indeed, Lesley Rogers [46,56] pioneered studies on the ontogenetic establishment of visual asymmetries in chicks and could demonstrate that both functional and anatomical lateralized systems can be easily modified in early ontogeny, with a similar effect also observed in young pigeons [57,58]. In Japanese quails, a life-long potential for plasticity has been observed [7]. Hence, we cannot exclude that in robins and other birds the left eye/right hemisphere system can still be activated in later years, but this appears to require more time than the six hours for which we tested during the second autumn migration [29]. Possibly, if a bird is injured and loses its right eye, its brain proves flexible enough to eventually restore magnetoreception to the left eye system. Studies in humans make it likely that asymmetries that depend on lateralized commissural interactions can retain their plasticity up to late adulthood [59].

4. Material and Methods

The experiments were performed during spring migration of the years 2011 to 2013 in the garden of the Zoological Institute of the University of Frankfurt am Main (50°08′N, 8°40′E).

4.1. Experimental Birds

The test birds were European Robins, a passerine species that is distributed all over Europe. The northern populations are nocturnal migrants and spend the winter in the Mediterranean region. In September, juvenile birds were caught using mist nets in the Botanical Garden of Frankfurt am Main, right next to the test sites and were identified as transmigrants of Scandinavian origin by their wing lengths. They were housed in individual cages in a photoperiod simulating the natural one until early December, when it was decreased to L:D 8:16. Around New Year, it was increased in two steps to L:D 13:11. This induced premature migratory activity and allowed us to conduct spring experiments already in January and February. After the end of the experiments, the birds were released in the Botanical Garden in the beginning of April when the photoperiod outside had reached 13 h.

4.2. Covering One Eye

With all experimental test series, we ran control tests with the same individual birds, testing them binocularly (Bi) without any treatment, because previous tests proved any unspecific effects from covering one eye to be negligible. The methods used to cover one eye for monocular testing was identical with those used in earlier studies with migratory birds [11,12,29]: a small non-magnetic aluminum cap was placed over the eye to be covered, fixed with adhesive tape (Leukoplast), as shown in Figure 1 in [11]. This was done either immediately before the tests started or at predetermined intervals before tests began; in some treatments, the eye-cover was removed before tests started and the other eye was covered instead. The various test conditions are defined in Table 1. Immediately after each test, any eye cover was removed and the birds were returned to their housing cages.

4.3. Test Performance

Testing followed our standard procedure, see, e.g., [11,18,29]: the test sites were wooden houses in the garden of the Zoological Institute where the geomagnetic field (46 μT, 66° inclination) was largely undisturbed. The birds were tested individually once per day in funnel-shaped cages lined with thermo-paper [60] where they left scratches as they moved. The cage was lit with green light, our standard control light. Each test lasted about 1 h. The individual birds were mostly tested three times in each test condition, in one condition four times (see Table 2).

In two test conditions, the birds were exposed to a radio-frequency field of 1.315 MHz (the local Larmor frequency) and 480 nT for 3 h before they were tested. This field was produced by a coil antenna consisting of a single winding of coaxial cable with 2 cm of the screening removed. This antenna was mounted horizontally on a wooden frame and was fed by oscillating currents from a high frequency generator, generating the oscillating field vertically, i.e., at a 24° angle to the vector of the geomagnetic field (for details, see [18,19,61]); four birds at a time were exposed in this field in all-plastic housing cages. In another test series, the birds were pre-exposed to, and tested in a magnetic field of 92 μT, twice the strength of the local geomagnetic field. This field was produced by Helmholtz coils (2 m in diameter and 1 m clearance) arranged in the way that the induced field added to the geomagnetic field, increasing the intensity, but not altering magnetic North and inclination [31].

4.4. Data Analysis and Statistics

After each test, the thermo-paper was removed from the funnels, virtually divided into 24 uniform sectors, and the scratches in these 24 sectors were counted by a person blind to the test conditions. Tests with less than a total of 35 scratches were considered to be of too little activity and were discarded; these tests were repeated with the same bird at the end of the test period. From the distribution of the scratches, the heading of the bird in the respective test was determined. The headings of each bird in each test condition were added to calculate a vector with the heading α_b and the length r_b. From these headings α_b, we calculated second order grand mean vectors for the various test conditions, which were tested for significant directional preference using the Rayleigh test [30]. The data of monocular treatments were compared with the binocular control data and the data from the same birds in different treatments with the Mardia Watson Wheeler test for differences in distribution, and the Mann–Whitney U test was applied to the differences of the birds' mean bearings from the grand mean for differences in variance [30]. From the individual vector lengths r_b, medians were calculated for each test condition; they reflect the intra-individual variance.

Acknowledgments: O.G. was supported by the Deutsche Forschungsgemeinschaft through Sonderforschungbereich 874; R.W was supported by the Deutsche Forschungsgemeinschaft through the grant Wi 988/8-2. We thank the students of the advanced lab classes, E. Berger, E. Dylda, D. Kringel, M. Kubi, P. Slattery and M. Wellmann, who helped us in carrying out the experiments.

Author Contributions: D.G., O.G., W.W. and R.W. conceived and designed the experiments; D.G., R.W. and W.W. performed the experiments; D.G. analyzed the data; R.W. and O.G. wrote the paper, with O.G. contributing substantially to the discussion.

References

1. Ocklenburg, S.; Ströckens, F.; Güntürkün, O. Lateralisation of conspecific vocalisation in non-human vertebrates. *Laterality* **2013**, *18*, 1–31. [CrossRef]
2. Ströckens, F.; Güntürkün, O.; Ocklenburg, S. Limb preferences in non-human vertebrates. *Laterality* **2013**, *18*, 536–575. [CrossRef]
3. Güntürkün, O.; Diekamp, B.; Manns, M.; Nottelmann, F.; Prior, H.; Schwarz, A.; Skiba, M. Asymmetry pays: Visual lateralization improves discrimination success in pigeons. *Curr. Biol.* **2000**, *10*, 1079–1081. [CrossRef]
4. Dadda, M.; Bisazza, A. Does brain asymmetry allow efficient performance of simultaneous tasks? *Anim. Behav.* **2006**, *72*, 523–529. [CrossRef]
5. Hirnstein, M.; Hugdahl, K.; Hausmann, M. How brain asymmetry relates to performance—A large-scale dichotic listening study. *Front. Psychol.* **2014**, *4*, 997. [CrossRef]
6. Ventolini, N.; Ferrero, E.A.; Sponza, S.; Della Chiesa, A.; Zucca, P.; Vallortigara, G. Laterality in the wild: Preferential hemifield use during predatory and sexual behaviour in the black-winged stilt. *Anim. Behav.* **2005**, *69*, 1077–1084. [CrossRef]
7. Gülbetekin, E.; Güntürkün, O.; Dural, S.; Cetinkaya, H. Visual asymmetries in Japanese quail (*Coturnix japonica*) retain a lifelong potential for plasticity. *Behav. Neurosci.* **2009**, *123*, 815–821. [CrossRef] [PubMed]
8. Vallortigara, G.; Chiandetti, C.; Sovrano, V.A. Brain asymmetry (animal). *WIREs Cogn. Sci.* **2011**, *2*, 146–157. [CrossRef] [PubMed]
9. Rogers, L.J.; Zucca, P.; Vallortigara, G. Advantages of having a lateralized brain. *Proc. R. Soc. B* **2004**, *271* (Suppl. S6), S420–S422. [CrossRef] [PubMed]

10. Vallortigara, G. The evolutionary psychology of left and right: Costs and benefits of lateralization. *Dev. Psychobiol.* **2006**, *48*, 418–427. [CrossRef] [PubMed]
11. Wiltschko, W.; Traudt, J.; Güntürkün, O.; Prior, H.; Wiltschko, R. Lateralisation of magnetic compass orientation in a migratory bird. *Nature* **2002**, *419*, 467–470. [CrossRef]
12. Wiltschko, W.; Munro, U.; Ford, H.; Wiltschko, R. Lateralisation of magnetic compass orientation in Silvereyes, *Zosterops lateralis*. *Aust. J. Zool.* **2003**, *51*, 597–602. [CrossRef]
13. Rogers, L.; Munro, U.; Freire, R.; Wiltschko, R.; Wiltschko, W. Lateralized response of chicks to magnetic cues. *Behav. Brain Res.* **2008**, *186*, 66–71. [CrossRef] [PubMed]
14. Stapput, K.; Güntürkün, O.; Hoffmann, K.P.; Wiltschko, R.; Wiltschko, W. Magnetoreception of directional information requires non-degraded vision. *Curr. Biol.* **2010**, *20*, 1259–1262. [CrossRef] [PubMed]
15. Wilzeck, C.; Wiltschko, W.; Güntürkün, O.; Wiltschko, R.; Prior, H. Lateralization of magnetic compass orientation in pigeons. *J. R. Soc. Interface* **2010**, *7*, 235–240. [CrossRef] [PubMed]
16. Ritz, T.; Adem, S.; Schulten, K. A model for photoreceptor-based magnetoreception in birds. *Biophys. J.* **2000**, *78*, 707–718. [CrossRef]
17. Henbest, K.B.; Kukura, P.; Rodgers, C.T.; Hore, P.J.; Timmel, C.R. Radio frequency magnetic field effects on a radical recombination reaction: A diagnostic test for the radical pair mechanism. *J. Am. Chem. Soc.* **2004**, *126*, 8102–8103. [CrossRef] [PubMed]
18. Ritz, T.; Thalau, P.; Philllips, J.B.; Wiltschko, R.; Wiltschko, W. Resonance effects indicate a radical-pair mechanism for avian magnetic compass. *Nature* **2004**, *429*, 177–180. [CrossRef] [PubMed]
19. Thalau, P.; Ritz, T.; Stapput, K.; Wiltschko, R.; Wiltschko, W. Magnetic compass orientation of migratory birds in the presence of a 1.315 MHz oscillating field. *Naturwissenschaften* **2005**, *92*, 86–90. [CrossRef] [PubMed]
20. Wiltschko, W.; Freire, R.; Munro, U.; Ritz, T.; Rogers, L.; Thalau, P.; Wiltschko, R. The magnetic compass of domestic chickens, *Gallus gallus*. *J. Exp. Biol.* **2007**, *210*, 2300–2310. [CrossRef] [PubMed]
21. Keary, N.; Roploh, T.; Voss, J.; Thalau, P.; Wiltschko, R.; Wiltschko, W.; Bischof, H.J. Oscillating magnetic field disrupts magnetic orientation in Zebra finches, *Taeniopygia guttata*. *Front. Zool.* **2009**, *6*, 25. [CrossRef] [PubMed]
22. Kavokin, K.; Chernetsov, N.; Pakomov, A.; Bojarinova, J.; Kobylkov, D.; Namozov, B. Magnetic orientation of garden warblers (*Sylvia borin*) under 1.4 MHz radio frequency field. *J. R. Soc. Interface* **2014**, *11*, 20140451. [CrossRef] [PubMed]
23. Nießner, C.; Denzau, S.; Gross, J.C.; Peichl, L.; Bischof, H.J.; Fleissner, G.; Wiltschko, W.; Wiltschko, R. Avian ultraviolet/violet cones identified as probable magnetoreceptors. *PLoS ONE* **2011**, *6*, e20091. [CrossRef] [PubMed]
24. Nießner, C.; Denzau, S.; Stapput, K.; Ahmad, M.; Peichl, L.; Wiltschko, W.; Wiltschko, R. Magnetoreception: Activated cryptochrome 1a concurs with magnetic orientation in birds. *J. R. Soc. Interface* **2013**, *10*, 20130618.
25. Hein, C.M.; Zapka, M.; Heyers, D.; Kurzschbauch, S.; Schneider, N.-L.; Mouritsen, H. Night-migratory Garden Warblers can orient with their magnetic compass using the left, the right or both eyes. *J. R. Soc. Interface* **2010**, *7*, S227–S233. [CrossRef] [PubMed]
26. Hein, C.M.; Engels, S.; Kishkinev, D.; Mouritsen, H. Robins have a magnetic compass in both eye. *Nature* **2011**, *271*, E11–E12. [CrossRef] [PubMed]
27. Engels, S.; Hein, C.; Lefeldt, N.; Prior, H.; Mouritsen, H. Night-migratory songbirds possess a magnetic compass in both eye. *PLoS ONE* **2012**, *7*, e43271. [CrossRef] [PubMed]
28. Wiltschko, W.; Traudt, J.; Güntürkün, O.; Prior, H.; Wiltschko, R. Reply to Hein et al. *Nature* **2011**, *471*, E12–E13.
29. Gehring, D.; Wiltschko, W.; Güntürkün, O.; Denzau, S.; Wiltschko, R. Development of lateralization of the magnetic compass in a migratory bird. *Proc. R. Soc. B* **2012**, *279*, 4230–4235. [CrossRef] [PubMed]
30. Batschelet, E. *Circular Statistics in Biology*; Academic Press: London, UK, 1981.
31. Wiltschko, W.; Stapput, K.; Thalau, P.; Wiltschko, R. Avian magnetic compass: Fast adjustment to intensities outside the normal functional window. *Naturwissenschaften* **2006**, *93*, 300–304. [CrossRef] [PubMed]
32. Wiltschko, R.; Wiltschko, W. Sensing magnetic directions in birds: Radical pair processes involving cryptochrome. *Biosensors* **2014**, *4*, 221–242. [CrossRef] [PubMed]
33. Semm, P.; Demaine, C. Neurophysiological properties of magnetic cells in the pigeon's visual system. *J. Comp. Physiol. A* **1986**, *159*, 619–625. [CrossRef] [PubMed]

34. Heyers, D.; Manns, M.; Luksch, H.; Güntürkün, O.; Mouritsen, H. A visual pathway links brain structures active during magnetic compass orientation in migratory birds. *PLoS ONE* **2007**, *9*, e937. [CrossRef] [PubMed]
35. Zapka, M.; Heyers, D.; Hein, C.M.; Engels, S.; Schneider, N.L.; Hans, J.; Weiler, S.; Dreyer, D.; Kishkinev, D.; Wild, J.M.; et al. Visual but not trigeminal mediation of magnetic compass information in a migratory bird. *Nature* **2009**, *461*, 1274–1277. [CrossRef] [PubMed]
36. Mouritsen, H.; Heyers, D.; Güntürkün, O. The neural basis of long-distance navigation in birds. *Annu. Rev. Physiol.* **2016**, *78*, 133–154. [CrossRef] [PubMed]
37. Güntürkün, O. Morphological asymmetries of the *tectum opticum* in the pigeon. *Exp. Brain Res.* **1997**, *116*, 561–566. [CrossRef] [PubMed]
38. Güntürkün, O.; Hellmann, B.; Melsbach, G.; Prior, H. Asymmetries of representation in the visual system of pigeons. *Neuroreport* **1998**, *9*, 4127–4130. [CrossRef] [PubMed]
39. Ströckens, F.; Freund, N.; Manns, M.; Ocklenburg, S.; Güntürkün, O. Visual asymmetries and the ascending thalamofugal pathway in pigeons. *Brain Struct. Funct.* **2013**, *218*, 1197–1209. [CrossRef] [PubMed]
40. Manns, M.; Güntürkün, O. "Natural" and artificial monocular deprivation effects on thalamic soma sizes in pigeons. *Neuroreport* **1999**, *10*, 3223–3228. [CrossRef] [PubMed]
41. Folta, K.; Diekamp, B.; Güntürkün, O. Asymmetrical modes of visual bottom-up and top-down integration in the thalamic *nucleus rotundus* of pigeons. *J. Neurosci.* **2004**, *24*, 9475–9485. [CrossRef] [PubMed]
42. Güntürkün, O.; Hahmann, U. Visual acuity and hemispheric asymmetries in pigeons. *Behav. Brain Res.* **1994**, *60*, 171–175. [CrossRef]
43. Valencia-Alfonso, C.-E.; Verhaal, J.; Güntürkün, O. Ascending and descending mechanisms of visual lateralization in pigeons. *Philos. Trans. Roy. Soc. B* **2009**, *364*, 955–963. [CrossRef] [PubMed]
44. Freund, N.; Valencia-Alfonso, C.E.; Kirsch, J.; Brodmann, K.; Manns, M.; Güntürkün, O. Asymmetric top-down modulation of ascending visual pathways in pigeons. *Neuropsychologia* **2016**, *83*, 37–47. [CrossRef] [PubMed]
45. Yamazaki, Y.; Aust, U.; Huber, L.; Hausmann, M.; Güntürkün, O. Lateralized cognition: Asymmetrical and complementary strategies of pigeons during discrimination of the "human concept". *Cognition* **2007**, *104*, 315–344. [CrossRef] [PubMed]
46. Rogers, L.J. Asymmetry of brain and behavior in animals: Its development, function, and human relevance. *Genesis* **2014**, *52*, 555–571. [CrossRef] [PubMed]
47. Keysers, C.; Diekamp, B.; Güntürkün, O. Evidence for physiological asymmetries in the intertectal connections of the pigeon (*Columba livia*) and their potential role in brain lateralisation. *Brain Res.* **2000**, *852*, 406–413. [CrossRef]
48. Genç, E.; Ocklenburg, S.; Singer, W.; Güntürkün, O. Abnormal interhemispheric motor interactions in patients with callosal agenesis. *Behav. Brain Res.* **2015**, *293*, 1–9. [CrossRef] [PubMed]
49. Bailey, C.H.; Kandel, E.R.; Harris, K.M. Structural components of synaptic plasticity and memory consolidation. *Cold Spring Harb. Perspect. Biol.* **2015**, *7*. [CrossRef] [PubMed]
50. Liedvogel, M.; Feender, G.; Wada, K.; Troje, N.F.; Jarvis, E.D.; Mouritsen, H. Lateralized activation of cluster N in the brain of migratory songbird. *Eur. J. Neurosci.* **2007**, *25*, 116–1173. [CrossRef] [PubMed]
51. Nottelmann, F.; Wohlschläger, A.; Güntürkün, O. Unihemispheric memory in pigeons—Knowledge, the left hemisphere is reluctant to share. *Behav. Brain Res.* **2002**, *133*, 309–315. [CrossRef]
52. Xiao, Q.; Güntürkünn, O. Natural split brains? Lateralized memory for task contingencies in pigeons. *Neurosci. Lett.* **2009**, *458*, 75–78. [CrossRef] [PubMed]
53. Vallortigara, G.; Rogers, L.J. Survival with an asymmetrical brain: Advantages and disadvantages of cerebral lateralization. *Behav. Brain Sci.* **2005**, *28*, 575–589. [CrossRef] [PubMed]
54. Zapka, M.; Heyers, D.; Liedvogel, M.; Jarvis, E.D.; Mouritsen, H. Night-time neuronal activation of cluster N in a day- and night-migration songbird. *Eur. J. Neurosci.* **2010**, *32*, 619–624. [CrossRef] [PubMed]
55. Nießner, C.; Ernst Strüngmann Institut, Frankfurt am Main, Germany. Personal communication, 2013.
56. Rogers, L.J. Light input and the reversal of functional lateralization in the chicken brain. *Behav. Brain Res.* **1990**, *38*, 211–221. [CrossRef]
57. Manns, M.; Güntürkün, O. Monocular deprivation alters the direction of functional and morphological asymmetries in the pigeon's visual system. *Behav. Neurosci.* **1999**, *113*, 1–10. [CrossRef]

58. Skiba, M.; Diekamp, B.; Güntürkün, O. Embryonic light stimulation induces different asymmetries in visuoperceptual and visuomotor pathways of pigeons. *Behav. Brain Res.* **2002**, *134*, 149–156. [CrossRef]
59. Hausmann, M. Why sex hormones matter for neuroscience: A very short review on sex, sex hormones, and functional brain asymmetries. *J. Neurosci. Res.* **2017**, *95*, 40–49. [CrossRef] [PubMed]
60. Mouritsen, H.; Feender, G.; Hegemann, A.; Liedvogel, M. Thermopaer can replace typewriter correction paper in Emlen funnels. *J. Ornithol.* **2009**, *150*, 713–715. [CrossRef]
61. Wiltschko, R.; Thalau, P.; Gehring, D.; Nießner, C.; Ritz, T.; Wiltschko, W. Magnetoreception in birds: The effect of radio frequency fields. *J. R. Soc. Interface* **2015**, *12*, 20141103. [CrossRef] [PubMed]

7

Audition and Hemispheric Specialization in Songbirds and New Evidence from Australian Magpies

Gisela Kaplan

School of Science and Technology, University of New England, Armidale, NSW 2351, Australia; gkaplan@une.edu.au

Academic Editor: Sergei D. Odintsov

Abstract: The neural processes of bird song and song development have become a model for research relevant to human acquisition of language, but in fact, very few avian species have been tested for lateralization of the way in which their audio-vocal system is engaged in perception, motor output and cognition. Moreover, the models that have been developed have been premised on birds with strong vocal dimorphism, with a tendency to overlook species with complex social and/or monomorphic song systems. The Australian magpie (*Gymnorhina tibicen*) is an excellent model for the study of communication and vocal plasticity with a sophisticated behavioural repertoire, and some of its expression depends on functional asymmetry. This paper summarizes research on vocal mechanisms and presents field-work results of behavior in the Australian magpie. For the first time, evidence is presented and discussed about lateralized behaviour in one of the foremost songbirds in response to specific and specialized auditory and visual experiences under natural conditions. It presents the first example of auditory lateralization evident in the birds' natural environment by describing an extractive foraging event that has not been described previously in any avian species. It also discusses the first example of auditory behavioral asymmetry in a songbird tested under natural conditions.

Keywords: auditory perception; auditory lateralization; song production; extractive foraging; visual laterality; memory; Australian magpie

1. Introduction

Field studies of behavioural laterality in birds are still relatively rare, but the few undertaken so far have shown that laterality may play a role in vigilance behaviour [1,2], in predation and sexual behaviour [3,4] and even in tool manufacture, as shown in the New Caledonian crow, *Corvus moneduloides* [5]. In fact, in the special case of tool use and manufacture by crows, the activity appears to be strongly lateralized because birds were seen to use their right eye even when this posed some difficulties [6].

Asymmetries in avian species have been found in visual processing from sensory input to motor output, admittedly largely in domestic chickens [7,8] and pigeons [9]. Lateralized foot use has been shown in pigeons [10,11], the New Zealand kākā [12], some songbirds (sittellas and crested shrike-tits [13]), Japanese jungle crow [14] and also in cockatoos and some parrots [7,15–17]. This paper will explore whether such lateralities, as shown in the visual behavior of many vertebrate species [18], may also be present in auditory abilities and their behavioral expressions in birds.

Without a doubt, vision and audition are the most well-developed sensory abilities both in birds and in humans, and they are often used in conjunction: for example, there is plenty of evidence that learning is particularly effective and often more powerful when vision and audition are coupled [19,20]. In many oscine birds, song learning occurs in a visual context, suggesting that both auditory and visual perceptual systems could be involved in the acquisition process. Hultsch et al. [21] examined, in male juvenile nightingales, whether song performance improved after coupling visual with auditory stimuli. It did and did so convincingly [21]. In a study on chickens, Van Kampen and Bolhuis [22] demonstrated that learning is improved through compound training with simultaneous exposure to visual and auditory stimuli, showing that either modality has some facilitating effects on the memorization of features from the other modality. Such coupling has also worked in the combination of visual with aversive olfactory stimuli [23]. Additionally, there is evidence from research on zebra finches that visual stimuli activate auditory brain areas, e.g., the HVC, formerly called high vocal centre, now called HVC and used as a proper noun (see Figure 1 below) [24]. Given this interaction between auditory and visual processing and, since visual lateralization is widespread in avian species, it could be that auditory processing is also lateralized.

The importance of asymmetry in song production was identified early by Nottebohm [25]. He found that when the HVC in the left hemisphere was lesioned, male canaries could not produce song. When the HVC in the right hemisphere was lesioned, it had no effect on song production [25]. However, such lateralization does not apply to song production in all species, since it has been shown in zebra finches that some perceived manifestations of lateralization in the HVC during song production proved to be rapid switches between hemispheres and that the overall contributions of both sides were actually equal [26].

In research on memory formation, hemispheric dominance has been found in zebra finch males. Gobes and Bolhuis [27] showed that tutored-song memory and a motor program for the bird's own song have separate neural representations in the songbird brain. Lesions to the caudomedial nidopallium (NCM) of adult male zebra finches impaired tutor-song recognition, but did not affect the males' song production or their ability to discriminate calls. Lesions were bilateral, so any potential lateralization could not be measured. Moorman and colleagues [28] recently measured neuronal activation during sleep in juvenile zebra finch males that were still learning their songs from a tutor. They found that during sleep, there was learning-dependent lateralization of spontaneous neuronal activation in the NCM. Birds that imitated their tutors well were left dominant, whereas poor imitators were right dominant, similar to language proficiency-related lateralization in humans. Indeed, interest in comparative work in song production and perception and human speech [29] has increased substantially in the last decade, finding important similarities in the role of specific auditory nuclei between humans and birds [30,31].

Limitations: Species Investigated

The species most often chosen for detailed neurobehavioral research on auditory perception/song performance is the zebra finch. The choice makes sense on a number of levels: the song of this species is relatively simple and has a defined learning period, the birds are easy to keep in a laboratory setting (opportunistic breeders as they are, they reproduce easily in captivity and over short periods of time).

However, research of song in zebra finches has some limitations. The zebra finch is a sexually dimorphic bird in which only the male sings. This is not the case in all avian species. In fact, the zebra finch has model character only for songbirds with credentials similar to itself [32,33]; these include, for instance, migratory songbirds of high latitudes that need to fit a complete reproductive time-table into the shortest possible time frame: find a mate in spring, breed, raise offspring and migrate in autumn. Under such circumstances, offspring have to become independent rapidly. Juvenile males have to be taught how to be able to compete and win a female, relying on recall and a perfect memory of the song that an adult male tutor may have taught them in the previous year [34,35].

Having chosen such a model for research on bird song may have implied a questionable underlying assumption that song in all songbirds is purely a male activity (be this for courtship or territorial display) and may be exclusive to the breeding season. The zebra finch model also implies that song is mostly or always crystallized early in development with limited or non-existent ability for any ongoing learning/brain plasticity. However, as has always been known, there is a considerable number of songbirds with vast and flexible repertoires [36], and some of these live in complex social groups. Burish et al. [37] argued that telencephalic volume is strongly correlated with social complexity. This correlation, so they show, accounts for almost half of the observed variation in telencephalic size, more than any other behavioral specialization examined, including the ability to learn song. Moreover, female song is widespread and ancestral in birds [38–41]. In other words, as was recognized some time ago, relying on the zebra finch model in terms of broader questions of behavior could lead to ignoring the importance of social learning in non-reproductive contexts [42,43], the significance of variability in avian communication outside the breeding context and the possibility of different underlying mechanisms of brain activity [44–46] for hearing and vocal production, of which lateralization may be an important manifestation.

Since the discovery of mirror neurons in birds by Prather and colleagues [47], we also know that birds can learn song without being actively supervised and instructed by an adult. Tchernichovski and Wallman [48] explain that, on input, the motor signal is delayed, and this implies that the mirror neurons are providing a 'corollary discharge' signal: that is, a neural representation of the song being heard is available to the bird on first hearing it, and the bird can now check the encoded version against the song it later sings; or expressed differently, the bird has the same neuron activation whether it sings or just listens and gets a copy of the song in its memory against which it can judge its own output (performance) of the song.

Importantly, the mirror neurons identified by Prather et al. [47] belong to a population of neurons that is not replaced, as other neurons in the song system are [49], but is stable across song development. It is this stability that enables the juvenile to improve its song as the memory trace of the correct version remains present and can be accessed. It was established decades ago that amongst the network of nuclei involved in song perception and production, some are essential and some are not essential for song production [50], as discussed below.

2. Song Control System, the Auditory System and Lateralization

Song development and song production entail a set of complex interactions between neurological, physiological and behavioral events, and it has taken more than thirty years of research to begin to understand the nature, type and dynamics of these interactions.

Songbirds possess a network of interconnected nuclei in the fore-, mid- and hind-brain used in the perception and production of vocalizations (see Figure 1) [51]. Furthermore, feedback loops are essential for vocal learning, and these are found only in passerines and parrots (and two species of humming birds), cetaceans and humans. The HVC, the robust nucleus of the arcopallium (RA) and the tracheosyringeal component of the hypoglossal nucleus (nXIIts), are necessary for the acquisition and expression of learned song [50], whilst Area X and the lateral magnocellular nucleus of the anterior nidopallium (LMAN) are important feedback loops [52–54]. These main nuclei and some important auxiliary nuclei (Figure 1), represented on both sides of the brain, have been tested for lateralized expression. The budgerigar, a psittacine species, capable of vocal learning, but not classed as a songbird, has multiple forebrain areas for vocal production, but some of these, it appears, are not homologous to those of songbirds [55].

A link has been made sometimes between size of song nuclei and song complexity. It is said that song nuclei tend to be larger in those species that have more complex songs, and the HVC is larger in individuals with larger repertoires [56]. However, the relationship between presence and size of nuclei and actual song performance is not always matched. Gahr et al. [57] found that the male and the female of the African duetting bush shrike, *Laniarius funebris*, produce songs of similar complexity, but the HVC is, nevertheless, sexually dimorphic (larger in the male than in the female). The Australian magpie, *Gymnorhina tibicen*, also duets, and these findings are therefore relevant here. Gahr et al. [57] argued that their results show how misleading it can be to assume a causal relation between sex difference in vocal behaviour and in the size of brain areas involved in song production and learning.

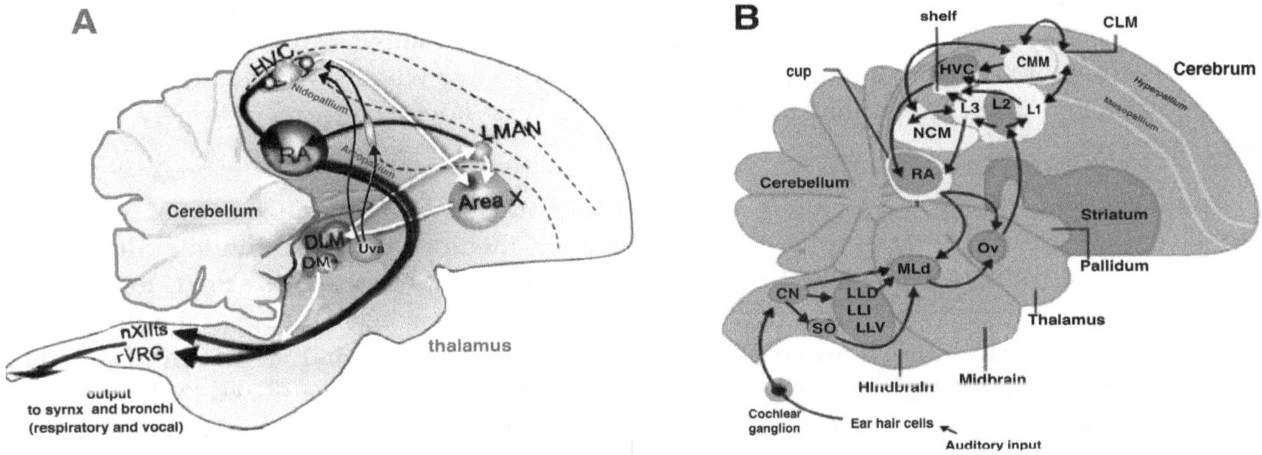

Figure 1. Song control system and auditory pathways. (**A**) The song control system. (**B**) Auditory pathways; simplified-arrows indicate flow of activations; right lateral view. (**A**) Song output via the main nuclei, the HVC of the nidopallium; RA, robust nucleus of the arcopallium; LMAN, lateral magnocellular nucleus of the anterior nidopallium; Area X of the striatum; DLM, medial subdivision of the dorsolateral nucleus of the anterior thalamus; DM, dorsomedial subdivision of nucleus intercollicularis of the mesencephalon; Uva, nucleus uvaeformis; nXIIts, tracheosyringeal portion of the nucleus hypoglossus (nucleus XII); rVRG, rostral ventral respiratory group. (**B**) Auditory input HVC of the nidopallium with HVC shelf (lightly shaded); CLM, caudolateral mesopallium; CMM, caudomedial mesopallium; Field L, large area (light grey) subdivided into L1, L2 and L3; NCM, caudomedial nidopallium; RA, robust nucleus of the arcopallium; Ov, nucleus ovoidalis; MLd, nucleus mesencephalicus lateralis, pars dorsalis; LL, lateral lemniscus subdivided into: LLD, dorsal nucleus; LLI, intermediate nucleus; LLV, ventral nucleus; CN, cochlear nucleus; SO, superior olive (adapted from [58]).

However, our own investigations of the song control system in magpies do not confirm those of Gahr and colleagues [57], as is summarized below. Moreover, unlike model species such as zebra finches, *Taeniopygia guttata*, Australian magpies do not use song as part of a reproductive strategy. Both males and females sing [59], and song in both males and females declines, not increases, during the breeding season and does not appear to play any known role in mate choice [60].

Exciting research in recent years has focused on specific areas of the brain and found intensity invariant neurons in Field L, important for distant conspecific recognition (temporal resolution of 30 ms) and noise invariant neurons for individuals at closer distance with a temporal resolution of just 10 ms [61]. While these areas (NCM and CM) were once just considered secondary auditory areas, they have now been recognized as important loci for conspecific song discrimination and individual song recognition and, as such, have behavioural significance [62–67]. Indeed, Woolley and colleagues [68] identified all nine functional areas in the forebrain and midbrain of the zebra finch (four in the midbrain alone), each of which was shown to play a specific role in extracting distinct complex sound features [68]. With the importance of these areas now identified, it should also be possible to ask whether any of these specific sound inputs activate neurons differentially in the left or the right hemisphere.

Indeed, a study by Poirier et al. [69] using functional magnetic resonance imaging (fMRI) discovered that, in zebra finches, the mid-brain shows neural activation in song recognition of both individual (own) and conspecific song, which is a crucial auditory and cognitive ability. These nuclei, called MLd (dorsal part of the lateral nucleus of the mesencephalon), are located in the midbrain, a subcortical region that, not so long ago, had been considered non-plastic and even 'primitive' [69]. They showed that there was a distinct right-side bias in the MLd, confirming a complex topography across the forebrain regions [70]. In other words, in perception of song, as distinct from song production, robust evidence is now emerging of lateralization of the mechanisms involved. In research on starlings, behaviourally-relevant song stimuli were used to test whether the NCM might be a site for categorizing complex communication signals, and it was indeed confirmed, largely on the right side of the brain [71,72].

There is no need here to catalogue all the various nuclei with lateralized functions in avian auditory perception and song output; in their review on memory-related brain lateralization [73], Moorman and Nicol (2015) published a very useful table listing nuclei concerned, together with the species and lateralized functions. Suffice it to say that avian species that are lateralized do not necessarily have the same side bias: chaffinches, song sparrows and canaries were found to be left lateralized for control of song, whereas the zebra finch is largely right lateralized [51]. The point is rather that the number of species tested is relatively limited and, except for the starling, they belong to a group of birds that are sexually dimorphic, may be short-lived, limited in repertoire and of varying brain plasticity. Each may have its own specific architecture with respect to how and what is lateralized.

It is a contention of this paper that lateralization may well be different, probably stronger and show more functional separation, the more complex a repertoire is and the greater the ability to learn. It is further a contention that in cases of functional changes of song, one might also expect changes in brain activation and different adaptations, particularly in species that, more like humans, show the same vocal capacities in male and female and are life-long learners. Although this hypothesis cannot be fully tested or confirmed in one paper, it would seem an important and necessary task to establish research on such a species, especially for comparative purposes with human vocal development. Australian magpies satisfy these criteria.

3. A Life-Long Learner as a Model Species

This paper reports new data and summarizes previous research obtained both in the laboratory and in the field concerned with auditory and visual hemispheric specialization in the Australian magpie, a species native to Australia. The magpie is one of Australia's foremost songbirds apart from the lyrebird. It is territorial, and residents consist of pairs with long-term bonds, their immediate offspring of one year and sometimes those of previous years.

The main reasons why magpies make a very useful model for perceptual research and memory formation is that in both males and females, song does not crystallize. With a lifespan of 25 or more years, they readily add new elements and sequences to their song, and they are also excellent mimics [74,75]. In these qualities, there are substantial overlaps with parrots and specifically with Australian cockatoos, as well as with ravens and crows. We know that they are amongst the most cognitively complex and long-lived birds (sulphur-crested cockatoos: 100 years; galahs: 80 years) [76]. These attributes are not odd anomalies in avian species, as may once have been believed, but may be significant in that these specific characteristics appeared early in avian evolution.

Some researchers concerned with hemispheric specialization have especially raised the question of evolution [77–79], but so far, little has been made of the geographic origin of modern birds. It has been known since the 1980s, but generally scientifically accepted since 2004, that a number of bird lineages and all modern songbirds in the world today arose in East Gondwana, now Australia [80–82], seemingly the only location where lineages survived the mass extinction events of 65 mya, including galliformes and anseriformes [83], to name a few among the precocial birds, although taxonomists still argue about dates [84], and all (altricial) songbirds. Songbirds radiated out from Gondwana to the rest of the world, a process that took tens of millions of years [85,86]. For reasons of similar climate and vegetation, those species that only went as far as the subtropical and tropical islands to the north of the supercontinent and to the tropical regions of northern hemispheric mainlands (the Indian subcontinent was once part of Gondwana) could presumably keep some of the traits they had acquired in Gondwana. Cockatoos probably arose in the Cretaceous [87,88], i.e., belong to the most ancient lineages of altricial land birds, and their highly lateralized footedness and its connection with complex cognition, a link that has been made only recently [16], gains significance given its very ancient origin.

As to songbirds, Sibley's and Ahlquist's broad taxonomical subdivision into Corvida and Passerida [89], although not necessarily used by taxonomists now, is still very useful to explain certain broad commonalities and traits. Corvida contain overwhelmingly birds with complex cognitive abilities (from problem solving, tool use, to measurably larger brain to body ratios) than the Passerida. Zebra finches (a native Australian species) belong to the Passerida, smaller songbirds that were the ones identified as among the main, probably first, 'escapees' from the Gondwanan continent. Magpies and crows belong to the Corvida, the group consisting of many species, in which we find most extant examples of complex vocal behaviour, learning and problem-solving abilities, qualities that significantly and overwhelmingly are present in species forming long-term bonds and/or engaging in cooperative breeding [76,90]. Most of these lineages, including magpies and lyrebirds [74,91,92], are capable of substantial and accurate mimicry. In summary, brain plasticity, large repertoires and often sophisticated vocal communication may require special architectural features in the brain. One could speculate that avian brains of songbirds of ancient lineages, and even of non-songbirds as cockatoos, might also be highly lateralized and be so for other functions [68].

3.1. Song Production in Australian Magpies

Magpies have an extraordinarily large repertoire. Strangely, 'repertoire size' in the literature, with a few exceptions [65], tends to mean the number of syllables in a song or total number of identifiably different songs a bird might sing, and is measured as such rather than as the sum total of vocalizations, not only song. To establish the true range of brain asymmetry or the lack thereof, it would seem important to consider the entire range of a bird's utterances (see Figure 2), since these are likely to represent different contexts and functions and may be under different neural control. In addition, there is the question of where and how the brain gets engaged when vocalizations are a matter of affect or are learned and/or intentional, such as in referential signalling [93]. To my knowledge, there is little to no research that has been done on any of these aspects, including any lateralization of their perception or production.

My own fieldwork on magpie vocal behavior identified as many as 27 different alarm calls [94], falling roughly into six distinct types, recognizable in sonograms as highly specific in profile. Field studies playing back alarm calls established that at least one of these calls is a referential alarm call, signalling the presence of an eagle [95]. We then also established the stability of such referentiality in different magpie subspecies and very different locations [96].

It would seem important to learn whether several categories of vocalizations have greater left or right hemisphere activation and what this might tell us. We already know from studies of song learning in zebra finches that new songs learned are memorized in the right hemisphere while the original song (long-term memory) is retrieved from and shows neural activity in the left hemisphere [27]. However, according to the results reported by Olsen et al. [97], direction and strength of laterality depend on how well each song is learned and by whom: The greater the retention of song from their first tutor, the more right-dominant the birds were when exposed to that song; but the more birds learned from their second tutor, the more left-dominant they were when exposed to the first song [97]. Lateralized memory strengthens the performance of well-learned song and presumably enables the bird to be competitive for females in the coming season. Since magpies are improvisers and have no tutors [75], it is likely that the quality of learning and recall determines whether the sounds are stored in long-term memory (left hemisphere) [98].

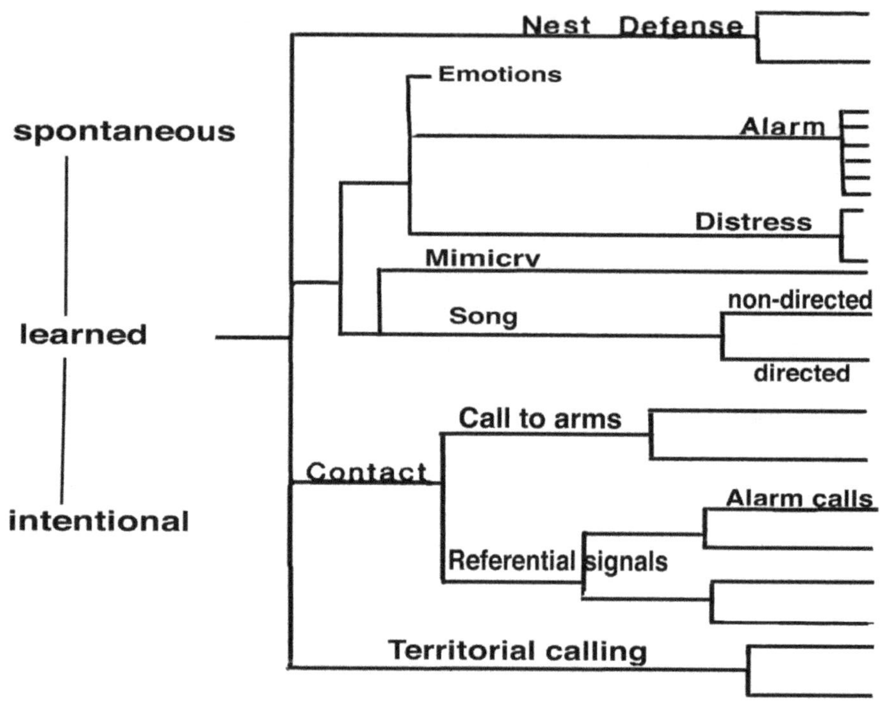

Figure 2. Range of vocalizations expressed by Australian magpies. These categories can roughly be subdivided as those that are a matter of affect, such as distress, fear and anger, but alarm calls, while also short, may involve forebrain regions (as in referential calls) or even in mobbing calls. Learned vocalizations in song, while not tutored, may have elements that are territorial or regional markers, and all mimicry is of course learned. Intentional vocalizations can be long or short, but they must have stereotyped characteristics, be uttered only in the presence of conspecifics and would usually lead to a change of behaviour in others (see [93,95]).

3.2. Song Control System in Magpies

When we sectioned magpie brains, albeit in a small sample ($N = 9$), we found that the female and male song nuclei of the magpie are about equal in volume and well developed and also well-developed in juvenile magpies (2–3 months post fledging), which is consistent with the vocal competence of juvenile magpies [99]. We also found the same song control nuclei and in the same topographical position in the forebrain of the Australian magpie, as present in canaries and zebra finches [50,52,99,100].

Our results indicate that, from juvenile to adult age, the volume of RA increases (10%), and the volume of the Area X decreases (19%). No such age-dependent change occurred in the HVC or LMAN (see Figure 1). The volume of mMAN (the medial magnocellular nucleus located adjacent to LMAN) was 40% smaller in juvenile females compared to a juvenile male and an adult female, but the volume of RA in the juvenile male was some 36% smaller than that of the juvenile females, suggesting that there may be both sex- and age-dependent differences in these nuclei. Interestingly, juvenile female magpies showed a fully-developed RA nucleus 2–3 months after fledging, whereas RA was developmentally delayed in the juvenile males, and the reverse applied to the nucleus mMAN [99]. Since all of the measurements were made on coronal sections and only one side of the brain was measured, no data examining lateralization were collected.

The Syrinx

The primary sound-producing organ in a bird is the syrinx, and the secondary system aiding sound production consists of the larynx, mouth, tongue and laryngeal muscles. Opening and closing of the beak may also affect the song produced [101–103].

The musculature controlling the syrinx is considered such a crucial anatomical feature that songbirds have been classified as such according to the absence or presence of these muscles [104]; or rather, the definition of a true songbird is based on the identification of the number of muscles present in the syrinx. Some avian species do not have a syrinx and produce sounds via clavicular sacs, and suboscines may have a syrinx with just one or two pairs of syringeal muscles. Certain suboscines, e.g., Tyranni, such as pittas, have a mesomyodian syrinx with either no or just one pair of syringeal muscles [105].

In the true oscines, as are magpies, the syrinx is equipped with four or more pairs of syringeal muscles, typically five pairs, important in the production of song. More recent research suggests that the syringeal muscles have mainly a modulatory function [106]. Furthermore, as some writers about psittacine vocalization have pointed out, the complexity of sound and a rich vocal repertoire may belie the simplicity of the sound-producing apparatus [107].

In early 19th century studies of the function of the syrinx, it was assumed that both sides of the syrinx always act together to produce one sound; but since the development of spectrographs, it could be shown that this was not the case, and birds could produce harmonically unrelated sounds simultaneously on both sides of the syrinx, giving rise to the 'two-voice' theory of song. Nottebohm [25] lesioned the hypoglossal nerve leading to the left side of the syrinx of male canaries, the consequence of which was that the bird's song was severely affected, losing the majority of its syllables, but sectioning the right side alone had relatively little effect on the postoperative song, a finding that was confirmed by testing other small songbirds, such as several species of sparrow and chaffinch [50,108]. The experiments have shown that the neural control of the syrinx is lateralized, with the left side being dominant. However, to assume that neural control and physiological adaptations come only in a fixed model for all songbirds would be incorrect.

Birds vocalize by expelling air over the elastic membranes of the syrinx housed within the inter-clavicular sac, an air sac in the pleural cavity. In songbirds, the syrinx consists of two parts, one in each bronchus, and each is innervated separately [50]. For a long time, sound was seen as being produced by the actions of lateral and medial labia, as well as the medial tympaniform membranes in the syrinx (see Figure 3). The actual sound-generating mechanism, however, appears to be located in the lateral tympaniform membranes (LTM) and not, as believed in classic theories, the medial tympaniform membranes (MTM). Goller and Larsen [106] showed in his sample of songbirds (a female crow, *Corvus brachyrhynchus*, wild-caught male Northern cardinals, *Cardinalis cardinalis*, and brown thrashers, *Toxostoma rufum*) that even the removal of the MTM did little to alter song performance. Instead, they concluded on experimental evidence that, since sound production is always accompanied by vibratory motions of both labia, the vibrations of the labia had to be the actual sound source. The onset and termination of vocalization (called phonation) is usually controlled by the syringeal muscles that open or close the lumen on each side of the syrinx. The elasticity and complexity of the membranes may determine the quality of sounds. The air pressure, the muscles and the internal membranes can interact to produce near pure tones (single frequency and similar to human whistles).

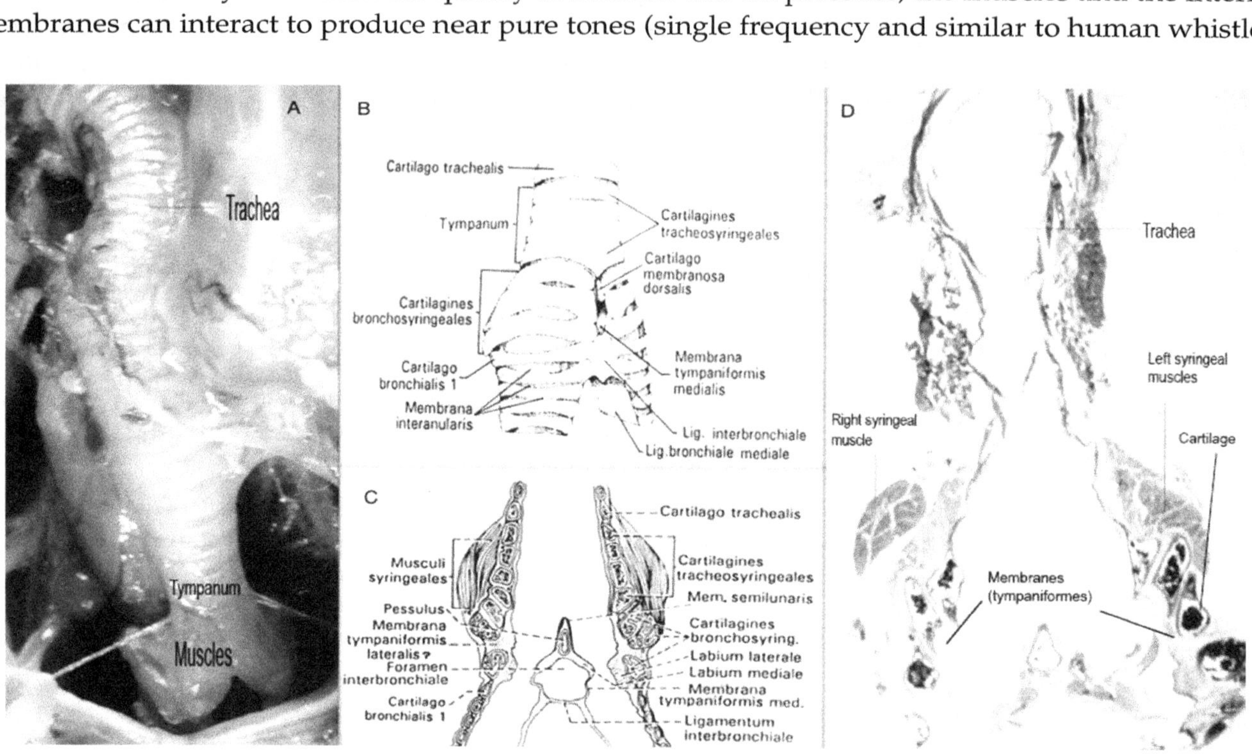

Figure 3. Syrinx anatomy. The syrinx of *Gymnorhina tibicen* (**A**,**D**). (**A**) The first panel shows the exposed syrinx deep in the chest of the Australian magpie (requiring sectioning the sternum), autopsied and photographed by the author. The two lips (musculature) at the bottom of the image are at the point of dividing into the two bronchial branches. The syrinx is connected to the trachea and the bronchial tubes below, but at the most vibratory section, just above the thick muscle belt, there are sinews and ligaments. (**B**) shows the syringeal cartilage, dorsal view (as (**A**), of the European black-billed magpie, *Pica pica*, a relative in name only of the Australian magpie, which was named after the European magpie. However, both are songbirds and of about equal size. In *Pica pica*, the four tracheosyringeal cartilages are fused to form the tympanum. The photograph of the Australian magpie syrinx in (**A**) shows the trachea, the tympanum and the tracheosyringeal cartilage. Where the cartilage splits into its bronchosyringeal arms, this is covered in the photograph by a layer of muscle flaps (inversely heart-shaped). (**C**) presents a diagram of a syrinx (horizontal plane) of a male European blackbird, *Turdus merula*, one of the most common European songbirds, diverse and musical in its song. (**D**) is a histologically-prepared horizontal cross-section of a syrinx of an adult male Australian magpie prepared by the author. Note the similarities of details of (**C**) with (**D**). The syrinx of the blackbird and the Australian magpie is arranged very similarly, particularly in the medial and lateral labia, the lateral and the medial tympaniform membranes and the asymmetrical arrangement of the syringeal muscles [75,108,109].

The production of sounds depends on a number of additional physiological features, called the peripheral auditory system. The length of the trachea is important since formant frequencies are inversely proportional to the length of the vocal tract; i.e., if this were halved, the formant frequencies would be doubled [110]. Nowicki's paper of 1987 [111] showed that not just the syrinx, but the vocal tract contributed to the sound quality, at least in filtering sound [112], although, as a singular tube, it would not contribute to our understanding of lateralization, but can explain certain auditory characteristics [113,114]. Indeed, Hoese and colleagues [101] provided evidence experimentally of an important coordination between beak and sound output (Figure 4), showing that restricting beak movement or closed beak vocalizations [115] changed the tonal quality of song and caused frequency-dependent changes in amplitude that may alter the message and, thus, require some instructional cues from the forebrain, and these may indeed be lateralized.

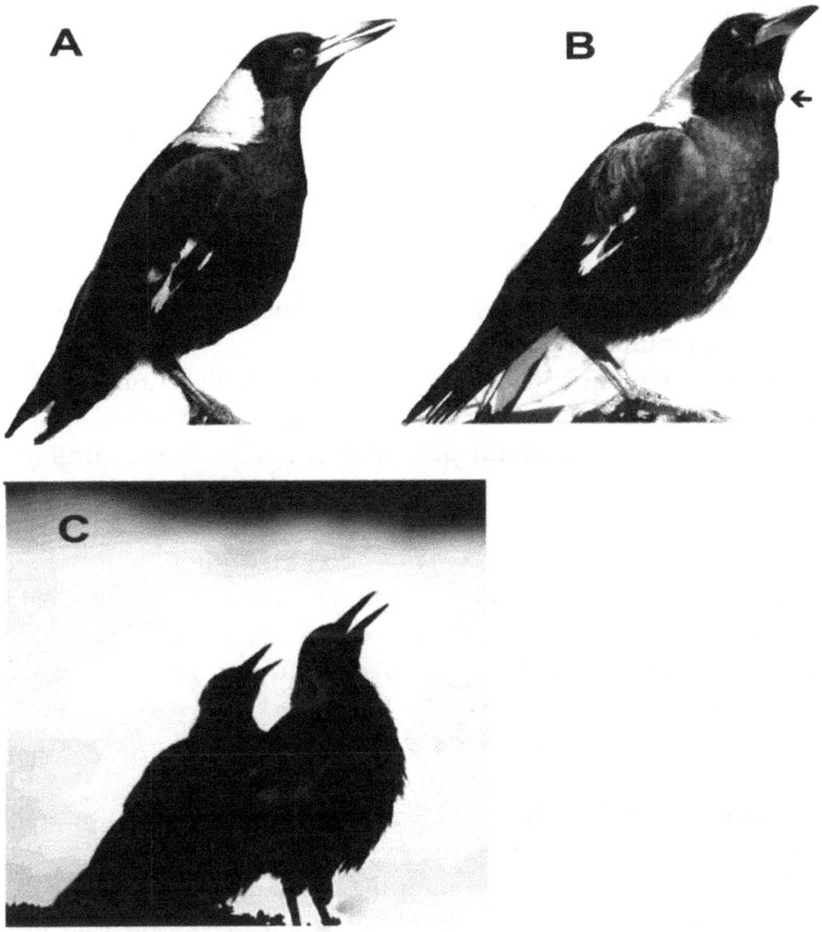

Figure 4. Body postures for specific phonations/song types in Australian magpies. The bird (**A**) is producing a low-level alarm call; posture erect and vigilant, and head raised slightly, beak open. (**B**) The same bird quietly singing. Note the bird is erect, but relaxed, and the beak is closed. The arrow points to the laryngeal area, and movement of feathers is clearly visible while the bird sings. (**C**) A pair carolling (i.e., using the territorial call). The birds arch their backs, extend their necks and throw their heads back, opening the beak widely to produce this loud and specialized call; chest and belly feathers tend to be ruffled as if major muscle groups are also involved in sustaining the call. Body posture and beak movement thus substantially differ from postures adopted in alarm calls or song.

3.3. Sound Production in the Magpie

Having identified the anatomy of the magpie's syrinx, our laboratory then proceeded to test phonation in wild magpies [116]. As in other songbirds, magpies have a tracheobronchial syrinx in which the cranial end of each primary bronchus contains a pair of vibratory structures, the medial and lateral labia, which vibrate in response to aerodynamic forces and produce sound when adducted into the expiratory airstream of the bronchial lumen (Figure 3 above). The muscles on each side of the syrinx are innervated by the ipsilateral tracheosyringeal branch of the hypoglossal nerve so that each side of the syrinx is under independent motor control by ipsilateral motor neurons that are in turn controlled by the central song system predominantly on the same side [116].

Lateralization of song production at the level of the syrinx (i.e., the contribution of the left and the right side of the syrinx) is relatively easy to ascertain either by syringeal nerve section or by measuring airflow on the left and right sides. If there is no airflow through one side of the syrinx, this indicates that the labial valve on the ipsilateral side of the syrinx is closed and silent. Vocalizations must therefore be generated by airflow through the contralateral side of the syrinx, and this was true of some magpie vocalizations, as described below [116].

We discovered during our investigation (see the details of the method in [116]) that in magpies, the left and right sides of the syrinx can simultaneously generate different, harmonically unrelated frequencies during some of these bilaterally-produced vocalizations. At first glance, this result fit into the 'two-voice' theory. However, in magpies, it was not a matter of syllables being produced on one side and some others on the other, but the distribution of activation was according to the frequency of sound. The higher frequency was consistently produced on the left side. The left/right distribution of frequencies explains why magpies can drop three or even four octaves of sound from one note to the next. Moreover, this lateralization of frequency range is in the opposite direction from other songbirds with very complex song or large repertoires studied previously, in which the right side of the syrinx produces the highest fundamental [116].

Another finding was that magpies sometimes sang syllables unilaterally while maintaining bilateral airflow through the syrinx. This motor pattern is rare in other songbirds so far studied, which nearly always silence the contralateral side of their syrinx during unilateral phonation [117]. The results also showed a number of nonlinear phenomena (such as biphonation, deterministic chaos, etc.) in which the two acoustic sources of the syrinx interact. Nowicki and Capranica [118] had found these in the black-capped chickadees, *Parus atricapillus*, and identified them as heterodyne frequencies (not harmonics), resulting from cross-modulation between the two syringeal sides. In magpies, we found such nonlinear phenomena in begging calls, and here, they were a prominent feature. Still, the workings of the syrinx in its detailed functions suggests that further investigation in species differences of lateralization may be important. Brenowitz [119] argued that revision may even be necessary especially for large songbirds or when songbirds with substantially larger song repertoires are being examined and concern the role hemispheric specialization may play.

Indeed, lateral specialization for different frequency ranges may, in fact, increase the range of frequencies that the bird can sing. There is some evidence of the advantages of lateralized control in so far as the magpies' patterns of syringeal lateralization are more similar to those in the brown thrasher, *Toxostoma rufum*, the grey catbird, *Dumetella carolinensis*, and the northern mockingbird, *Mimus polyglottos*, all of the family Mimidae, than to the motor patterns of other species that have been studied. In the northern mockingbird, two-voiced singing is achieved from a single side of the syrinx unlike the magpie's dual use of different frequency ranges on each side of the syrinx [120]. The comparison with the Mimidae species is useful because they are amongst the most prolific singers and thus invite comparison with the Australian magpie. We know of none of these prolific singers, including our own study, as to whether they are lateralized consistently in one direction or whether lateralization changes over time since the method permits only seven days of testing of awake and relatively confined birds. The thermistors that had been implanted were removed after a week and the birds released [116]. Perhaps even more important is the possibility that, if the syringeal activation is lateralized consistently in the same direction, one might surmise that this could contribute to versatility and complexity in song repertoire.

4. Testing Sound Perception and Laterality in Field and Laboratory Studies

So far, some of the areas of interest in lateralization in song/vocal production have been raised. The last section of this paper will now be devoted to auditory perception in magpies as gleaned from scores in field observations and some specific elements of foraging behaviour, pertinent to lateralization, discussed.

We have a good and representative sample of hearing ranges of non-songbirds, raptors and songbirds [121], and one can infer from the magpie's own vocalizations that their auditory range is likely to fit in well into the average range of hearing in songbirds so far tested (see Figure 5).

It is important to know this hearing range well because without this biological evidence, it would be difficult to argue for auditory perception and lateralization at extreme upper and lower ends of hearing capabilities, unless there is some evidence, as one of the following field observations will show.

Audible sounds perceived by magpies may range from 0.5 kHz to 7 kHz, requiring higher sound pressure levels (SPL) for the very low frequencies (below 1 kHz), as well as for sounds above 5 kHz, at least judging by the range of sounds they can produce. At the low frequency end is a call that magpie females make. It is a particularly low frequency call emitted near or in the nest and typically directed at offspring (see Figure 5C). Its function seems to be both affiliative, as well as mildly punitive. The latter has been recorded in contexts when the offspring were still begging for food in the nest after the mother had fed them; a reassuring 'growl' (sometimes referred to as purrs) immediately stopped all begging (personal observation).

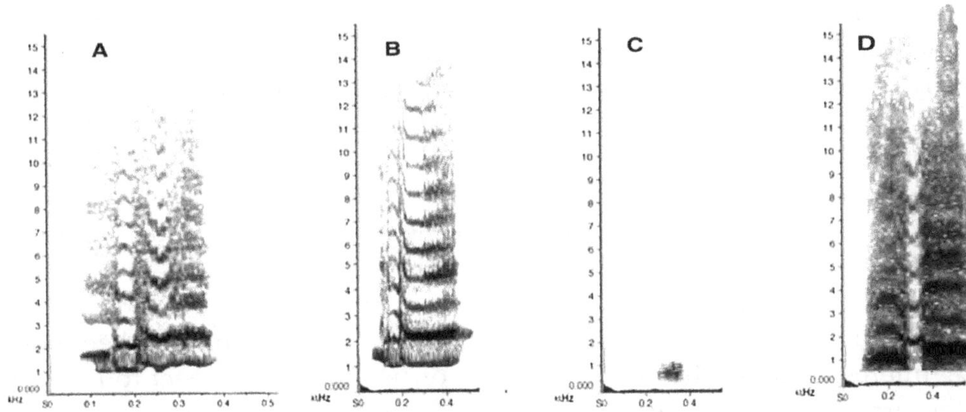

Figure 5. Magpie range of vocalizations. The figure shows the wide range of frequencies produced in magpie vocalizations, not included here is an actual song/warble sequence typically in the range of 1.5–2.2 kHz. y axis: frequencies in kilohertz (kHz); x axis: time in seconds. (**A**) is a complex single alarm call (type that is often a precursor to the eagle alarm call); (**B**) a sharp high amplitude alarm call; (**C**) a 'purr', discussed below; (**D**) is a mobbing call, containing a good deal of noise (grey); note that the mobbing call, stretched here for better visibility, has a characteristic midsection, which clearly distinguishes this category of call from alarm calls; that midsection being of less than 1 ms can at best be identified by a human ear as a faint 'click' sound, but with better temporal resolution of hearing in birds, it is likely to be unmistakable for conspecifics. Note that (**A**,**B**,**D**) are very high amplitude sounds, and (**A**,**B**) have frequency ranges (audible harmonics with considerable energy, darker horizontal lines/regular intervals) from 2 to 6 kHz and in some special calls, as (**B**), even maintaining some energy at 7–8 kHz. (**C**) By contrast, a very low amplitude 'purr' vocalization, is even lower (400–500 Hz) than the fundamentals of alarm calls and below the magpie's typical song and is usually delivered at 35–40 dB. Every example presents just one sound, but the darker harmonics indicate that the call has some energy at that frequency level, well above the first formant (**A**) at 6 kHz; (**B**,**D**) at approximately 5–6 kHz), and accordingly, one may assume that magpies can also hear most of the sounds they produce, even if the very upper limit harmonics (at 7 kHz and beyond) may become inaudible to magpies).

Anatomical differences between mammalian and avian audition have often been called upon to possibly explain differences in perception. Cohen [122] suggested that the hearing threshold of humans is generally about 18 dB lower than that of passerines, and the lesser hearing capacity in songbirds has been attributed to some main factors, although they have been questioned. King and McLelland [103] had shown that the basilar membrane of the cochlea of birds is restricted in size by head size. In pigeons, for example, this membrane is a mere 3 mm long, less than a tenth of that in the human ear. However, while this membrane carries the neuro-epithelial receptor cells, cells are far more densely packed in avian than in human ears, and so, King and McLelland [103] point out that the 'crista basilaris', in its cross-section, has about ten-times more receptor cells than the mammalian organ of Corti. A counter-argument made by Henry and Lucas [123] is that the avian middle ear has just a single ossicle, the columella, that transfers acoustic energy to the cochlea, while mammals possess three middle ear ossicles, and these ossicles improve high-frequency efficiency. Several studies of columellar middle ear systems indicate that efficiency is greatest from 2 to 3 kHz and declines sharply above 3–4 kHz (reviewed in [124]).

However, there is apparently another level at which avian audition is different and, in this case, arguably better than the human ear, and this is in the temporal resolution of sounds, which, according to King and McLelland [103], was alleged to be 10-times faster in songbirds than in human ears, but if true, would provide a substantial auditory advantage and possible specialized ability to focus on specific sounds. By 2002, a study by Dooling and colleagues [125] tackled this question of temporal resolution. They found that birds were capable of discriminations between two sounds that differed in fine structure over time intervals as small as 1 ms, much faster than any estimate of the monaural temporal resolution capacity of humans. The researchers were thus able to demonstrate that the temporal resolution in the processing of acoustic communication signals in birds was well beyond the limits typically reported for humans; with the correction of King and McLelland's [103] claims, however, that a bird's discrimination of the temporal fine structure of complex sounds is two- to three-times, not ten-times, better than the limits shown for humans [125]. Henry and Lucas [123] speculated that taxa with lower temporal resolution may compensate for this with greater frequency resolution. They base this on theoretical models of cochlear tuning that predicts a trade-off between temporal resolution and frequency resolution [126].

Whether or not any of these very specific aspects of audition in birds are lateralized remains largely unchartered territory. Studies in temporal resolution have been undertaken mostly on aquatic mammals [127]. Interest had also been particularly consistent with respect to localizing sound by establishing interaural time differences (ITDs) and interaural level differences (ILDs). The puzzle is how birds with small heads can identify the direction of sounds [128–130]. A more recent study suggests that budgerigars may be able to localize pure tones as high as 4 kHz based solely on ITD information and that small birds generally may be able to enhance directional hearing by using the acoustic coupling of the middle ear cavities and so perform well above expectations [131]. In larger birds, one suspects that head turning, studied in the context of visual perception, may be useful to identify sounds, and these could reveal side biases.

Indeed, several such studies of auditory laterality have been undertaken by placing the sound sources behind the test birds, some purely for establishing threshold levels [122]. The playback method, placing specific auditory stimuli to the side or behind an animal, is a technique that is usually used in larger animals as, for instance, a study on dogs that tested hemispheric specializations for processing auditory stimuli [132]. Dogs turned their head to the right side (left hemisphere) in response to conspecific vocalizations, but to the left side (right hemisphere) in response to the sound of a thunderstorm. In birds, because of their small heads, it usually becomes a little more difficult although not insurmountable to test auditory responses. One study, for instance, tested experienced and young, inexperienced harpy eagles and exposed them to sounds of pure tones, of a bird (tinamous) and of a potential prey item (howler monkey calls) and of a conspecific from a speaker placed behind the bird. Both young and adult harpy eagles turned their head to the left when exposed to irrelevant sounds, such as pure tones or peeps of the tinamous, and both turned right on hearing the calls of another harpy eagle. On hearing the calls of the howler monkey, however, the captive young harpy eagle without hunting experience oriented to the left, whereas the eagle experienced in hunting oriented significantly to the right, clearly an example of purely auditory orienting asymmetry [133]. This suggests that socially-relevant information and potential food items are identified by sound alone and processed by the left hemisphere.

In humans, a behavioral method used to establish hemispheric dominance in auditory perception is dichotic listening in which subjects have earphones in both ears and similar sounding consonants (such as Da/Ta) are delivered to each ear separately and simultaneously, and the subjects then tell the experimenter which consonant/syllable they mostly heard. Research in those cases have shown a clear right ear/left hemisphere dominance [134,135].

The same method (in principle) has been successfully employed in studying the ability of budgerigars to identify cues of interaural time differences (ITDs) and interaural level differences (ILDs) by implanting headphones [131], a technique also used to test left-right identification of sounds [136]. Interestingly, in humans, ITD performance drops off markedly for frequencies above 1.5 kHz, but budgerigars maintained sensitivity up to 4 kHz. The method could be used to also establish ear preference. Possible methods of auditory lateralization testing for lateralized brain functions have recently (2017) been discussed by Rogers and invite further study [137].

5. Field Studies Concerning Audition in Australian Magpies

5.1. Introduction

Very few field studies have shown lateralization of auditory processing in birds. There has been one study that meticulously established that some prey search by magpies is based purely on audition. Floyd and Woodland [138] hypothesized that magpies can forage for scarab larvae purely by listening to the chewing sounds they make in the soil. These sounds are so faint that the experimenters were unable to hear what the magpies heard under the same field conditions.

Magpies feed regularly on scarab larvae, and they are a prized food owing to their size (2–3 cm) and the high protein content and fluids they provide. Some studies confirmed that, in some cases, grubs retrieved from below the surface could be found by visual means. In heavily infested areas in England, rooks, *Corvus frugilegus*, and starlings, *Sturnus vulgaris*, feeding on scarab larvae, *Phyllopertha horticola*, were able to do so because of visual cues, for instance when turf had died off, i.e., had changed colour, or the soil surface was loose and could be lifted and pulled aside [139]. The American robin, *Turdus migratorius*, was also shown to use visual surface cues (worm casts) for locating earthworms [140]. Similarly, it was known that in Australia the currawong, *Strepera graculina*, closely related to the Australian magpie, both belonging to the family of Artamidae, used a similar visual guidance system in years of severe infestation of scarab beetles of the species *Seriesthis pruinosa* [141].

However, not all scarab larva species leave identifying marks on the surface. Floyd and Woodland [136] wanted to know how magpies could find larvae that leave no visual cues. First, they established that there were no visual or other cues by which the magpies could identify where the larvae were, and they then conducted a series of auditory tests, finally pre-recording the chewing sounds the larvae made while feeding underground and playing back these sounds to magpies through micro-speakers. Under well-controlled experimental conditions, they could then test whether the magpies found the sound source. They did.

The speakers they used for playback in the field had a frequency response of 50–12,000 Hz [138]. Most of the sounds played backed to the magpies were at frequencies between 50 and 800 Hz, but there was a small high frequency component in the 1700–3000-Hz range. The scarabs produced sounds at an intensity of 30–38 dB. As tape hiss intensity was 30 dB, the subjects were offered a choice of playback of scarab noises or tape hiss alone (at 30 dB); the former resulted in immediate and successful responses; the latter did not elicit responses. Playback intensities were measured at 2 cm above ground level [138].

5.2. Foraging for Scarab Beetles by Magpies Is Lateralized

My own field observations on foraging behaviour in magpies (specifically for scarab larvae) are based on recordings made over a three-year period using several of our well-established research field sites on the Northern Tableland, near the city of Armidale, New South Wales (30°32′ S, 148°29′ E). All sites were permanent magpie territories of 3–7 residents, consisting of one breeding pair, juveniles and also some young adults (daughters from the previous year). Each territory was at least 2.5 hectares in size, flat grassland dotted with the occasional mature gum trees, some pine trees and shrubs, an environment in which scarab larvae flourish. Two of the territories were adjacent to each other while the visits to two others were separated from each other by at least 2 km and 5 km, respectively.

On this Northern Tableland, largely sheep-grazing country, at altitudes of about 1000 m, three species of scarab beetles were strongly represented [142]. The larvae may pupate and emerge as beetles any time between November and March, i.e., larvae reach their full size at exactly the time when magpie offspring fledge (around September, sometimes earlier-depending on weather conditions) and make the greatest protein and food demands on the parent birds.

Magpies feed exclusively on the ground, and they walk, putting one foot before another, while foraging, sometimes referred to as 'walk-foraging' [143]. Their ground feeding habits make them easy to watch and follow their foraging in open fields especially. Moreover, magpies forage very systematically and according to a time-plan. They will reliably be at one specific transect of their territory at a certain time of day and will generally walk diagonally and in half a meter to meter distance from one another (Figure 6). No matter how large the territory, once their habits and time frame were known, observations could be made at set times in the morning and in the afternoon (changing the hour of day weekly to cover the times of their most vigorous foraging in the morning and the later afternoon).

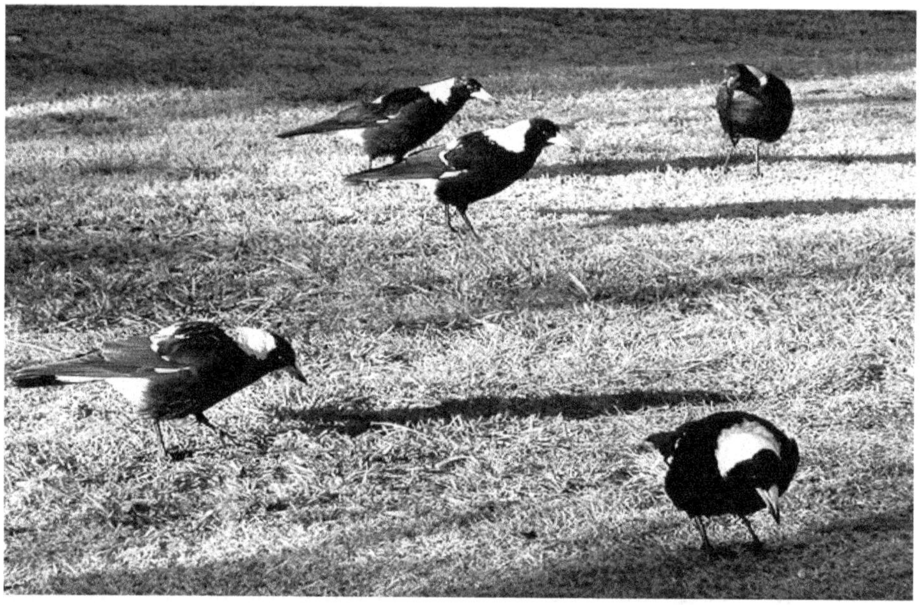

Figure 6. Directionality and spacing in magpie foraging. Magpies tend to walk slowly and steadily in a direct line and in parallel to each other, taking transect after transect in a methodical way.

Each territory was visited daily for five days a week between September and March for three consecutive seasons, and all observable incidents of extractive foraging were recorded. Individual magpies could not be identified.

In the first weeks of watching foraging behavior closely, it became clear that the steps in all successful extractive foraging events were the same; the foraging bird was: (1) scanning the ground walking slowly; (2) then stopping and seemingly looking closely at the ground binocularly; (3) holding absolutely still; (4) in the last moment, turning the head so that the left side of the head/ear was close to the ground; (5) straightening up, the bird then executed a powerful jab into the ground; (6) then retrieving a large scarab larva from the grassy surface; and (7) expertly removing the hard head and the biting mandibles before swallowing it or feeding it to an offspring. Steps 3–7 typically lasted less than 30 s.

5.3. Results: Extractive Foraging

The sheer consistency of the foraging sequence and the changed posture of the bird observed made it possible to recognize the special extractive foraging strategy and made it clear, especially in some years with greater abundance of scarab larvae, that this was not an unusual and rare event, but a seasonal and integral part of the foraging behaviour of the territorial magpies, at least in a region where scarab larvae were often abundant.

A total number of observations accounted for 446 attempts at extractive foraging, but only 135 observations were ultimately included. One reason for the exclusion of a substantial number of seemingly successful extractions was the consequence of the behaviour of juveniles. Young juveniles (a month old or less post fledging) walked with the parent bird, but had the tendency to intervene in the process of foraging, by posting themselves in front of the adult to block the path, just so as to ensure that the morsel was fed to them as shown in Figure 7.

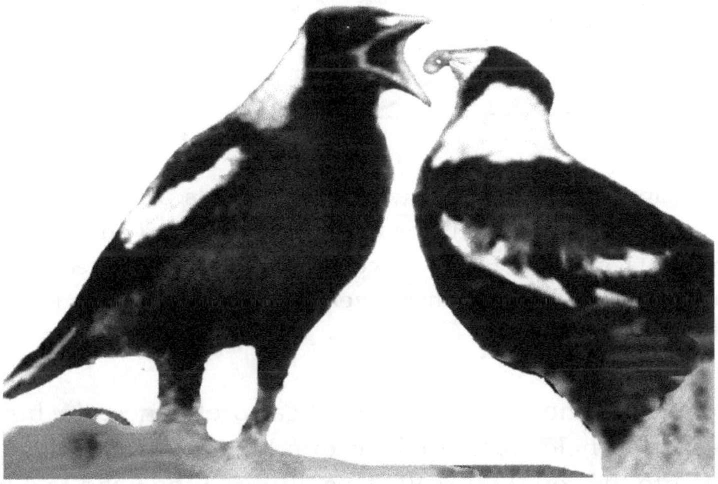

Figure 7. Parent feeding scarab larvae to magpie juvenile. Female magpie feeding a larva to a young fledgling. Such an example was not included in the analysis, and this method of feeding, the juvenile right in front of the parent bird, was limited in time and dependent on the juvenile's development. Blocking the path of the female walking was observed only in juveniles one month post-fledging. By two months post-fledging, most juveniles walked next to the adult (usually on the right side) and actively started observing the processes of the adult's food acquisition.

The most common reason for exclusion, however, concerned problems for the observer regarding distance or terrain. The most obvious problem occurred when the magpies foraged with their backs turned towards the observer and often at some distance, and in such cases, it made it difficult to be certain of the direction of head movements prior to extraction. Hence, such sequences were excluded even when the actual retrieval of larvae was seen.

The instances included were based on the foraging data obtained from four different territories. In an area of over 18 hectares traversed daily, the total number of resident magpies observed seems small ($N = 16$), and hence, it is very possible that, in some cases, the same magpies were scored repeatedly if they happened to be the successful ones in extracting the larvae, and this may partially account for the consistency of the findings. Relatedness is unlikely to be an issue in these results since juveniles forced out by the parents tend to roam in bachelor groups for at least four years and feed in non-dedicated, usually inferior, sites before some of them succeed in finding a suitable territory and a partner. There is no evidence that a daughter or son might secure a neighbouring territory.

Equally, the number of juveniles observed, at least in the first month of the season (September), typically made no contribution to extractive foraging, but were keen consumers: they often did not commence making successful extractions of larvae on their own until nearly the middle of the observation period. Hence, although some magpies may have contributed several scores of extractions of larvae over the observation period of three months, this does not invalidate the observations because each event was a new event and an individual magpie could have approached the excavation site differently on each occasion.

Most incidents of successful extractive foraging were observed in October and November, the observed incidents sharply declining after mid-December when the ground became very dry and compacted and most scarab beetles might have emerged (see Figure 8).

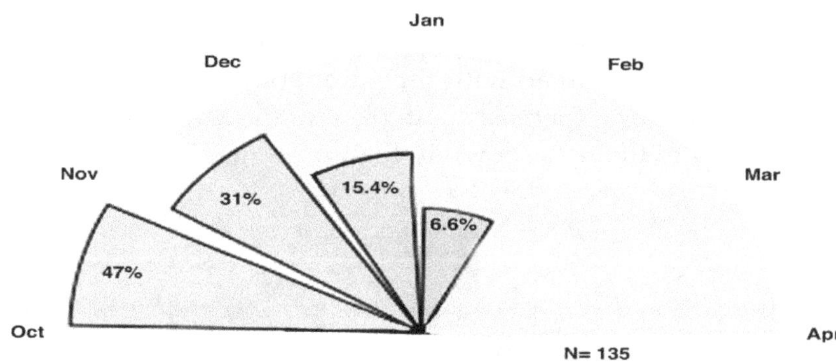

Figure 8. Walk-foraging and successful extractive foraging events. The majority of scarab larvae were retrieved in October, decreasing substantially by December and found only scarcely thereafter and not at all by February (percentage figures refer to successful retrievals counted). The large light-shaded semi-circle shows the months and hours when juveniles started searching for scarab larvae on their own, mostly with relatively little success.

All 135 recorded sequences showed the same left ear preference: the bird being observed tilted the head so that the left ear was held closer to the ground before straightening up and delivering the successful jab of its beak into the soil (Figure 9). This tilting of the head to a left position was clearly visible in each of the incidents. One would expect to find that not all scores of extractive foraging used the left ear (i.e., at least some magpies might have tilted the head in the other direction), but this was not so. Even though some of the scores were likely repeats for the same individual, the total absence of right ear use means that the bias is significant at the population level.

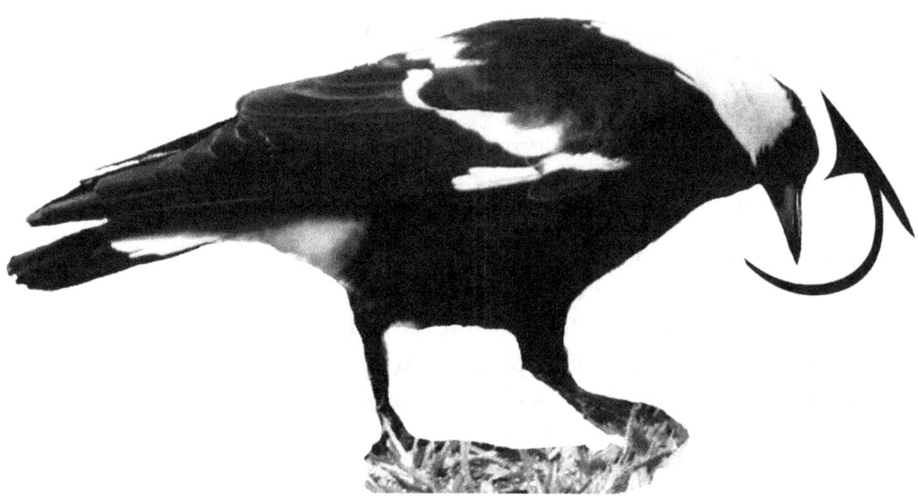

Figure 9. Lateralized auditory detection of prey item. The image of the magpie shows Step 4 in the extractive foraging sequence, moving the head from a 90° angle, binocular viewing, to a 45° angle, moving the beak to the right and up so that the left ear is closer to the ground.

5.4. Discussion

To my knowledge, this is the first example of auditory lateralization in the field describing an extractive foraging event that has not been described in any avian species. It is also the first example of auditory behavioural asymmetry under natural conditions.

The point made here is that the foraging strategy was not based on visual scanning, but crucially on auditory examination of a potential prey item and that it was consistently performed by the left ear. In the image shown above (Figure 9), the bird is walking leftwards, and the right ear would have been nearer for auditory inspection than the left, but the bird turned the head right around in order to listen to the underground larva with its left ear. In all cases included in the sample, the birds turned to position their left ear close to the ground.

It seems highly unlikely that this head tilt related to improving visual scanning. The visual field of magpies in the binocular field at close range is about 28–34° [4], and any fixation of a potential prey item is therefore most accurate when the beak points at about 90° to the ground (for binocular viewing). Since scarab larvae create no visual surface cues, as Floyd and Woodland (1981) had so convincingly shown [138], the only way magpies are able to identify the location of the underground prey item is by auditory means. Hence, regarding the head tilt prior to grasping the grub, we are left with only one explanation, namely that the bird obtained confirmation of the presence of a scarab larva exclusively by aural means.

In retrospect, watching magpie groups combing through their territories in such an orderly fashion (Figure 6 above) and doing so grid-by-grid every day may well be a result of having acquired the skill of extractive foraging. Clearly, the sounds that larvae make are so faint that they would be easily missed unless a group spaces out in such a way that every part of the ground can actually be scanned by listening to sounds at very close proximity.

5.5. Additional Field Results in Magpie Foraging

The results of foraging raise the question why this auditory behaviour is left-biased (right hemisphere) and significant at the population level and how this may fit the results in other and related studies we had conducted.

The extractive foraging results of lateralized listening follow from the results obtained on lateralized foraging behaviour in magpies in a series of additional field studies conducted by members of our laboratory [4,144]. One tested head turning during foraging (visual scanning); another scored eye preferences for tracking moving prey (for both, see [4], called Study 2 in the summarizing table below); and a third scored the side of begging behaviour of juveniles walk-foraging with a parent bird [144] (see the results summarized in Table 1 below).

Head turning during visual foraging (pecking food from the ground) was found to favour the right eye/left hemisphere. There was a slight, but significant bias at the population level for the bird to turn its head so that the right eye monocular field was directed towards the ground.

In a third study (eye preference for moving prey [4]), we supplied the magpies with food by purposely throwing mince-meat pieces in their direction and then scoring which eye they last used before taking and consuming it. Of 155 scores, 97 percent were left-eye dominant, meaning they involved left-eye viewing the moving target before food retrieval.

Later that year (also published in [4]), we had the opportunity to observe magpies dealing with moving prey items and watching the magpies trying to capture them. There was a locust plague, and locust were either jumping or flying up from the grass. Under natural conditions, we received the same results as in the food-supplementation experiment, finding a strong left-eye/right hemisphere preference. The results are consistent with use of the right hemisphere processing spatial information as known from studies in chicks [145].

In another field study (called Study 4 here; see also Table below [144]), it was recorded on which side juveniles approached the parent birds and begged for food while walk-foraging, and a significant group-level bias for begging on the right side of the parent was found. Juveniles were 2.46-times more likely to beg on the right side than on the left [144]. By begging on the right side of a parent, a juvenile uses its left eye to view the adult and is in the parent's right visual field. Hoffman et al. [144] pointed out that visual inputs from the right visual field are processed by the left hemisphere, which is known to inhibit conspecific aggression, as found in chickens [146]. By approaching in the right hemifield, a juvenile magpie may also avoid being scolded by the parent bird [144]. Alternatively, and more likely, as a recent comparison across species indicates [147], the infant is positioning itself so that it can monitor the parent's behavior using its left visual field and right hemisphere, specialized for processing social behaviour.

Table 1. Hemispheric specializations in five field studies on foraging and vigilance in magpies.

Study	No. (Subjects)	No. Scores (Behavioral) Total/Bracket: Majority of Responses	Left Eye or Ear/Right Hemisphere	Right Eye or Ear/Left Hemisphere	Authors
(1) Extractive foraging	16	135 (135)	Left ear dominant		Kaplan, this paper,
(2) Head-turning during foraging	20	266 (116)		Right eye dominant	Rogers and Kaplan 2006 [4]
(3) Tracking moving prey	12	159 (155)	Left eye dominant		Rogers and Kaplan 2006 [4]
(4) Begging position of juveniles during foraging	6 parent-juvenile pairs	16/64 scores	Left eye dominant (begging juveniles)	Right eye dominant (feeding adult)	Hoffman et al. and Rogers 2006 [144]
(5) Inspecting predator	55	270 (compound score/various behaviors)	Left eye dominant		Koboroff, Kaplan and Rogers 2008 [148]

Brackets give the number of subjects/behavior showing eye/ear bias.

A fifth field study, not on foraging, but on eye preference in magpies when viewing a predator, scored eye use when presented with taxidermic models of a potential predator, a lace monitor [148]. We established by scoring monocular fixations from video footage that magpies used their left eye in the majority of instances while inspecting the potential predator, such as jumping (73%), prior to circling (65%), as well as during circling (58%) and for high alert inspection of the predator (72%), and we concluded that mobbing and perhaps circling are likely agonistic responses controlled by the left eye/right hemisphere [148].

The results of the second field study are consistent with preferred use of the left hemisphere and right eye in control of feeding responses as has also been shown in other species, including the zebra finch [149]. In the third field study, magpies show a left eye/right hemisphere preference reflecting a specialization for spatial information using global cues and also for rapid responding. It is thus noteworthy that of the three foraging tasks, two were controlled by the right hemisphere or expressed differently; it would be odd if two foraging tasks, looking for prey on the ground and listening for prey under the ground, were managed by different hemispheres. One is consistent with feeding responses generally, while the other method (extractive foraging using the left ear) is based on spatial information and auditory cues. Hence, these two foraging methods do not only require different strategies, but are also under the control of different hemispheres. While three of the findings for four field studies relate to visual lateralization in magpies (see Table 1), there may also be an auditory element to them.

My field study of foraging for scarab larvae showed a very strong bias towards the left ear to pinpoint the larvae's presence under the ground, leaving the right ear free to respond to the begging or other calls of an offspring. This may allow the magpie to attend to two tasks at once. Rogers et al. [148] showed in chicks that the performance of two tasks simultaneously, such as foraging and attending to a predator overhead, is undertaken effectively in strongly-lateralized chicks in which visual search is processed by the left hemisphere and predator detection by the right hemisphere [150].

Furthermore, agonistic responses are processed by the right hemisphere, consistent with research results in chicks [146] and other species [151]. Chicks also use the left eye to examine novel objects and the details of a stimulus detecting small changes in familiar stimuli, whereas the right eye detects large changes that represent categories rather than details [152]. It is conceivable and even probable that the same hemispheric specializations that apply to eye use apply also to ear use.

6. Conclusions

This paper has presented evidence of lateralized behaviour in phonation and listening in one songbird species. Motor output and the way magpies produce song were shown to involve an entire range of techniques that enable an individual magpie not only to maintain singing for hours, but allow for a range of extraordinary modulations at a wide range of frequencies by using unusual techniques of lateralized frequency use (higher on left, lower on right side of syrinx). Paradoxically, so far, specific functions for their varied song have not been discovered. It is clear that their song can identify individuals one from another [75], but such individual recognition is conceivably achieved by just listening to their territorial call, referred to as carolling. There appears to be no territorial advantage for having a larger or smaller repertoire. It is possible, given that magpies form auditory maps of other species in their territory (they mimic only heterospecific sounds pertaining to their territory [74,76]), that the auditory memory, in this case of heterospecific sounds, is lateralized on the left side, as in other songbirds, but this has not been studied. It is also possible that such auditory 'maps' may be linked to other brain regions.

The substantial and innovative neuroscientific research in avian vocal production and vocal perception over the last decades notwithstanding, it pertains largely to a few small songbird species. Ocklenburg and Güntürkün in their paper [153] published a telling 'cladogram' showing that we have no information at all on lateralization in vocal production (central and peripheral) and vocal perception on any of the 28 clades of extant non-songbirds. Although Passeriformes are just one clade in this cladogram [153], Passeriformes, i.e., the true songbirds, actually make up the majority of all extant birds (over 5000 species). Additionally, while we know plenty about the zebra finch and a few other songbird species in this regard, there is little to no information available on almost all other extant songbirds either. It would help to understand whether large repertoires and flexible/plastic brains have developed other or additional neural mechanisms for song production and perception and whether this is achieved via specific hemispheric specializations. The magpie is certainly a representative of this kind of songbird. With an evolutionary history of likely more than 20 million years and in an evolutionary context of substantial speciation pre- and post the mass extinction of 65 mya, the emergence of a major songbird at that time may be as fascinating genetically as it is in its current performance.

Here, results of several field studies were presented. The results of lateralization in the field have been telling us that there are behaviours that are clearly highly lateralized in magpies. Extractive foraging has a particular place in ethological-cognitive research and, in primates, has been identified as one of the very complex cognitive behaviours and, when reported, relies usually on vision or on experience, but not purely on audition (the very specialized adaptations of the aye-aye being one of the few known exceptions).

This is the first paper that reports this auditory behaviour in a songbird and, furthermore, shows that the success of it may depend on a highly lateralized neuronal aspect in the auditory system. The results of the other field studies on foraging behaviour make a powerful point that the bird has to handle very different experiences and tackle potential dangers while foraging or encountering predators. Here, it has been shown that these key functions are lateralized, which may have substantial advantages for survival.

Acknowledgments: The research on magpies was largely funded by the Australian Research Council and also by an annual personal bequest to Kaplan (The Cardigan Fund) made to our Research Centre of Neuroscience and Animal Behaviour and these funding sources are gratefully acknowledged.

Author Contributions: This is the original contribution by the author and any reference to previously published materials, be this by the author or other researchers, is fully acknowledged.

References

1. Franklin, W.E.; Lima, S.L. Laterality in avian vigilance: Do sparrows have a favourite eye? *Anim. Behav.* **2001**, *62*, 879–885. [CrossRef]
2. Koboroff, A.; Kaplan, G.; Rogers, L.J. Clever strategists: Australian Magpies vary mobbing strategies, not intensity, relative to different species of predator. *PeerJ* **2013**, *56*, 1–14. [CrossRef] [PubMed]
3. Ventolini, N.; Ferrero, E.A.; Sponza, S.; Chiesa, A.D.; Zucca, P.; Vallortigara, G. Laterality in the wild: P, hemifield use during predatory and sexual behaviour in the black-winged stilt. *Anim. Behav.* **2005**, *69*, 1077–1084. [CrossRef]
4. Rogers, L.J.; Kaplan, G. An eye for a predator: Lateralisation on birds, with particular reference to the Australian magpie. In *Behavioral and Morphological Asymmetries in Vertebrates*; Malashichev, Y., Deckel, W., Eds.; Landes Bioscience: Georgetown, TX, USA, 2006; pp. 47–57.
5. Hunt, G.R. Manufacture and use of hook-tools by New Caledonian crows. *Nature* **1996**, *379*, 249–251. [CrossRef]
6. Hunt, G.R.; Corballis, M.C.; Gray, R.D. Laterality in tool manufacture by crows—Neural processing and not ecological factors may influence 'handedness' in these birds. *Nature* **2001**, *414*, 707. [CrossRef] [PubMed]
7. Rogers, L.J. Lateralisation in the avian brain. *Bird Behav.* **1980**, *2*, 1–12. [CrossRef]
8. Rogers, L.J. Development of functional lateralization in the avian brain. *Brain Res. Bull.* **2007**, *76*, 304–306.
9. Güntürkün, O.; Ocklenburg, S. Ontogenesis of Lateralization. *Neuron* **2017**, *94*, 256–262. [CrossRef] [PubMed]
10. Fisher, H.I. Footedness in domestic pigeons. *Wilson Bull.* **1957**, *69*, 170–177.
11. Davies, M.O.; Green, P.R. Footedness in pigeons, or simply sleight of foot? *Anim. Behav.* **1991**, *42*, 311–312. [CrossRef]
12. McGavin, S.H. Footedness in north island kākā (Nestor meridionalis septentrionalis). *Notornis* **2009**, *56*, 139–143.
13. Noske, R.A. Left-footedness and tool-using in the varied sittella Daphoenositta chrysoptera and crested shrike-tit Falcunculus frantatus. *Corella* **1985**, *9*, 63–64.
14. Izawa, E.I.; Kusayama, T.; Watanabe, S. Foot-use laterality in the Japanese jungle crow (Corvus macrorhynchos). *Behav. Proc.* **2005**, *69*, 357–362. [CrossRef] [PubMed]
15. Harris, L. Footedness in parrots: Three centuries of research, theory, and mere speculation. *Can. J. Physiol.* **1989**, *43*, 369–396.
16. Brown, C.; Margat, M. Cerebral lateralization determines hand preferences in Australian parrots. *Biol. Lett.* **2011**, *7*, 496–498. [CrossRef] [PubMed]
17. Randler, C.; Braun, M.; Lintker, S. Foot preferences in wild-living ring-necked parakeets (Psittacula krameri, Psittacidae). *Laterality* **2011**, *16*, 201–206. [CrossRef] [PubMed]
18. Rogers, L.J.; Vallortigara, G.; Andrew, R.J. *Divided Brains: The Biology and Behaviour of Brain Asymmetries*; Cambridge University Press: Cambridge, UK, 2013; ISBN 978-1-107-00535-8.
19. Eales, L.A. The influences of visual and vocal interactions on song learning in zebra finches. *Anim. Behav.* **1989**, *37*, 507–508. [CrossRef]
20. West, M.J.; King, A.P. Female visual displays affect the development of male song in the cowbird. *Nature* **1988**, *334*, 244–246. [CrossRef] [PubMed]
21. Hultsch, H.; Schleuss, F.; Todt, D. Auditory-visual stimulus pairing enhances perceptual learning in a songbird. *Anim. Behav.* **1999**, *58*, 143–150. [CrossRef] [PubMed]
22. Van Kampen, H.S.; Bolhuis, J.J. Auditory learning and filial imprinting in the chick. *Behaviour* **1991**, *117*, 303–319. [CrossRef]
23. Rowe, C.; Guilford, T. Hidden colour aversions in domestic chicks triggered by pyrazine odours of insect warning displays. *Nature* **1996**, *383*, 520–522. [CrossRef]
24. Bischof, H.J.; Engelage, J. Flash evoked responses in a song control nucleus of the zebra finch (Taeniopygia guttata castanotis). *Brain Res.* **1985**, *326*, 370–374. [CrossRef]
25. Nottebohm, F. Asymmetries in neural control of vocalization in the canary. In *Lateralization in the Nervous System*; Harnard, S.R., Ed.; Academic Press: London, UK, 1977; pp. 23–44, ISBN 0-12-325750-6.

26. Wang, C.Z.H.; Herbst, J.A.; Keller, G.B.; Hahnloser, R.H.R. Rapid interhemispheric switching during vocal production in a songbird. *PLoS Biol.* **2008**, *6*, 1–9. [CrossRef] [PubMed]
27. Gobes, S.M.; Bolhuis, J.J. Birdsong memory: A neural dissociation between song recognition and production. *Curr. Biol.* **2007**, *17*, 789–793. [CrossRef] [PubMed]
28. Moorman, S.; Gobes, S.M.H.; van de Kamp, F.C.; Zandbergen, M.A.; Bolhuis, J.J. Learning-related brain hemispheric dominance in sleeping songbirds. *Sci. Rep.* **2015**, *5*, 9041. [CrossRef] [PubMed]
29. Doupe, A.J.; Kuhl, P.K. Birdsong and human speech: Common themes and mechanisms. *Annu. Rev. Neurosci.* **1999**, *22*, 567–631. [CrossRef] [PubMed]
30. Ohms, V.R.; Escudero, P.; Lammers, K.; ten Cate, C. Zebra finches and Dutch adults exhibit the same cue weighting bias in vowel perception. *Anim. Cogn.* **2012**, *15*, 155–161. [CrossRef] [PubMed]
31. Pfenning, A.R.; Hara, E.; Whitney, O.; Rivas, M.V.; Wang, R.; Roulhac, P.L.; Howard, J.T.; Wirthlin, M.; Lovell, P.V.; Ganapathy, G.; et al. Convergent transcriptional specializations in the brains of humans and song-learning birds. *Science* **2014**, *346*, 1256846. [CrossRef] [PubMed]
32. Avey, M.T.; Phillmore, L.S.; MacDougall-Shackleton, S.A. Immediate early gene expression following exposure to acoustic and visual components of courtship in zebra finches. *Behav. Brain Res.* **2005**, *165*, 247–253. [CrossRef] [PubMed]
33. Meyer, C.C.; Boroda, E.; Nick, T.A. Sexually dimorphic perineuronal net expression in the songbird. *Basal Ganglia* **2014**, *3*, 229–237. [CrossRef]
34. Weary, D.; Krebs, J. Birds learn song from aggressive tutors. *Nature* **1987**, *329*, 485. [CrossRef]
35. Zann, R.A. *The Zebra Finch: A Synthesis of Field and Laboratory Studies*; Oxford University Press: Oxford, UK, 1996.
36. Catchpole, C.K.; Slater, P.L.B. *Bird Song: Biological Themes and Variations*; Cambridge University Press: Cambridge, UK, 2008.
37. Burish, M.J.; Kueh, H.Y.; Wang, S.H. Brain architecture and social complexity in modern and ancient birds. *Brain Behav. Evolut.* **2004**, *63*, 107–124. [CrossRef] [PubMed]
38. Odom, K.J.; Hall, M.L.; Riebel, K.; Omland, K.E. Female song is widespread and ancestral in birds. *Nat. Commun.* **2014**, *5*, 3379. [CrossRef] [PubMed]
39. Price, J.J. Rethinking our assumptions about the evolution of bird song and other sexually dimorphic signals. *Front. Ecol. Evolut.* **2015**. [CrossRef]
40. Cain, K.E.; Langmore, N.E. Female and male song rates across breeding stage: Testing for sexual and nonsexual functions of female song. *Anim. Behav.* **2015**, *109*, 65–71. [CrossRef]
41. Lobato, M.; Vellema, M.; Gahr, C.; Gahr, M. Mismatch in sexual dimorphism of developing song and song control system in blue-capped cordon-bleus, a songbird species with singing females. *Front. Ecol. Evolut.* **2015**, *3*, 117. [CrossRef]
42. Eens, M.; Pinxten, R.; Verheyen, R.F. Song learning in captive European starlings, Sturnus vulgaris. *Anim. Behav.* **1992**, *44*, 1131–1143. [CrossRef]
43. Hausberger, M. Social influences on song acquisition and sharing in the European starling (Sturnus vulgaris). In *Social Influences on Vocal Development*; Snowdon, C.T., Hausberger, M., Eds.; Cambridge University Press: Cambridge, UK, 1997; pp. 128–156.
44. Kroodsma, D.E.; Vielliard, J.M.E.; Stiles, F.G. Study of Bird Sounds in the Neotropics: Urgency and Opportunity. In *Ecology and Evolution of Acoustic Communication in Birds*; Kroodsma, D.E., Miller, E.H., Eds.; Cornell University Press Comstock: London, UK, 1996; pp. 269–281.
45. Slater, P.J.B.; Mann, N.I. Why do the females of many bird species sing in the tropics. *J. Avian Biol.* **2004**, *35*, 289–294. [CrossRef]
46. Schwabl, H.; Dowling, J.; Baldassarre, D.T.; Gahr, M.; Lindsay, W.R.; Webster, M.S. Variation in song system anatomy and androgen levels does not correspond to song characteristics in a tropical songbird. *Anim. Behav.* **2015**, *104*, 39–50. [CrossRef]
47. Prather, J.F.; Peters, S.; Nowicki, S.; Mooney, R. Precise auditory–vocal mirroring in neurons for learned vocal communication. *Nature* **2008**, *451*, 305–310. [CrossRef] [PubMed]
48. Tchernichovski, O.; Wallman, J. Neurons of imitation. *Nature* **2008**, *451*, 249–250. [CrossRef] [PubMed]
49. Nottebohm, F. From bird song to neurogenesis. *Sci. Am.* **1989**, *260*, 74–79. [CrossRef] [PubMed]
50. Nottebohm, F.; Nottebohm, M.E. Left hypoglossal dominance in the control of canary and white-crowned sparrow song. *J. Comp. Physiol.* **1976**, *108*, 171–192. [CrossRef]

51. Nottebohm, F.; Alvarez-Buylla, A.; Cynx, J.; Kirn, J.; Ling, C.Y.; Nottebohm, M.; Suter, R.; Tolles, A.; Williams, H. Song learning in birds: The relation between perception and production. *Philos. Trans. R. Soc. B* **1990**, *329*, 115–124. [CrossRef] [PubMed]
52. Bottjer, S.W.; Halsema, K.A.; Brown, S.A.; Miesner, E.A. Axonal connections of a forebrain nucleus involved with vocal learning in zebra finches. *J. Comp. Neurol.* **1989**, *279*, 312–326. [CrossRef] [PubMed]
53. Farries, M.A. The oscine song system considered in the context of the avian brain: Lessons learned from comparative neurobiology. *Brain Behav. Evolut.* **2001**, *58*, 80–100. [CrossRef]
54. Schmidt, M.F.; Wild, J.M. The respiratory-vocal system of songbirds: Anatomy, physiology, and neural control. *Prog. Brain Res.* **2014**, *212*, 297–335. [CrossRef] [PubMed]
55. Striedter, G. The vocal control pathways in budgerigars differ from those in songbirds. *J. Comp. Neurol.* **1994**, *343*, 35–56. [CrossRef] [PubMed]
56. DeVoogd, T.J.; Krebs, J.R.; Healy, S.D.; Purvis, A. Relations between song repertoire size and the volume of brain nuclei related to song—Comparative evolutionary analyses amongst oscine birds. *Proc. R. Soc. Lond. B* **1993**, *254*, 75–82. [CrossRef] [PubMed]
57. Gahr, M.; Sonnenschein, E.; Wickler, W. Sex difference in the size of the neural song control regions in a duetting songbird with similar song repertoire size of males and females. *J. Neurosci.* **1998**, *18*, 1124–1131. [PubMed]
58. Moorman, S.; Gobes, S.M.; Kuijpers, M.; Kerkhofs, A.; Zandbergen, M.A.; Bolhuis, J.J. Human-like brain hemispheric dominance in birdsong learning. *Proc. Nat. Acad. Sci. USA* **2012**, *109*, 12782–12787. [CrossRef] [PubMed]
59. Sanderson, K.; Crouche, H. Vocal Repertoire of the Australian Magpie Gymnorhina tibicen in South Australia. *Aust. Bird Watcher* **1993**, *15*, 162–164.
60. Kaplan, G. The Australian Magpie (Gymnorhina tibicen): An alternative model for the study of songbird neurobiology. In *The Neuroscience of Birdsong*; Zeigler, P., Marler, P., Eds.; Cambridge University Press: Cambridge, UK, 2008; pp. 153–170.
61. Mouterde, S.C.; Elie, J.E.; Mathevon, N.; Theunissen, F.E. Single Neurons in the Avian Auditory Cortex Encode Individual Identity and Propagation Distance in Naturally Degraded Communication Calls. *J. Neurosci.* **2017**, *37*, 3491–3510. [CrossRef] [PubMed]
62. Billimoria, C.P.; Kraus, B.J.; Narayan, R.; Maddox, R.K.; Sen, K. Invariance and sensitivity to intensity in neural discrimination of natural sounds. *J. Neurosci.* **2008**, *28*, 6304–6308. [CrossRef] [PubMed]
63. Chew, S.J.; Vicario, D.S.; Nottebohm, F. A large-capacity memory system that recognizes the calls and songs of individual birds. *Proc. Natl. Acad. Sci. USA* **1996**, *93*, 1950–1955. [CrossRef] [PubMed]
64. Gentner, T.Q.; Margoliash, D. Neuronal populations and single cells representing learned auditory objects. *Nature* **2003**, *424*, 669–674. [CrossRef] [PubMed]
65. Elie, J.E.; Theunissen, F.E. Meaning in the avian auditory cortex: Neural representation of communication calls. *Eur. J. Neurosci.* **2015**, *41*, 546–567. [CrossRef] [PubMed]
66. Gaucher, Q.; Huetz, C.; Gourevitch, B.; Laudanski, J.; Occelli, F.; Edeline, J.M. How do auditory cortex neurons represent communication sounds? *Hear Res.* **2013**, *305*, 102–112. [CrossRef] [PubMed]
67. Menardy, F.; Touiki, K.; Dutrieux, G.; Bozon, B.; Vignal, C.; Mathevon, N.; Del Negro, C. Social experience affects neuronal responses to male calls in adult female zebra finches: Call familiarity affects neuronal responses in NCM. *Eur. J. Neurosci.* **2012**, *35*, 1322–1336. [CrossRef] [PubMed]
68. Woolley, S.M.N.; Gill, P.R.; Fremouw, T.; Theunissen, F.E. Functional Groups in the Avian Auditory System. *J. Neurosci.* **2009**, *29*, 2780–2793. [CrossRef] [PubMed]
69. Poirier, C.; Boumans, T.; Verhoye, M.; Balthazart, J.; Van der Linden, A. Own-song recognition in the songbird auditory pathway: Selectivity and lateralization. *J. Neurosci.* **2009**, *29*, 2252–2258. [CrossRef] [PubMed]
70. Voss, H.U.; Tabelow, K.; Polzehl, J.; Tchernichovski, O.; Maul, K.K.; Salgado-Commissariat, D.; Ballon, D.; Helekar, S.A. Functional MRI of the zebra finch brain during song stimulation suggests a lateralized response topography. *Proc. Natl. Acad. Sci. USA* **2007**, *104*, 10667–10672. [CrossRef] [PubMed]
71. George, I.; Cousillas, H.; Richard, J.-P.; Hausberger, M. Perception of song in the European starling is lateralized. *Adv. Ethol.* **2001**, *36*, 163.
72. Cousillas, H.; Leppelsack, H.J.; Leppelsack, E.; Richard, J.P.; Mathelier, M.; Hausberger, M. Functional organization of the forebrain auditory centres of the European starling: A study based on natural sounds. *Hear Res.* **2005**, *207*, 10–21. [CrossRef] [PubMed]

73. Moorman, S.; Nicol, A.U. Memory-related brain lateralisation in birds and humans. *Neurosci. Biobehav. Rev.* **2015**, *5*, 86–102. [CrossRef] [PubMed]
74. Kaplan, G. Song structure and function of mimicry in the Australian magpie (Gymnorhina tibicen) compared to the lyrebird (Menura ssp.). *Int. J. Comp. Psychol.* **2000**, *12*, 219–241.
75. Kaplan, G. *Australian Magpie: Biology and Behaviour of an Unusual Songbird. Natural History Series*; CSIRO Publishing: Melbourne, Australia, 2004; ISBN 0-643-09068-1.
76. Kaplan, G. *Bird Minds. Cognition and Behaviour of Australian Native Birds*; CSIRO Publishing: Melbourne, Australia, 2015.
77. Vallortigara, G. Comparative neuropsychology of the dual brain: A stroll through animals' left and right perceptual worlds. *Brain Lang.* **2000**, *73*, 189–219. [CrossRef] [PubMed]
78. Rogers, L.J. Lateralization in its many forms, and its evolution and development. In *The Evolution of Hemispheric Specialization in Primates*; Special Topics in Primatology; Hopkins, W.D., Ed.; Elsevier: Amsterdam, The Netherlands, 2007; pp. 23–56, ISBN 978-0-12-374197-4.
79. Chakraborty, M.; Jarvis, E.D. Brain evolution by brain pathway duplication. *Philos. Trans. R. Soc. Lond. B* **2015**, *370*, 20150056. [CrossRef] [PubMed]
80. Cracraft, J. Avian evolution, Gondwana biogeography and the Cretaceous-Tertiary mass extinction event. *Proc. R. Soc. B* **2001**, *268*, 459–469. [CrossRef] [PubMed]
81. Cracraft, J.; Barker, F.K.; Braun, M.; Harshman, J.; Dyke, G.J.; Feinstein, J.; Stanely, S.; Cibois, A.; Schikler, P.; Beresford, P.; et al. Phylogenetic relationships among modern birds (Neornithes): Towards an avian tree of life. In *Assembling the Tree of Life*; Cracraft, J., Donoghue, M.J., Eds.; Oxford University Press: Oxford, UK, 2004; pp. 468–489, ISBN 9780195172348.
82. Barker, K.F.; Cibois, A.; Schikler, P.; Feinstein, J.; Cracraft, J. Phylogeny and diversification of the largest avian radiation. *Proc. Natl. Acad. Sci. USA* **2004**, *101*, 11040–11045. [CrossRef] [PubMed]
83. De Pietri, V.L.; Scofield, R.P.; Zelenkov, N. The unexpected survival of an ancient lineage of anseriform birds into the Neogene of Australia. The youngest record of Presbyornithidae. *R. Soc. Open Sci.* **2016**, *3*, 150635. [CrossRef] [PubMed]
84. Mayr, G. The fossil record of galliform birds: Comments on Crowe et al. (2006). *Cladistics* **2008**, *24*, 74–76. [CrossRef]
85. Boles, W.E. The world's oldest songbird. *Nature* **1995**, *374*, 21–22. [CrossRef]
86. Edwards, S.V.; Boles, W.E. Out of Gondwana: The origin of passerine birds. *Trends Ecol. Evol.* **2002**, *17*, 347–349. [CrossRef]
87. White, N.E.; Phillips, M.J.; Gilbert, M.T.; Alfaro-Núñez, A.; Willerslev, E.; Mawson, P.R.; Spencer, P.B.; Bunce, M. The evolutionary history of cockatoos (Aves: Psittaciformes: Cacatuidae). *Mol. Phylogen. Evol.* **2011**, *59*, 615–622. [CrossRef] [PubMed]
88. Wright, T.F.; Schirtzinger, E.E.; Matsumoto, T.; Eberhard, J.R.; Graves, G.R.; Sanchez, J.J.; Capelli, S.; Müller, H.; Scharpegge, J.; Chambers, G.; et al. A multilocus molecular phylogeny of the parrots (Psittaciformes): Support for a Gondwanan origin during the Cretaceous. *Mol. Biol. Evol.* **2008**, *25*, 2141–2156. [CrossRef] [PubMed]
89. Sibley, C.G.; Ahlquist, J.E. *Phylogeny and Classification of Birds: A Study in Molecular Evolution*; Yale University Press: New Haven, CT, USA, 1990.
90. Cockburn, A. Why do so many Australian birds cooperate: Social evolution in the Corvida? In *Frontiers of Population Ecology*; Floyd, R.B., Sheppard, A.W., De Barro, P.J., Eds.; CSIRO Publishing: Melbourne, Australia, 1996; pp. 451–472.
91. Robinson, F.N. Vocal mimicry and the evolution of birdsong. *EMU* **1975**, *75*, 23–27. [CrossRef]
92. Robinson, F.N.; Curtis, H.S. The vocal displays of the lyrebirds (Menuridae). *EMU* **1996**, *96*, 258–275. [CrossRef]
93. Kaplan, G. Animal Communication. Advanced Review. *Wiley Interdiscip. Rev.: Cogn. Sci.* **2014**, *5*, 661–677. [CrossRef] [PubMed]
94. Kaplan, G. Vocal Behaviour of Australian Magpies (Gymnorhina tibicen): A Study of Vocal Development, Song Learning, Communication and Mimicryctio 3.2 in the Australian Magpie. Ph.D. Thesis, University of Queensland, Brisbane, Australia, 2005.
95. Kaplan, G.; Johnson, G.; Koboroff, A.; Rogers, L.J. Alarm calls of the Australian magpie (Gymnorhina tibicen): I. predators elicit complex vocal responses and mobbing behaviour. *Open Ornithol. J.* **2009**, *2*, 7–16. [CrossRef]

96. Kaplan, G.; Rogers, L.J. Stability of referential signalling across time and locations: Testing alarm calls of Australian magpies (Gymnorhina tibicen) in urban and rural Australia and in Fiji. *PeerJ* **2013**, *1*, e112. [CrossRef] [PubMed]
97. Olson, E.M.; Maeda, R.K.; Gobes, S.M.H. Mirrored patterns of lateralized neuronal activation reflect old and new memories in the avian auditory cortex. *Neuroscience* **2016**, *330*, 395–402. [CrossRef] [PubMed]
98. Bolhuis, J.J.; Gahr, M. Neural mechanisms of birdsong memory. *Nat. Rev. Neurosci.* **2006**, *7*, 347–357. [CrossRef] [PubMed]
99. Deng, C.; Kaplan, G.; Rogers, L.J. Similarity of the song control nuclei of male and female Australian magpies (Gymnorhina tibicen). *Behav. Brain Res.* **2001**, *123*, 89–102. [CrossRef]
100. Fortune, E.S.; Margoliash, D. Parallel pathways and convergence onto HVC and adjacent neostriatum of adult zebra finches (Taeniopygia guttata). *J. Comp. Neurol.* **1995**, *360*, 413–441. [CrossRef] [PubMed]
101. Hoese, W.J.; Podos, J.; Boetticher, N.C.; Nowicki, S. Vocal tract function in birdsong production: Experimental manipulation of beak movements. *J. Exp. Biol.* **2000**, *203*, 1845–1855. [PubMed]
102. Elemans, C.P. The singer and the song: The neuromechanics of avian sound production. *Curr. Opin. Neurobiol.* **2014**, *28*, 172–178. [CrossRef] [PubMed]
103. Elemans, C.P.; Rasmussen, J.H.; Herbst, C.T.; Düring, D.N.; Zollinger, S.A.; Brumm, H.; Srivastava, K.; Svane, N.; Ding, M.; Larsen, O.N.; et al. Universal mechanisms of sound production and control in birds and mammals. *Nat. Commun.* **2015**, *8978*, 1–13. [CrossRef] [PubMed]
104. King, A.S.; McLelland, J. *Birds: Their Structure and Function*; Bailliere Tindall: London, UK, 1984.
105. Miskimen, M. The syrinx in certain tyrant flycatchers. *Auk* **1963**, *80*, 156–165. [CrossRef]
106. Goller, F.; Larsen, O.N. A new mechanism of sound generation in songbirds. *Proc. Natl. Acad. Sci. USA* **1997**, *94*, 14787–14791. [CrossRef] [PubMed]
107. Nu, M.M. Vocal and Auditory Communication in Parrots: Some Anatomical and Behavioural Aspects. Ph.D. Thesis, Zoology, University of New England, Armidale, NSW, Australia, 1974.
108. Nottebohm, F. Ontogeny of bird song. *Science* **1970**, *167*, 950–956. [CrossRef] [PubMed]
109. King, A.S. Apparatus Respiratorius (Systema Respiratorium). In *Handbook of Avian Anatomy: Nomina Anatomica Avium*; Baumel, J.J., Ed.; The Nuttall Ornithological Club: Cambridge, MA, USA, 1993.
110. Klatt, D.H.; Stefanski, R.A. How does a mynah bird imitate human speech? *J. Acoust. Soc. Am.* **1974**, *55*, 822–832. [CrossRef] [PubMed]
111. Nowicki, S. Vocal tract resonance in oscine bird sound production: Evidence from birdsongs in a helium atmosphere. *Nature* **1987**, *325*, 53–55. [CrossRef] [PubMed]
112. Baker, M.C. Bird song research: The past 100 years. *Bird Behav.* **2001**, *14*, 3–50.
113. Podos, J.; Sherer, J.K.; Peters, S.; Nowicki, S. Ontogeny of vocal tract movements during song production in song sparrows. *Anim. Behav.* **1995**, *50*, 1287–1296. [CrossRef]
114. Beckers, G.J.L.; Nelson, B.S.; Suthers, R.S. Vocal-tract filtering by lingual articulation in a parrot. *Curr. Biol.* **2004**, *14*, 1592–1597. [CrossRef] [PubMed]
115. Riede, T.; Eliason, C.M.; Miller, E.H.; Goller, F.; Clarke, J.A. Coos, booms, and hoots: The evolution of closed-mouth vocal behavior in birds. *Evolution* **2016**, *70*, 1734–1746. [CrossRef] [PubMed]
116. Suthers, R.; Wild, M.; Kaplan, G. Mechanisms of song production in the Australian magpie. *J. Comp. Phys. A* **2011**, *197*, 45–59. [CrossRef] [PubMed]
117. Wild, J.M.; Williams, M.N.; Suthers, R.A. Neural pathways for bilateral vocal control in songbirds. *J. Comp. Neurol.* **2000**, *423*, 413–426. [CrossRef]
118. Nowicki, S.; Capranica, R.R. Bilateral syringeal coupling during phonation of a songbird. *J. Neurosci.* **1986**, *6*, 3595–3610. [PubMed]
119. Brenowitz, E.A. Comparative approaches to the avian song system. *J. Neurobiol.* **1997**, *33*, 517–531. [CrossRef]
120. Zollinger, S.A.; Riede, T.; Suthers, R.A. Two-voice complexity from a single side of the syrinx in northern mockingbird Mimus polyglottos vocalizations. *J. Exp. Biol.* **2008**, *211*, 1978–1991. [CrossRef] [PubMed]
121. Dooling, R.J.; Lohr, B.; Dent, M.L. Hearing in birds and reptiles. In *Comparative Hearing: Birds and Reptiles*; Dooling, R.J., Fay, R.R., Popper, A.N., Eds.; Springer: New York, NY, USA, 2000; pp. 308–359.
122. Cohen, S.M.; Stebbins, W.C.; Moody, D.B. Auditory thresholds of the blue jay. *Auk* **1978**, *95*, 563–568.
123. Henry, K.S.; Lucas, J.R. Auditory sensitivity and the frequency selectivity of auditory filters in the Carolina chickadee, Poecile carolinensis. *Anim. Behav.* **2010**, *80*, 497–507. [CrossRef]

124. Saunders, J.C.; Duncan, R.K.; Doan, D.E.; Werner, Y.L. The middle ear of reptiles and birds. In *Comparative Hearing: Birds and Reptiles*; Dooling, R.J., Fay, R.R., Popper, A.N., Eds.; Springer: New York, NY, USA, 2000; pp. 13–69.
125. Dooling, R.J.; Leek, M.R.; Gleich, O.; Dent, M.L. Auditory temporal resolution in birds: Discrimination of harmonic complexes. *J. Acoust. Soc. Am.* **2002**, *112*, 748–759. [CrossRef] [PubMed]
126. Joris, P.X.; Schreiner, C.E.; Rees, A. Neural processing of amplitude-modulated sounds. *Physiol. Rev.* **2004**, *84*, 541–577. [CrossRef] [PubMed]
127. Mooney, T.A.; Yamato, M.; Branstetter, B.K. Hearing in cetaceans: From natural history to experimental biology. *Adv. Mar. Biol.* **2012**, *63*, 197–246. [PubMed]
128. Larsen, O.N.; Dooling, R.J.; Michelsen, A. The role of pressure difference reception in the directional hearing of budgerigars (Melopsittacus undulatus). *J. Comp. Physiol. A* **2006**, *192*, 1063–1072. [CrossRef] [PubMed]
129. Schnyder, H.A.; Vanderelst, D.; Bartenstein, S.; Firzlaff, U.; Luksch, H. The avian head induces cues for sound localization in elevation. *PLoS ONE* **2014**, *9*, e112178. [CrossRef] [PubMed]
130. Ohmori, H. Neuronal specializations for the processing of interaural difference cues in the chick. *Front. Neural Circuits* **2014**, *8*, 47. [CrossRef] [PubMed]
131. Welch, T.E.; Dent, M.L. Lateralization of acoustic signals by dichotically listening budgerigars (Melopsittacus undulatus). *Acoust. Soc. Am.* **2011**, *130*, 2293–2301. [CrossRef] [PubMed]
132. Siniscalchi, M.; Quaranta, A.; Rogers, L.J. Hemispheric specialization in dogs for processing different acoustic stimuli. *PLoS ONE* **2008**, *3*, e3349. [CrossRef] [PubMed]
133. Palleroni, A.M.; Hauser, M. Experience-dependent plasticity for auditory processing in a raptor. *Science* **2003**, *299*, 1195. [CrossRef] [PubMed]
134. Tervaniemi, M.; Hugdahl, K. Lateralisation of auditory-cortex functions. Brain Research. *Brain Res. Rev.* **2003**, *43*, 231–246. [CrossRef] [PubMed]
135. Ocklenburg, S.; Arning, L.; Hahn, C.; Gerding, W.M.; Epplen, J.T.; Güntürkün, O.; Beste, C. Variation in the NMDA receptor 2B subunit gene GRIN2B is associated with differential language lateralisation. *Behav. Brain Res.* **2011**, *255*, 284–289. [CrossRef] [PubMed]
136. Osmanski, M.S.; Dooling, R.J. The effect of altered auditory feedback on control of vocal production in budgerigars (Melopsittacus undulatus). *J. Acoust. Soc. Am.* **2009**, *126*, 911–919. [CrossRef] [PubMed]
137. Rogers, L.J. Eye and ear preferences. In *Lateralized, Brain Functions. Methods in Human and Non-Human Species*; Rogers, L.J., Vallortigara, G., Eds.; Humana Press: New York, NY, USA, 2017; pp. 79–102, ISBN 978-1-4939-6723-0.
138. Floyd, R.B.; Woodland, D.J. Localization of soil dwelling scarab larvae by the black-backed magpie, Gymnorhina tibicen (Latham). *Anim. Behav.* **1981**, *29*, 510–517. [CrossRef]
139. Raw, F. The ecology of the garden chafer, Phyllopertha horticola (L.), with preliminary observations on control measures. *Bull. Entomol. Res.* **1952**, *42*, 605–646. [CrossRef]
140. Heppner, F. Sensory mechanisms and environmental cues used by the American robin in locating earthworms. *Condor* **1965**, *67*, 247–256. [CrossRef]
141. Carne, P.B.; Chinnick, L.J. The pruinose scarab (Sericesthis pruinose Dalman) and its control in turf. *Austral J. Agric. Res.* **1957**, *8*, 604–616. [CrossRef]
142. Goodyer, G.J.; Nicholas, A. Scarab grubs in northern tableland pastures. *Primefact* **2007**, *512*, 1–8.
143. Brown, E.D.; Veltman, C.J. Ethogram of the Australian magpie (Gymnorhina tibicen) in comparison to other cracticidae and corvus species. *Ethology* **1987**, *76*, 309–333. [CrossRef]
144. Hoffman, A.M.; Robakiewicz, A.; Tuttle, E.M.; Rogers, L.J. Behavioural lateralisation in the Australian magpie (Gymnorhina tibicen). *Laterality* **2006**, *11*, 110–121. [CrossRef] [PubMed]
145. Tommasi, L.; Vallortigara, G. Hemispheric processing of landmarks and geometric information in male and female domestic chicks (Gallus gallus). *Behav. Brain Res.* **2004**, *155*, 85–96. [CrossRef] [PubMed]
146. Vallortigara, G.; Cozzutti, C.L.; Tommasi, L.; Rogers, L.J. How birds use their eyes; opposite left–right specialisation for the lateral and frontal visual hemifield in the domestic chick. *Curr. Biol.* **2001**, *1*, 29–33. [CrossRef]
147. Karenina, K.; Giljov, A.; Ingram, J.; Rowntree, V.J.; Malashichev, Y. Lateralization of mother–infant interactions in a diverse range of mammal species. *Nat. Ecol. Evol.* **2017**, *1*, 1–30. [CrossRef]

148. Koboroff, A.; Kaplan, G.; Rogers, L.J. Hemispheric specialization in Australian magpies (Gymnorhina tibicen) shown as eye preferences during response to a predator. *Brain Res. Bull.* **2008**, *76*, 304–306. [CrossRef] [PubMed]
149. Alonso, Y. Lateralization of visual guided behaviour during feeding in zebra finches (Taeniopygia guttata). *Behav. Process.* **1998**, *43*, 257–263. [CrossRef]
150. Rogers, L.J.; Zucca, P.; Vallortigara, G. Advantages of having a lateralized brain. *Proc. R. Soc. Lond. B* **2004**, *271*, S420–S422. [CrossRef] [PubMed]
151. Rogers, L.J. Advantages and disadvantages of lateralization. In *Comparative Vertebrate Lateralization*; Rogers, L.J., Andrew, R.J., Eds.; Cambridge University Press: Cambridge, UK, 2002; pp. 126–155.
152. Vallortigara, G.; Andrew, R.J. Differential involvement of right and left hemisphere in individual recognition in the domestic chick. *Behav. Proc.* **1994**, *33*, 41–58. [CrossRef]
153. Ocklenburg, S.; Ströckens, F.; Güntürkün, O. Lateralisation of conspecific vocalisation in non-human vertebrates. *Laterality* **2013**, *18*, 1–31. [CrossRef] [PubMed]

8

Early- and Late-Light Embryonic Stimulation Modulates Similarly Chicks' Ability to Filter out Distractors

Cinzia Chiandetti [1,*], Bastien S. Lemaire [2,3], Elisabetta Versace [3] and Giorgio Vallortigara [3]

1 Department of Life Sciences, University of Trieste, I-34127 Trieste, Italy
2 Institute of applied biology (IBFA), University of Caen, 14000 Caen, France; lemaire.bas@gmail.com
3 Center for Mind/Brain Sciences, University of Trento, I-38068 Rovereto, Italy; elisabetta.versace@unitn.it (E.V.); giorgio.vallortigara@unitn.it (G.V.)
* Correspondence: cchiandetti@units.it

Academic Editor: Lesley Rogers

Abstract: Chicks (*Gallus gallus*) learned to run from a starting box to a target located at the end of a runway. At test, colourful and bright distractors were placed just outside the starting box. Dark incubated chicks (maintained in darkness from fertilization to hatching) stopped significantly more often, assessing more the left-side distractor than chicks hatched after late (for 42 h during the last three days before hatching) or early (for 42 h after fertilization) exposure to light. The results show that early embryonic light stimulation can modulate this particular behavioural lateralization comparably to the late application of it, though via a different route.

Keywords: attention; functional lateralization; cerebral lateralization; embryo; light; fish; chicks; birds

---

1. Introduction

It is now well established that environmental light stimulation interplays with a genetic cascade of events in promoting brain specialization in two different classes of vertebrates, fish and birds (reviews in [1–3]).

A complex chain of developmental steps leads to brain lateralization in zebrafish starting with an asymmetrical expression of a gene network that controls the development of structural left-right differences within the epithalamus, including asymmetric parapineal migration [4–7]. As a secondary consequence, in the transparent eggs of the zebrafish an early action of light prompts functional brain asymmetries including motor and sensory processing. Fry hatched from eggs exposed to the photic input during the first week after fertilization prefer to attend to conspecifics with the left eye, whereas fries whose embryonic development happened in darkness do not display the same asymmetry [8]. If the light fails to reach the embryos in two distinct moments within the first week post-fertilization, the normal development of some lateralized behaviours is either compromised or prevented. For instance, darkness during the first day results in an inversion of the reaction to a dummy predator: after normal light regimes, zebrafish avoid the predator appearing on the left side, whereas after darkness they respond more intensely to a predator coming from the right side [9]; in contrast, darkness during the third day prevents the appearance of any asymmetric response to the predator [10]. However, the role of light stimulation on brain structural asymmetry has not been conclusively clarified in zebrafish, as no effect of light has been shown on the asymmetry of molecular markers [11], and some behaviours are lateralized while some others are not, independently of the neuroanatomical asymmetries [12].

Embryonic light application influences also the neurodevelopment of cerebral lateralization in the avian brain, but via a different pathway, i.e., by the asymmetric stimulation of one eye. For more than three decades, it has been repeatedly shown that an asymmetrical embryonic positioning before hatching (due to unilateral expression of Nodal signals responsible for the body torsion [13]) allows light penetration of the egg during the final days of incubation to act selectively on one side of the chick's head and to trigger anatomical and functional brain asymmetries via right eye stimulation [14]. In response to the asymmetric light input to the retinal cells, brain regions in the left hemisphere fed by the right eye develop earlier than their counterparts in the right hemisphere and a higher number of fibers crosses from the left side of the thalamus to the right hemisphere via the supraoptic decussation [15–17]. Such structural asymmetry is functionally detectable in several visually-guided behaviours, such as the advantage of the right eye in preventing pecks to not edible elements when searching for food [18]. Furthermore, chicks presenting such an asymmetry outperform chicks hatched in darkness in dual tasks [19] or when they have to combine different kinds of information to master a correct discrimination [20]. The multifaceted role of light is apparent in the fact that light exposure affects not only abilities related to the stimulated right eye but also functions of the left eye related to attack, copulation, predator detection [15], and visuospatial abilities [21]. Moreover, reversing the eye exposed to light by untwisting the embryo's head and applying a patch to the right eye causes the pattern of asymmetries to be inverted [15,22]. Note, however, that although light exerts such an important role in the establishment of lateralization, some forms of asymmetries as those associated with unilateral eye used during sleep [23] or with the neural mechanisms of social recognition and imprinting [24–26] develop even if the incubation process takes place in darkness [27,28].

The depicted scenario shows a composite set of mechanisms at play in the development of brain asymmetries and the common thread to birds and fish seems to indicate that, following two different anatomical routes, light moulds a similar functional cerebral specialization in the two taxa [29]. Broadly speaking, the right hemisphere orchestrates a form of primitive avoidance and wariness while the left-hemisphere complements brain specialization with the control of routine behaviours of feeding and analysis in familiar contexts, counteracting distraction and irrelevant response to novelty credited to the right hemisphere [1,30]. Thus, apparently similar behavioural asymmetries can be generated by different neural asymmetric systems [31,32].

To check whether a different critical period for the application of the light input could be part of the asymmetric neurodevelopment of cerebral functions also in the chick, Chiandetti et al. [33] exposed eggs to light for a brief period after fertilization, when other photosensitive regions are developing but no retinal photoreceptors have been differentiated yet [34,35], and thereafter maintained them in the dark. Chicks hatched under this condition performed in a comparable fashion to chicks hatched from eggs light-stimulated in the canonical time-window, i.e., during the last three days of incubation [33]. The testing condition required chicks to avoid an obstacle placed midway between the starting box and the target at the other end. In such a situation, the two light-stimulated groups showed no preference to detour the obstacle by circumventing it well as much from the left as the right side. By contrast, chicks hatched in darkness showed a pronounced bias to detour the obstacle systematically on the left side. In that case, a motoric difference between stimulated and unstimulated individuals was insufficient to explain the pattern of behaviour observed because all the chicks showed the same motor bias to run slightly toward the left side of the environment when tested without any obstacle on their way to the target (for the specificity of light effect, see reviews in [2,31]). Rather, unstimulated chicks' selective bias emerged only when an obstacle was on the way to the target. It is possible that, when freely running, chicks previously kept in darkness are less able to sustain attention toward the target and need the right eye to view the obstacle in order to keep track of it while running toward the target, and avoiding the obstacle.

Here, in the attempt to widen the comprehension of when and how light stimulation is effective in shaping visually-driven asymmetric responses, we assessed stimulated (early and late) and unstimulated chicks and compared the performance of the three groups of animals in a further testing situation. Briefly, two days old domestic chicks (*Gallus gallus*) first learned to run from one end of a runway to a target located at the opposite end; then, at day 5 of age, colourful and bright distractors were placed close to the starting area and we scored whether the chicks pecked at the distractor, how many times and whether preferentially on the one positioned on the left, assuming that the novelty would have engaged mainly the left eye (right hemisphere). The task was chosen as a replication of a previous one with a change in the type of distractor that could provide an incremental knowledge about the observed phenomenon.

2. Materials and Methods

The study was carried out in compliance with the European Community and the Italian law on animal experiments by the Ministry of Health, under the authorization of the Ethical Committee of the University of Trieste (protocol number 385 pos II/9 dd 16.03.2012).

2.1. Subjects

Chicks of the Ross 308 (Aviagen) broiler strain hatched in our laboratory under controlled conditions. The eggs were collected from a local commercial hatchery immediately after fertilization and, thereafter, kept in a FIEM snc, MG 100 H incubator under controlled temperature (37.7 °C) and humidity (about 50–60%) conditions, in a darkened room so that no further incidental light could reach the eggs. Fifty eggs were incubated in complete darkness from the arrival to the laboratory and until the hatching day (Di-chicks = 38); fifty eggs were exposed to light from their arrival to the lab and for 42 h and thereafter remained in the dark (EarlyLi-chicks = 39); fifty eggs were maintained in darkness and exposed to light from day 18 and for 42 h before hatching (LateLi-chicks = 36). A 60 W incandescent light bulb or 15 LEDs (18 lumens per LED) provided homogeneous light of about 250 lux within the incubator. As reviewed in [2], high intensity and prolonged exposure to light can exert various effects (from hatchability to interlimb coordination) and this applies to LEDs too; however, the light regime adopted in our protocol is not proven to have comparable side-effects (and see [33] for an analysis of the identical running trajectories in Di-, EarlyLi-, and LateLi-chicks). Immediately after hatching, each chick was reared singly in a metal home-cage (28 cm wide × 32 cm high × 40 cm deep) illuminated by LED (12 L: 12 D cycle) and located in a separate room at 30 °C. Food and water were available *ad libitum*.

2.2. Apparatus

A white rectangular enclosure (40 cm wide × 50 cm high × 160 cm deep) with sawdust (5 cm in depth) on the floor served as training apparatus. A red conspicuous plastic beacon was placed at the middle of the smaller end of the apparatus and 7 cm above the floor, indicating the presence of a plastic feeder (target) exactly below it. Two lamps of 50 W centered on the top of the smaller ends provided uniform illumination to the apparatus. For the testing, two slanted walls were adjusted close to the starting point on both the left and the right (see Figure 1) and decorated with salient shiny beads placed at about chick's head height, functioning as distractors.

In order to keep track of the chick's movements within the apparatus, a black removable sticky paper was temporarily attached on the chick's back. The behaviour was videorecorded from above and scored offline by an independent observer blind with respect to the hatching conditions of the animals.

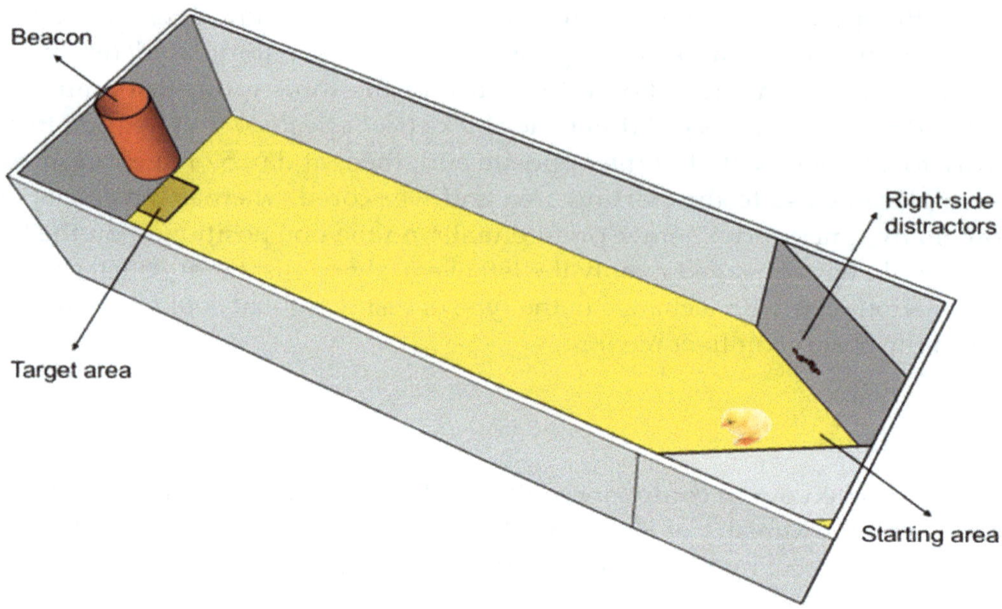

Figure 1. Schematic layout of the experimental apparatus as prepared for the test, with exemplifier distractors placed on both the left and the right side of the starting point and the red beacon signalling the presence of the plate with the mealworms (available only during training). A chick is inspecting the distractors located on the left of the starting point.

2.3. Procedure

On day 2 of age, after 3 h of food deprivation, each chick was first accustomed to the training apparatus by letting it free to explore the environment for about 30 min and reach the target where some mealworm larvae (*Tenebrio molitor*) were placed. The next two days, each chick was placed within the apparatus at the opposite end in front of the target and left free to run toward the feeder. This procedure was repeated 20 times (10 times per day).

On day 5, each chick was given one trial as used during training to reinstate motivation and immediately after it was tested only once with the distractors. In the single testing trial, no mealworm was available under the target. This procedure was chosen to rule out any potential influence of the presence of the reward. The trial ended as soon as the chick reached the feeder. The positions of the starting point and the target were counterbalanced between subjects in order to control for any undesired asymmetry within the environment. As a dependent measure, we scored the number of pecks directed at right and left distractors.

3. Results

After having verified that the assumption of homogeneity of variances was not satisfied with the Levene's test, we ran the non-parametric test Kruskal-Wallis on the overall number of pecks, which showed a significant difference between the three hatching groups ($\chi^2_{(2)} = 10.194$, $p = 0.006$): Di-chicks were more distracted than the two stimulated groups on the pecks toward the left distractor ($\chi^2_{(2)} = 9.352$, $p = 0.009$), but not to the right distractor ($\chi^2_{(2)} = 2.844$, $p = 0.241$), as visible in Figure 2. Di-chicks pecked more at the distractor placed on the left side than both EarlyLi- ($Z = -2.271$, $p = 0.023$) and LateLi-chicks ($Z = -2.588$, $p = 0.010$), whereas no difference emerged between the two light-stimulated groups ($Z = -0.368$, $p = 0.713$, Mann-Whitney Post Hoc test).

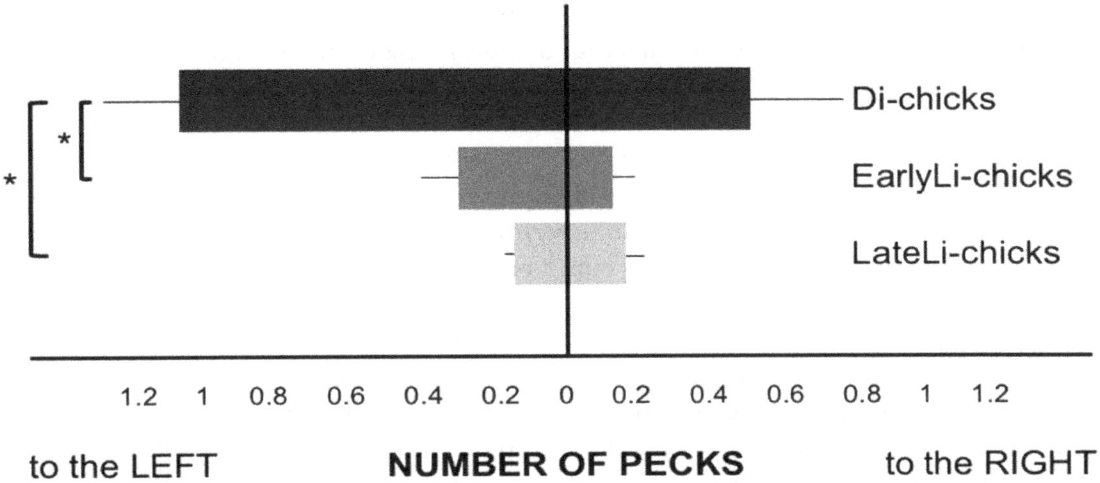

Figure 2. Plot of the performance (average number of pecks and S.E.M.) of the three groups of chicks in the presence of the distractor (* $p < 0.05$).

4. Discussion

In this investigation of the time windows in which embryonic light stimulation affects the development of functional brain asymmetries, we replicated previous findings showing that chicks hatched from eggs exposed to environmental illumination for 42 h, at either an early or a late stage of embryonic development, display a comparable behaviour. Specifically, both EarlyLi- and LateLi-chicks were not distracted by the novel elements placed in proximity of the starting area. Conversely, Di-chicks, hatched from eggs maintained for the whole developmental period in complete darkness, were significantly attracted by the novel elements and could not restrain from pecking at these items before reaching the target, and especially at those placed on their left side. Note that the procedure used here matches the one used in our previous work [33], where we showed a specific effect of light stimulation on hemispheres' functionality with no detriment of dark incubation condition on a typical motor and cognitive development (see also [36] for comparable results on pigeons).

The observed pattern of chicks' performance confirms that embryonic application of light stimulation modulates the ability to sustain attention. EarlyLi- and LateLi-chicks ignored the novel elements and focused on the target, directly approaching it in a routine-like behaviour as learned during the familiarization trials without distractors. Both the left and the right eyes seemed equally good in targeting the goal and avoiding the salient distractor elements presented at test. By contrast, Di-chicks were strongly biased toward the distractors. The fact that the distractors placed on the left side resulted more attractive than those placed on the right side, uncovers the brain asymmetry at play in Di-chicks: the right eye is engaged in sustaining attention to the target, while the left eye mediates attention deployment to the novel and salient elements located on the left side. Our findings suggest that in Di-chicks the separation of the two hemispheres also maintains segregated the processing of the target and the distractor. While the left hemisphere would control the routine running behaviour toward the target, the right hemisphere is engaged by novelty and the chicks stop their running to assess the distractor located on the left, as they do when they monitor the predator [19,37].

In LateLi-chicks, instead, it appears that the right hemispheric involvement in response to novelty is modulated by the asymmetric embryonic light stimulation. The cross-talk between the two halves of the brain makes the left hemisphere capable of inhibitory control over the compulsory attention directed toward the novelty, similarly to the testing situation in which the right eye (left hemisphere) inhibits pecks at irrelevant elements spread among grains [19].

What remains to be understood is how light induces a comparable performance in LateLi- and EarlyLi-chicks, considering that only on LateLi-chicks light acts asymmetrically on the fully-formed eye. In zebrafish, the involvement of both habenulae in the control of behaviour is shown by the fact that selective inactivation of these nuclei induces a persistent freezing response [38]; furthermore, the use of the right eye to target the food implies that the left hemisphere is engaged in sustained control, with the enrollment of the left lateral habenulae, reducing the probability of being distracted [39,40]. Although the fact that there is no clear evidence that the role of light on the lateralized behaviour depends directly on a stimulation of the parapineal, this could account for the performance observed in both fish and EarlyLi-chicks. This hypothesis requires further investigation: indeed, in fish, other photosensitive areas than the eye participate in determining lateralization [41,42] and one may wonder whether the involvement of the same regions could be extended to explain chicks' performance, since analogous cells are developing in the chick embryo at the early stages when we applied the light stimulation [43]. Due to the common differentiation of the diencephalic areas in birds and fish, the involvement of the ephyphysis-habenula axis could be the target for a further window in which light may be operating in chicks as well. A further complication may derive from the fact that the habenular nuclei are asymmetric in several species [44,45] and hence might be differentially stimulated by the action of light. By contrast, in birds the habenulae are assumed to be symmetric, despite the fact that one study on chicks showed that there can be individual asymmetries and males tend to present a larger right medial habenula [46]; unfortunately, there was no mention of the incubation condition in this study and hence whether it applies to our results or not is open to speculation. On the basis of atlases of different avian species, it appears that the pineal gland, projecting to the habenulae, is larger in absolute size in chicks than, for instance, in pigeons. The cytochemical characterization of the avian pineal organ demonstrates many structural, functional and biochemical analogies between the retinal and the pineal photoreceptors [47,48]. Furthermore, other brain regions involved in lateralization may have been simply overlooked in previous histological assessments of light stimulation effects. There might also be a further extra-retinal photoreceptive candidate in birds outside the pineal gland. As shown in quails, in the avian ventral thalamus and septal region there are so-called deep photoreceptors that seem to participate in the regulation of seasonal cycles of reproduction [49,50]. These further photosensitive receptors respond to light in the quail and might be activated in domestic chicks as well. Certainly, this hypothesis paves the way to further investigations addressing specifically the neural substrates enrolled by light at precocious stages of the chick's embryonic development.

5. Conclusions

Here we documented that an early application of light during incubation modulates a particular functional asymmetry in chicks in a similar way to the well-known late stimulation. Light seems to operate on a genetically determined asymmetry by mediating a better cooperation between the two hemispheres. The asymmetrical light stimulation experience does not simply affect hemispheric specialization (like a left-hemispheric dominance of visuomotor control (discussed for instance in [32])) but also how efficiently the hemispheres can interact or cooperate [36,51].

The mechanisms responsible for the early modulation remain to be investigated, however a broader consideration on the effects of light stimulation before birth is worth discussing. Despite it is controversial whether the human foetus is reached by asymmetric light to one eye (it is attested that 2/3 of the embryos are rotated with the right eye toward the external abdominal wall in the latest stages of gestation), in principle the light reaches the intrauterine environment [52]. Indeed, at about 36–40 weeks, the foetus responds to flashes of light to the maternal abdomen with an increment in cardiac frequency and eye and body movements [53]. There are also indications that light can affect the development of cerebral lateralization in human foetuses by modulating the available hormonal levels [54]. Although assessing this hypothesis has proven to be very difficult, seasonal anisotropy has been recently shown with respect to the distribution of handedness as related to gender: longer photoperiods experienced during the first 14–18 weeks are associated with left-handed males [55]. Hence, at present, a hormonal modulation cannot be ruled out.

Asymmetries induced by genetic factors are shaped by environmental illumination, as indicated by previous results on zebrafish and chicks, but here we showed that in an avian species this takes place in two different time-windows. If light entails two different processes in the two time-windows, a more sensitive test could reveal a specific involvement of each hemisphere. For instance, an investigation of the performance under monocular testing condition [56] could reasonably refine the enrolment of each hemisphere depending on the specific genetic-environment route, since monocular and binocular performances could differ profoundly (e.g., [57]).

Acknowledgments: Thanks are extended to Margherita Lucadello and Eliana Boschetti for supporting data collection and off-line scoring, and to the anonymous reviewers for the thoroughness with which they evaluated our manuscript. C.C. was partially funded by a UniTs-FRA2015 grant.

Author Contributions: C.C. and G.V. conceived the experiment; C.C., B.L. and E.V. designed the procedure; B.L. and C.C. performed the experiments; C.C. analyzed the data and prepared the figures; C.C. drafted the paper; C.C., G.V., E.V. and B.L. revised and approved the final version of the paper.

References

1. Rogers, L.J.; Vallortigara, G.; Andrew, R.J. *Divided Brains: The Biology and Behaviour of Brain Asymmetries*; Cambridge University Press: Cambridge, UK, 2013.
2. Chiandetti, C. Manipulation of strength of cerebral lateralization via embryonic light stimulation in birds. In *Lateralized Brain Functions. Methods in Human and Non-Human Species*; Rogers, L.J., Vallortigara, G., Eds.; Humana Press: New York, NY, USA, 2017; pp. 611–631.
3. Vallortigara, G.; Versace, E. Laterality at the Neural, Cognitive, and Behavioral Levels. In *APA Handbook of Comparative Psychology: Vol. 1. Basic Concepts, Methods, Neural Substrate, and Behavior*; Call, J., Ed.; American Psychological Association: Washington DC, USA, 2017; pp. 557–577.
4. Kuan, Y.-S.; Gamse, J.T.; Schreiber, A.M.; Halpern, M.E. Selective asymmetry in a conserved forebrain to midbrain projection. *J. Exp. Zool. B Mol. Dev. Evol.* **2007**, *308*, 669–678. [CrossRef] [PubMed]
5. Roussigné, M.; Blader, P.; Wilson, S.W. Breaking symmetry: The zebrafish as a model for understanding left-right asymmetry in the developing brain. *Dev. Neurobiol.* **2012**, *72*, 269–281. [CrossRef] [PubMed]
6. Gamse, J.T.; Thisse, C.; Thisse, B.; Halpern, M.E. The parapineal mediates left-right asymmetry in the zebrafish diencephalon. *Development* **2003**, *130*, 1059–1068. [CrossRef] [PubMed]
7. Concha, M.L.; Bianco, I.H.; Wilson, S.W. Encoding asymmetry within neural circuits. *Nat. Rev. Neurosci.* **2012**, *13*, 832–843. [CrossRef] [PubMed]
8. Andrew, R.J.; Osorio, D.; Budaev, S. Light during embryonic development modulates patterns of lateralization strongly and similarly in both zebrafish and chick. *Philos. Trans. R. Soc. Lond. B Biol. Sci.* **2009**, *364*, 983–989. [CrossRef] [PubMed]
9. Budaev, S.; Andrew, R.J. Patterns of early embryonic light exposure determine behavioural asymmetries in zebrafish: A habenular hypothesis. *Behav. Brain Res.* **2009**, *200*, 91–94. [CrossRef] [PubMed]
10. Budaev, S.; Andrew, R. Shyness and behavioural asymmetries in larval zebrafish (*Brachydanio rerio*) developed in light and dark. *Behaviour* **2009**, *146*, 1037–1052. [CrossRef]
11. De Borsetti, N.H.; Dean, B.J.; Bain, E.J.; Clanton, J.A.; Taylor, R.W.; Gamse, J.T. Light and melatonin schedule neuronal differentiation in the habenular nuclei. *Dev. Biol.* **2011**, *358*, 251–261. [CrossRef] [PubMed]
12. Barth, K.A.; Miklósi, A.; Watkins, J.; Bianco, I.H.; Wilson, S.W.; Andrew, R.J. Fsi zebrafish show concordant reversal of laterality of viscera, neuroanatomy, and a subset of behavioral responses. *Curr. Biol.* **2005**, *15*, 844–850. [CrossRef] [PubMed]
13. Levin, M.; Johnson, R.L.; Stern, C.D.; Kuehn, M.R.; Tabin, C. A molecular pathway determining left-right asymmetry in chick embryogenesis. *Cell* **1995**, *82*, 803–814. [CrossRef]
14. Rogers, L.J. Light experience and asymmetry of brain function in chickens. *Nature* **1982**, *297*, 223–225. [CrossRef] [PubMed]
15. Rogers, L.J. Light input and the reversal of functional lateralization in the chicken brain. *Behav. Brain Res.* **1990**, *38*, 211–221. [CrossRef]
16. Rogers, L.J.; Deng, C. Light experience and lateralization of the two visual pathways in the chick. *Behav. Brain Res.* **1999**, *98*, 277–287. [CrossRef]

17. Ströckens, F.; Güntürkün, O. Cryptochrome 1b: A possible inducer of visual lateralization in pigeons? *Eur. J. Neurosci.* **2016**, *43*, 162–168. [CrossRef] [PubMed]
18. Rogers, L.J.; Anson, J.M. Lateralisation of function in the chicken fore-brain. *Pharmacol. Biochem. Behav.* **1979**, *10*, 679–686. [CrossRef]
19. Rogers, L.J.; Zucca, P.; Vallortigara, G. Advantages of having a lateralized brain. *Proc. R. Soc. B Biol. Sci.* **2004**, *271*, S420–S422. [CrossRef] [PubMed]
20. Chiandetti, C.; Vallortigara, G. Effects of embryonic light stimulation on the ability to discriminate left from right in the domestic chick. *Behav. Brain Res.* **2009**, *198*, 240–246. [CrossRef] [PubMed]
21. Chiandetti, C. Pseudoneglect and embryonic light stimulation in the avian brain. *Behav. Neurosci.* **2011**, *125*, 775–782. [CrossRef] [PubMed]
22. Manns, M.; Güntürkün, O. Monocular deprivation alters the direction of functional and morphological asymmetries in the pigeon's (*Columba livia*) visual system. *Behav. Neurosci.* **1999**, *113*, 1257–1266. [CrossRef] [PubMed]
23. Mascetti, G.G.; Vallortigara, G. Why do birds sleep with one eye open? Light exposure of the chick embryo as a determinant of monocular sleep. *Curr. Biol.* **2001**, *11*, 971–974. [CrossRef]
24. Vallortigara, G.; Andrew, R.J. Lateralization of response by chicks to change in a model partner. *Anim. Behav.* **1991**, *41*, 187–194. [CrossRef]
25. Vallortigara, G.; Andrew, R.J. Olfactory lateralization in the chick. *Neuropsychologia* **1994**, *32*, 417–423. [CrossRef]
26. Vallortigara, G. Right hemisphere advantage for social recognition in the chick. *Neuropsychologia* **1992**, *30*, 761–768. [CrossRef]
27. Andrew, R.J.; Johnston, A.N.B.; Robins, A.; Rogers, L.J. Light experience and the development of behavioural lateralisation in chicks. II. Choice of familiar versus unfamiliar model social partner. *Behav. Brain Res.* **2004**, *155*, 67–76. [CrossRef] [PubMed]
28. Johnston, A.N.B.; Rogers, L.J. Light exposure of chick embryo influences lateralized recall of imprinting memory. *Behav. Neurosci.* **1999**, *113*, 1267–1273. [CrossRef] [PubMed]
29. Andrew, R.J. Origins of asymmetry in the CNS. *Semin. Cell Dev. Biol.* **2009**, *20*, 485–490. [CrossRef] [PubMed]
30. MacNeilage, P.F.; Rogers, L.J.; Vallortigara, G. Origins of the left & right brain. *Sci. Am.* **2009**, *301*, 60–67. [PubMed]
31. Rogers, L.J. Asymmetry of Brain and Behavior in Animals: Its Development, Function, and Human Relevance. *Genesis* **2014**, *52*, 555–571. [CrossRef] [PubMed]
32. Manns, M.; Ströckens, F. Functional and structural comparison of visual lateralization in birds—Similar but still different. *Front. Psychol.* **2014**, *5*, 1–10. [CrossRef] [PubMed]
33. Chiandetti, C.; Galliussi, J.; Andrew, R.J.; Vallortigara, G. Early-light embryonic stimulation suggests a second route, via gene activation, to cerebral lateralization in vertebrates. *Sci. Rep.* **2013**, *3*, 2701. [CrossRef] [PubMed]
34. Hamburger, V.; Hamilton, H. A series of normal stages in the development of the chick embryo. *J. Morphol.* **1951**, *88*, 49–92. [CrossRef] [PubMed]
35. Tomonari, S.; Takagi, A.; Akamatsu, S.; Noji, S.; Ohuchi, H. A non-canonical photopigment, melanopsin, is expressed in the differentiating ganglion, horizontal, and bipolar cells of the chicken retina. *Dev. Dyn.* **2005**, *234*, 783–790. [CrossRef] [PubMed]
36. Manns, M.; Römling, J. The impact of asymmetrical light input on cerebral hemispheric specialization and interhemispheric cooperation. *Nat. Commun.* **2012**, *3*, 696. [CrossRef] [PubMed]
37. Rogers, L.J. The two hemispheres of the avian brain: Their differing roles in perceptual processing and the expression of behavior. *J. Ornithol.* **2012**, *153*, 61–74. [CrossRef]
38. Agetsuma, M.; Aizawa, H.; Aoki, T.; Nakayama, R.; Takahoko, M.; Goto, M.; Sassa, T.; Amo, R.; Shiraki, T.; Kawakami, K.; et al. The habenula is crucial for experience-dependent modification of fear responses in zebrafish. *Nat. Neurosci.* **2010**, *13*, 1354–1356. [CrossRef] [PubMed]
39. Miklósi, A.; Andrew, R.J. Right eye use associated with decision to bite in zebrafish. *Behav. Brain Res.* **1999**, *105*, 199–205. [CrossRef]
40. Miklósi, A.; Andrew, R.J.; Gasparini, S. Role of right hemifield in visual control of approach to target in zebrafish. *Behav. Brain Res.* **2001**, *122*, 57–65. [CrossRef]

41. Omura, Y.; Oguri, M. Early development of the pineal photoreceptors prior to the retinal differentiation in the embryonic rainbow trout, *Oncorhynchus mykiss* (Teleostei). *Arch. Histol. Cytol.* **1993**, *56*, 283–291. [CrossRef] [PubMed]
42. Östholm, T.; Brännäs, E.; van Veen, T. The pineal organ is the first differentiated light receptor in the embryonic salmon, *Salmo salar* L. *Cell Tissue Res.* **1987**, *249*, 641–646. [CrossRef] [PubMed]
43. Harris, J.A.; Guglielmotti, V.; Bentivoglio, M. Diencephalic asymmetries. *Neurosci. Biobehav. Rev.* **1996**, *20*, 637–643. [CrossRef]
44. Braitenberg, V.; Kemali, M. Exceptions to bilateral symmetry in the epithalamus of lower vertebrates. *J. Comp. Neurol.* **1970**, *138*, 137–146. [CrossRef] [PubMed]
45. Bianco, I.H.; Wilson, S.W. The habenular nuclei: A conserved asymmetric relay station in the vertebrate brain. *Philos. Trans. R. Soc. B Biol. Sci.* **2009**, *364*, 1005–1020. [CrossRef] [PubMed]
46. Gurusinghe, C.J.; Ehrlich, D. Sex-dependent structural asymmetry of the medial habenular nucleus of the chicken brain. *Cell. Tissue Res.* **1985**, *240*, 149–152. [CrossRef] [PubMed]
47. Fejér, Z.; Röhlich, P.; Szél, Á.; Dávid, C.; Zádori, A.; Manzano, M.J.; Vígh, B. Comparative ultrastructure and cytochemistry of the avian pineal organ. *Microsc. Res. Tech.* **2001**, *53*, 12–24. [CrossRef] [PubMed]
48. Vígh, B.; Röhlich, P.; Görcs, T.; Maria, M.J.; Szél, Á.; Fejér, Z.; Vígh-Teichmann, I. The pineal organ as a folded retina: Immunocytochemical localization of opsins. *Biol. Cell* **1998**, *90*, 653–659. [PubMed]
49. Nakane, Y. Intrinsic photosensitivity of a deep brain photoreceptor. *Curr. Biol.* **2014**, *24*, R596–R597. [CrossRef] [PubMed]
50. Nakane, Y.; Ikegami, K.; Ono, H.; Yamamoto, N.; Yoshida, S.; Hirunagi, K.; Ebihara, S.; Kubo, Y.; Yoshimura, T. A mammalian neural tissue opsin (Opsin 5) is a deep brain photoreceptor in birds. *Proc. Natl. Acad. Sci. USA* **2010**, *107*, 15264–15268. [CrossRef] [PubMed]
51. Letzner, S.; Patzke, N.; Verhaal, J.; Manns, M. Shaping a lateralized brain: Asymmetrical light experience modulates access to visual interhemispheric information in pigeons. *Sci. Rep.* **2014**, *4*, 4253. [CrossRef] [PubMed]
52. Del Giudice, M. Alone in the dark? Modeling the conditions for visual experience in human fetuses. *Dev. Psychobiol.* **2011**, *53*, 214–219. [CrossRef] [PubMed]
53. Kiuchi, M.; Nagata, N.; Ikeno, S.; Terakawa, N. The relationship between the response to external light stimulation and behavioral states in the human fetus: How it differs from vibroacoustic stimulation. *Early Hum. Dev.* **2000**, *58*, 153–165. [CrossRef]
54. Geschwind, N.; Galaburda, A.M. *Cerebral Lateralization: Biological Mechanisms, Associations and Pathology*; MIT Press: Cambridge, MA, USA, 1987.
55. Tran, U.S.; Stieger, S.; Voracek, M. Latent variable analysis indicates that seasonal anisotropy accounts for the higher prevalence of left-handedness in men. *Cortex* **2014**, *57*, 188–197. [CrossRef] [PubMed]
56. Andrew, R.J. *Neural and Behavioural Plasticity: The Use of the Domestic Chick as a Model*; Oxford University Press: Oxford, UK, 1991.
57. Vallortigara, G.; Regolin, L.; Zucca, P. Secondary imprinting in the domestic chick: Binocular and lateralized monocular performance. *Int. J. Comp. Psychol.* **2000**, *13*, 119–136.

9

Does Brain Lateralization Affect the Performance in Binary Choice Tasks? A Study in the Animal Model *Danio rerio*

Maria Elena Miletto Petrazzini [1,*], Alessandra Pecunioso [2], Marco Dadda [2] and Christian Agrillo [2,3]

1 Department of Biomedical Sciences, University of Padova, Via Bassi 58-b, 35131 Padova, Italy
2 Department of General Psychology, University of Padova, Via Venezia 8, 35131 Padova, Italy; alessandra.pecunioso@studenti.unipd.it (A.P.); marco.dadda@unipd.it (M.D.); christian.agrillo@unipd.it (C.A.)
3 Padua Neuroscience Center, University of Padova, Via 8 Febbraio 2, 35122 Padova, Italy
* Correspondence: m.e.milettopetrazzini@qmul.ac.uk or mariaelena.milettopetrazzini@gmail.com

Abstract: Researchers in behavioral neuroscience commonly observe the behavior of animal subjects in the presence of two alternative stimuli. However, this type of binary choice introduces a potential confound related to side biases. Understanding whether subjects exhibit this bias, and the origin of it (pre-existent or acquired throughout the experimental sessions), is particularly important to interpreting the results. Here, we tested the hypothesis according to which brain lateralization may influence the emergence of side biases in a well-known model of neuroscience, the zebrafish. As a measure of lateralization, individuals were observed in their spontaneous tendencies to monitor a potential predator with either the left or the right eye. Subjects also underwent an operant conditioning task requiring discrimination between two colors placed on the left–right axis. Although the low performance exhibited in the operant conditioning task prevents firm conclusions from being drawn, a positive correlation was found between the direction of lateralization and the tendency to select the stimulus presented on one specific side (e.g., right). The choice for this preferred side did not change throughout the experimental sessions, meaning that this side bias was not the result of the prolonged training. Overall, our study calls for a wider investigation of pre-existing lateralization biases in animal models to set up methodological counterstrategies to test individuals that do not properly work in a binary choice task with stimuli arranged on the left–right axis.

Keywords: lateralization; side bias; fish; methodological artefacts; symmetry

---

1. Introduction

In the last three decades, an increasing number of studies have been reported in the field of behavioral neuroscience that are based on animal models. The observation of spontaneous behavior assessed through the use of free choice tests [1,2] or the study of learned abilities as a result of operant conditioning studies [3–5] shed light on the perceptual–cognitive mechanisms of vertebrates. For both methodological approaches, animals typically undergo binary choices with stimuli presented on the left–right axis [6–9]. These are usually either two biologically relevant stimuli (e.g., pieces of food or conspecifics, in the case of free choice tests [7,10,11]) or two sets of neutral stimuli (e.g., two-dimensional figures or pictures, in the case of operant conditioning studies [8,9,12]). In both types of studies, it is not rare to find subjects that repeatedly select the stimulus presented on one specific side (e.g., always the right one). This effect is referred to as side bias or side preference [13,14], which is the tendency to select one alternative stimulus over others even though there is not any identified reason, and belongs to the category of idiosyncratic choice biases [15]. Such biases have also been widely observed in human research (e.g., [15]) and may represent a potential confounding factor that affects the conclusions of an experiment. For instance, Andrade et al. [16] found that rats commonly show left or right bias in spontaneous arm preference in a T-maze, a fact that might have impacted the conclusions of several studies on spatial abilities, learning, and memory in rats tested with this type of apparatus. Understanding the reason for a consistent preference for a stimulus placed on the same side of the apparatus is fundamental. A random choice between two stimuli, whose presentation is counterbalanced across trials between left and right, might be due to two opposite reasons: subjects might not have the cognitive abilities to discriminate between the two stimuli, or they might display such cognitive skills but have side biases that prevent the experimenters from testing their hypotheses. Dissociating between these two alternative explanations is necessary for interpreting subjects' performance.

Side biases might have at least two different origins. First, they might be the result of the experimental context. For instance, due to a repeated number of stimulus presentations used in operant conditioning studies, animals might have started to develop a preference for one side of the apparatus (e.g., [17,18]) because this strategy permits obtaining food rewards approximately 50% of the time (avoiding any need to understand which is the discriminative cue between two stimuli). Second, side biases may be present at the onset of the training because of an intrinsic side preference of the subjects [19–23]. Recently, it has been suggested that, at least in human participants, this type of bias might emerge regardless of the peculiarity of the experimental context or procedure, or any kind of pre-existing side preferences of the individuals. By investigating computational models of decision-making, Lebovich et al. [15] found that idiosyncratic choice biases may emerge naturally from the neural circuits underlying decision-making. In this sense, they would represent a virtually inevitable side effect of all binary choice tasks. A recent study requiring rhesus monkeys to choose between two colors by making saccadic movements [24] suggested that when the reward is unpredictable (for instance, when food items are randomly assigned to the two colors), animals may start to exhibit sub-optimal exploratory behaviors, which would be the result of very slow learning, or reward memory, in the attempt to face the unpredictability of non-stationary environments.

Side biases related to the experimental context or procedure can be partially adjusted, for instance, by adopting a correction procedure, such as presenting the target stimulus on the non-preferred side of the subject, to correct their acquired tendency to turn in one direction. On the contrary, side biases related to pre-existing preferences of subjects might be more difficult to modify if stimuli are exclusively arranged on the left–right axis. Therefore, it becomes fundamental to discriminate the type of side bias (spontaneous vs. acquired) observed in a binary choice task.

Intrinsic side bias is believed to be the result of brain lateralization. Functional brain asymmetries were initially thought to be a human peculiarity, but evidence collected in the last few decades has shown that the asymmetries are a widespread principle of nervous system organization. Functional right–left brain asymmetries have been found in a wide range of species [25–31]. For instance, when exploring a predator, some fish species exhibit a preference for monitoring it with a specific eye [32], as a result of a brain specialization that allows them to encode predators' features with one particular side of the brain (the one contralateral to the eye used to inspect the predator). The possibility exists that strongly lateralized individuals are more susceptible to side biases in binary choices than poorly lateralized ones [33].

In the last few decades, the teleost fish *Danio rerio*—also known as zebrafish—has become one of the most adopted models in genetics, neuroscience, and developmental biology [34,35]. Despite the wide range of neurobiological investigations, the cognitive skills of this species remain largely unknown. Only recently, the methodology for the study of cognition in zebrafish has been improved, a fact that permitted the discovery of the existence of numerical [36,37], spatial [38,39], and perceptual [40,41] abilities in this species. Zebrafish also exhibit a wide range of lateralized behaviors, including conspecifics inspection [42], escape response [43], and foraging behavior [44]. However, no study has directly focused on the relation between brain lateralization and side bias in binary choices of this important animal model.

Here, we tested the hypothesis according to which lateralized individuals are more likely to exhibit side biases than poorly lateralized ones in a binary choice test. To achieve this goal, we observed zebrafish behavior in both a spontaneous choice task and an operant conditioning task. To assess the degree of lateralization of subjects, we used a test known as a detour test [32,45,46] that sheds light on the spontaneous preference for the use of one eye (and, hence, one side of the brain) in the presence of a potential predator. The same subjects were observed in a color discrimination task. They were required to discriminate between two rectangles differing in color, one placed on the right and one placed on the left, to obtain a food reward. Unlike many other training studies on cold-blooded vertebrates [47,48], here we used an automated procedure to guarantee extensive training comparable to that used with mammals and birds. This permitted us to establish whether side biases are acquired throughout the experimental sessions because of the prolonged presentation of stimuli. We correlated the behavior in the detour test to the choices for one side of the experimental tank of the color discrimination task to see whether there was any significant link between brain lateralization and performance in the operant conditioning task.

2. Methods

2.1. Subjects

We tested 16 adult zebrafish (9 females, with approximate ages of 8–14 months). Fish were maintained at the comparative psychology laboratory of the Department of General Psychology (University of Padova) in mixed-sex groups of 20–30 individuals (150 L in each tank). The aquaria each had a 14:10 h light to dark (L:D) photoperiod and an 18 W fluorescent light. Aquaria were provided with air filters, natural gravel, and live plants at a temperature of 25 ± 1 °C. Fish were fed daily twice: once with commercial food flakes and once with live brine shrimps (*Artemia salina*). Each subject was singly moved into a 50 × 19 × 32 cm tank in the week preceding our experiment. Four smaller conspecifics were inserted in the tank to reduce the possibility that social isolation might have affected the subjects' behavior in the two tasks. The local ethics committee of the University of Padova approved the study (permit number: 37/2016).

Fish were observed in two different tasks (presented according to a pseudorandom order): (a) a detour test to assess the degree of each subject's lateralization, and (b) a color discrimination task to assess their ability to learn a conditioned rule.

2.2. Lateralization Test: Detour Test

In this test, subjects typically swim along a runway until they encounter a dummy predator behind a barrier (Figure 1). Eye preference—and the corresponding left or right hemisphere that preferentially encodes the potential predator—is inferred by the subject's direction when leaving the runway [17,34,35].

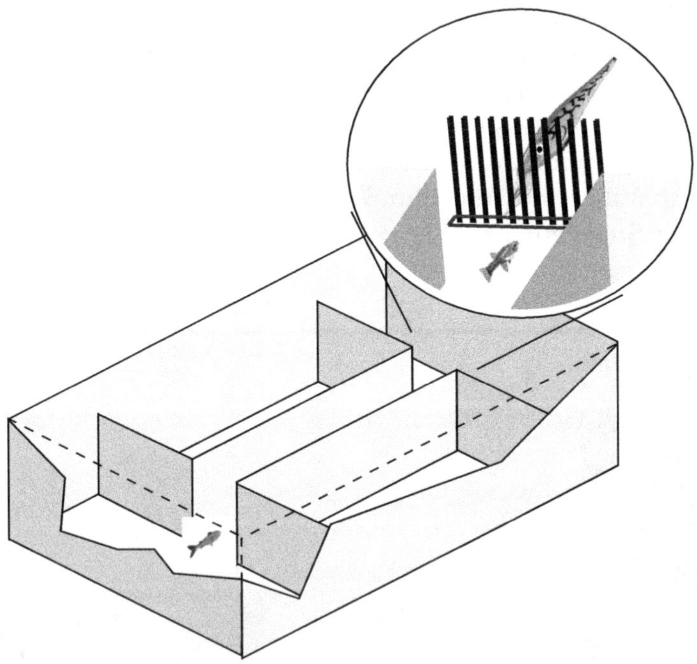

Figure 1. Detour test. A dummy predator was visible behind a barrier at both ends of the runway. The lateralization index was based on 20 observations for each subject.

2.2.1. Stimuli and Apparatus

The apparatus was a modified version used in previous studies of fish [27,33] and consisted of a glass tank (60 × 94 × 36 cm) filled with 10 cm of water. A plastic runway (7 × 40 cm) was placed in the middle, permitting subjects to encounter a barrier. Behind the barrier—a series of vertical yellow cylindrical plastic bars (0.05 cm in diameter, spaced at 0.25 cm intervals) that occupied 17 × 17 cm—a dummy predator (Rapala lure no.18, 18 × 2.5 cm) was visible at both ends of the runway. At the two short sides of the apparatus, we placed two 18 W fluorescent lamps to maximize the visibility of the dummy predators.

2.2.2. Procedure

A single subject was inserted in the middle of the runway. Then, by using a pair of fishnets, the subject was gently pushed toward the starting point. In this way, the subject started to swim along the runway until the dummy predator was visible. We recorded twenty consecutive trials. We used the percentage of left and right turns taken by the subject when leaving the runway as an index of lateralization, based on the following formula: (([number of rightward turns − number of leftward turns]/total number of turns) × 100). This index is a continuous variable and fish with a positive score were classified as subjects with a right detour preference whereas individuals with a negative score were classified as subjects with a left detour preference. In the case of individuals turning rightward half of the time, we classified them as non-lateralized [27,33].

2.3. Color Discrimination Task

Color discrimination tasks are commonly used in operant conditioning studies to assess learning abilities [49–51]. Zebrafish were required to reach the positive stimulus (e.g., a green square), instead of the negative one (e.g., a blue square), to obtain a food reward.

2.3.1. Apparatus and Stimuli

We used an automated operant conditioning apparatus developed for zebrafish (Zantiks AD, Figure 2). The whole unit's size included the experimental chamber (22 × 30 × 50 cm, width × length ×

height), a computer, and the software (C++ language). The chamber (14 × 20 × 15 cm) was made up of white plastic walls; the floor was made of transparent plastic. The chamber was filled with 8 cm of water. A computer screen (16 × 10 cm) placed beneath the tank presented the stimuli in correspondence with one of the short walls. A wireless router allowed us to use a laptop to run the experiment and collect data. The integrated computer automatically detected the subject's position through an infrared camera placed above the chamber and an infrared source placed below the chamber. Zantiks scripts of the task are available in the Supplementary Materials.

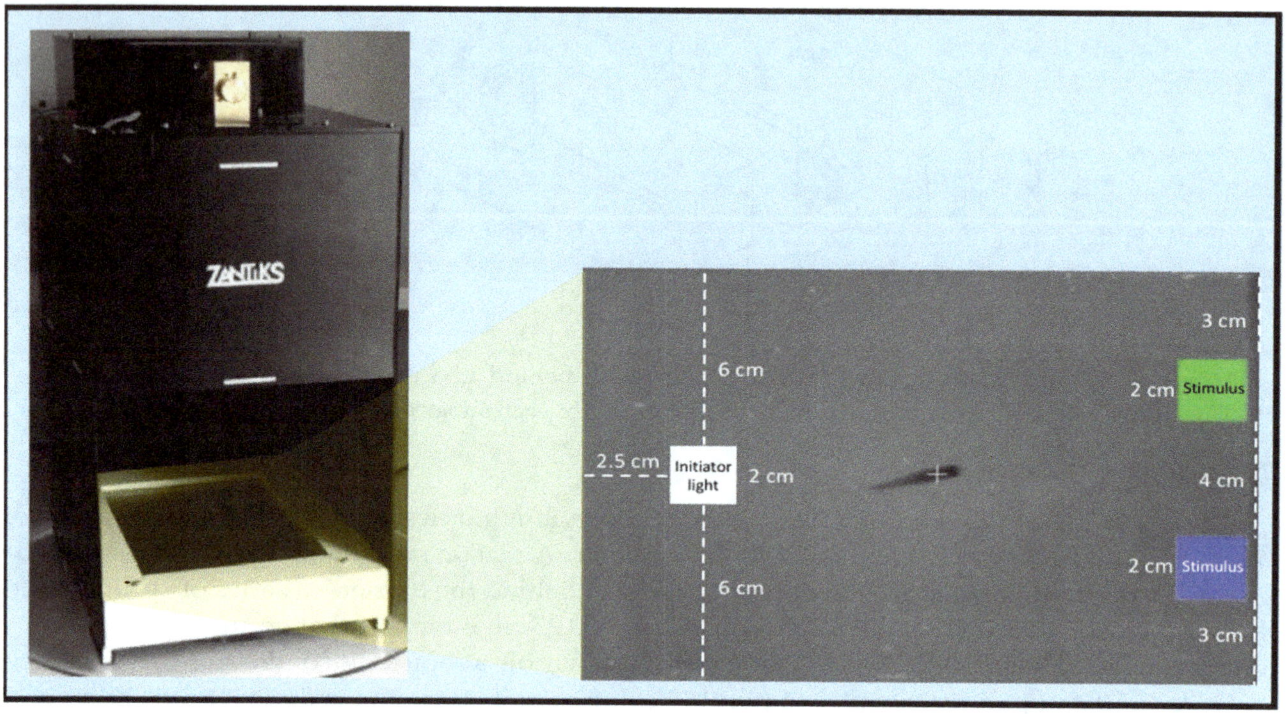

Figure 2. Operant conditioning chamber (Zantiks©) used in the color discrimination task. Stimuli were presented on the bottom of the tank. On the opposite side, we presented two rectangles differing in color (e.g., blue and green). A correct choice triggered the release of a food reward.

Stimuli (2 × 2 cm) consisted of colored rectangles: red (RGB: 255, 0, 0), yellow (RGB: 255, 255, 0), green (RGB: 0, 255, 0), and blue (RGB: 0, 0, 255). An initiator white light rectangle (RGB: 255, 255, 255) appeared at the beginning of each trial.

2.3.2. Procedure

Pre-training: In this stage, we needed to ensure that the zebrafish learned how to trigger the presentation of the stimuli, select one stimulus, and then swim to the feeder and eat the reward. This phase enabled us to eliminate any eventual lack of color discrimination as a general failure to understand the sequence of events composing the trial.

Subjects were moved from their home tanks to the experimental chamber. The pre-training session started after 5 min of habituation and was characterized by 80 overall trials. Each trial started with a white rectangle (2 × 2 cm) that served as an initiator light. This light was presented in correspondence with one short end of the chamber. The initiator light remained visible for a maximum of 10 s; if not selected, the initiator light disappeared for the next 10 s. As soon as a fish approached the initiator light by swimming above the white rectangle, a colored rectangle appeared on the opposite short wall.

In the case of the discrimination of yellow vs. red, the colored rectangle was green; in the case of the discrimination of green vs. blue, the colored rectangle was red. The colored rectangle remained visible for a maximum of 10 s. The food reward consisted of a 2 mg portion of commercial flake food, GVG Sera©, and was released above the initiator light every time the subject swam above the colored light. In the event of no selection of the colored square, the trial was not considered for the analysis and a time-out of 10 s was presented. Subjects completing at least 25 out of 80 trials in a single session started the next step.

Training: Fifty percent of the subjects were trained in yellow and red discrimination (50% with red as a positive stimulus); and 50% of them were trained in blue and green discrimination (50% with blue as a positive stimulus). These specific contrasts were chosen because previous studies showed that zebrafish successfully discriminate between yellow and red, and between blue and green [49].

The experiment was run in a dark environment. As soon as the white initiator light appeared, the trial began. If a fish swam above the light within 10 s, a choice between two different colored squares was given on the opposite side of the tank (see Figure 2 for measures). The interstimulus distance was equal to 4 cm. As the stimuli appeared when subjects triggered the initiator light, placed at 15.5 cm from the stimuli, optical refraction might not have significantly affected the hue, saturation, or brightness of our target colors in any position of the experimental chamber [52]. In the case of the correct choice, we delivered the same food reward used in the pre-training phase in correspondence with the initiator light. On the contrary, if a fish selected the wrong alternative, the two stimuli disappeared, and the bottom of the tank became white until the beginning of next trial. If subjects did not select the initiator light within 10 s, or did not select either stimulus, the stimuli disappeared, and the trial was considered to be an omission. Each training session included 100 trials. The stimulus position on the left–right axis was switched across trials according to a random sequence. The task ended when the fish reached 500 valid trials. (No omissions were included.)

As the data were normally distributed, we used parametric statistics (Kolmogorov–Smirnov on the overall performance of the training, $p = 0.138$).

3. Results

Color discrimination task: a generalized linear mixed model (GLMM) was used to assess whether the performance differed among subjects. A significant inter-individual difference was found ($\chi^2(15) = 529.57$, $p < 0.001$). In particular, binomial tests on the frequency of correct choices showed that 5 subjects out of 16 (31%) selected the color associated with the food reward ($p < 0.05$). No difference in the proportion of choice towards the positive stimulus was found between fish tested in the discrimination between yellow and red and those tested in the discrimination between green and blue (yellow vs. red: 0.424 ± 0.151, blue vs. green: 0.498 ± 0.118; independent t-test, t (14) = −1.096, p = 0.292, d = 0.274). Therefore, we pooled the two groups for the subsequent analyses. To measure whether any side bias emerged throughout the training, we calculated the proportion of choices for the stimulus presented on the right side. The proportion of choice for the stimulus on the right side did not change as a function of trials (repeated measures of ANOVA, Greenhouse–Geisser correction, $F(2.515, 37.719) = 1.788$, $p = 0.173$, partial eta squared $\eta_p^2 = 0.106$, Figure 3), meaning that the repeated presentation of stimuli on the left–right axis did not lead to the development of side biases per se.

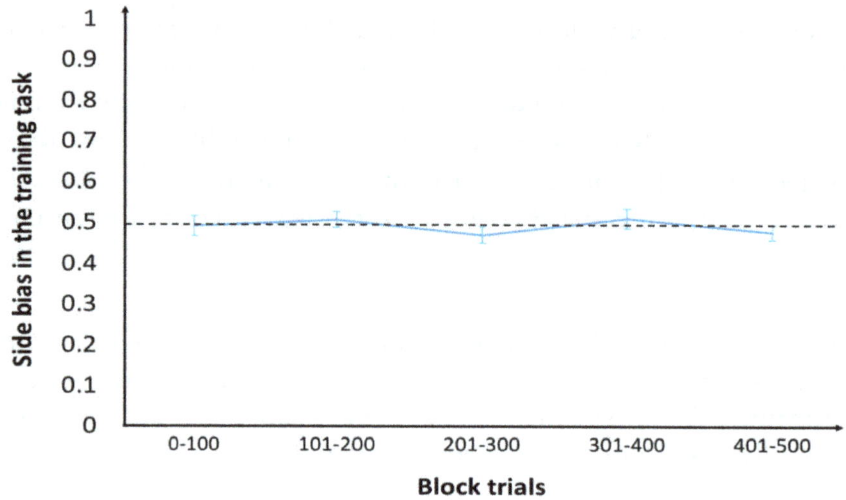

Figure 3. Proportion of choices for the right side of the tank in the color discrimination task. No side bias was developed throughout the 500 trials of the color discrimination task.

Correlation between the detour test and the color discrimination task: a positive correlation was observed between the performance in the detour test and the proportion of choices for the stimulus presented on the right in the color discrimination task (r (14) = 0.921, $p < 0.001$, Bayes factor < 0.001, Figure 4), meaning that the side bias observed in the training task was related to the subject's brain lateralization observed in the detour test. However, no correlation was found between the performance in the detour test and the proportion of correct choices in the training task (r (14) = 0.181, $p = 0.503$, Bayes factor = 4.228, Figure 5), meaning that non-lateralized individuals did not outperform lateralized ones in the present operant conditioning task.

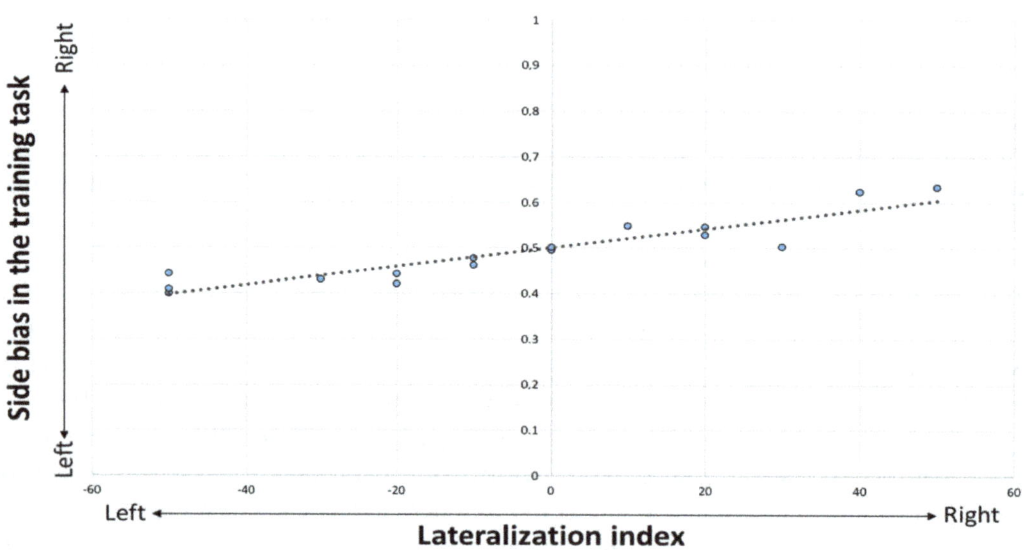

Figure 4. Positive correlation between the lateralization index and the proportion of choices for the right side in the operant conditioning task. Right detour fish tended to select the stimuli of the color discrimination task presented on the right; left detour fish tended to select the opposite stimulus (left).

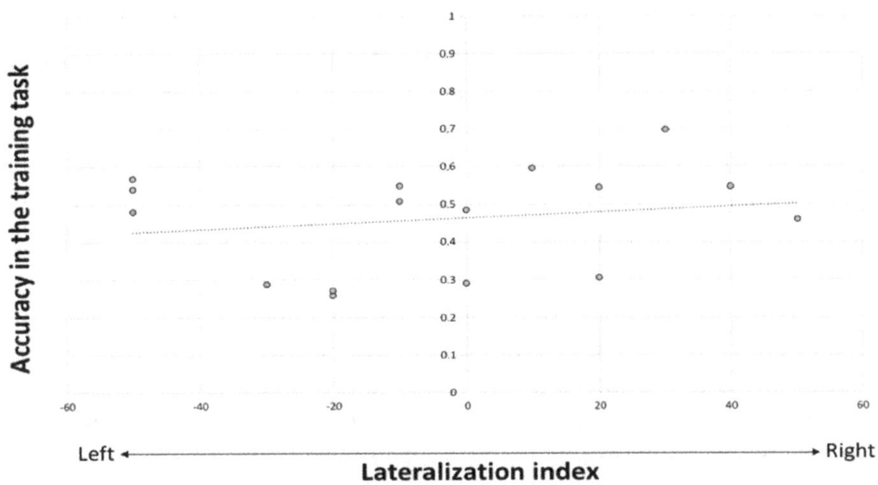

Figure 5. Correlation between the lateralization index and the overall accuracy in the operant conditioning task. Despite a clear side bias of lateralized fish, non-lateralized fish did not statistically outperform lateralized fish.

4. Discussion

We wondered whether brain lateralization impacts the performance of laboratory animals that undergo operant conditioning tasks based on binary choices. To achieve this goal, we used the detour test, one of the most established tests, to assess the direction and degree of brain lateralization, and correlated zebrafish behavior with the performance exhibited in an operant conditioning task requiring selection between one of two colors presented on the left–right axis. We found a strong positive correlation between brain lateralization and the tendency to select repeatedly the stimulus presented on one side of the tank. Our conclusion is supported by two different statistical perspectives: the *p*-value and Bayesian approaches.

Our result has important methodological implications for animal studies based on binary choices. Indeed, most of these studies do not preliminarily assess the degree of hemispheric specialization of their subjects. Therefore, the performance in binary choice tasks may be interpreted because of cognitive abilities or inabilities. We showed that lateralized individuals exhibit this bias from the beginning of the training, a fact that indicates a pre-existing bias rather than an acquired bias developed throughout the trials. Interestingly, we found that zebrafish could not inhibit their tendencies to swim to the preferred side of the experimental chamber even after an extensive training of 500 trials, in which the positive and the negative stimuli were presented randomly on the left–right axis. These subjects may have had the cognitive abilities to solve the color discrimination task, but they might not have been able to perform the correct choice when the correct stimulus was placed on the non-preferred side. This result calls for a cautious interpretation of binary choice tasks, particularly in the case of those studies in which animals are tested only once or twice, such as in free choice tests with subjects observed in their spontaneous preferences for biologically relevant stimuli [53–55]. In this case, it is difficult to establish whether the subjects have a lateralization bias, making data interpretation ambiguous.

The results of our study may be important in behavioral neuroscience because zebrafish are one of the most adopted animal models in genetics, neuroscience, and developmental biology [34,35]. To assess their performance in perceptual–cognitive tasks, many studies used free choice tests [37,43,56] or operant conditioning studies [36,39]. In either case, binary choices are often presented to subjects and the differential performance has been read as the existence of inter-individual variability in the perceptual–cognitive skill under investigation [36,40].

The use of a preliminary test on the brain lateralization of subjects could solve this issue. We suggest two potential solutions. One consists of discarding those subjects who exhibit a robust lateralization bias in the detour test. This would lead to including in the final sample only those fish that could respond to the stimuli. However, this would bring researchers to test a specific subsample of fish: the poorly lateralized ones. There is evidence that strongly and poorly lateralized fish differ for several cognitive factors, including the capacity to perform dual tasks [57], numerical discrimination [58], and spatial tasks [33]. In this sense, testing a sample made by non-lateralized individuals would prevent researchers from generalizing the conclusions to the whole population of zebrafish. Alternatively, detour tests might be useful to identify if there is a large percentage of strongly lateralized individuals. If so, subjects could undergo binary choices with stimuli arranged on the vertical axis (one above and the other below). This experimental strategy, of course, would skip the left–right bias, but could be adopted only after ensuring that the species under investigation does not have a spontaneous preference for selecting a stimulus placed on either the top or bottom of the experimental apparatus (a fact that might represent another side bias that affects the validity of the binary choice tasks).

If strongly lateralized individuals are expected to exhibit strong side bias choice, we should expect non-lateralized individuals to be advantaged in tasks that require learning a discriminative rule between stimuli arranged on the left–right axis. There is indeed evidence that, in some cases, non-lateralized fish outperform lateralized ones; non-lateralized goldbelly topminnows are more accurate when required to bisect a line or to transfer visual information quickly between the two halves of the brain before choosing which shoal to join [33]. We have not found a correlation between the degree of lateralization and the accuracy in the operant conditioning task, but we cannot exclude that an advantage for non-lateralized ones may emerge in other cognitive tasks or other experimental conditions. We must note that a large inter-individual variability in the subjects' performance of the color discrimination task was found, and the overall performance of subjects in our color discrimination task was low. We cannot exclude the possibility that the results of the correlational analyses reported here would not persist in a population of well-trained fish. Developing finer procedures for testing perceptual–cognitive skills in zebrafish is fundamental, given the brain imaging possibilities available in larvae. Such investigation would permit, for instance, mapping behavioral lateralization (such as the one tested here) onto the neural circuits of a zebrafish brain, or to determine neural circuits underlying the emergence of side biases. However, it is worth noting that the subjects' percentage for selecting the positive stimulus at the end of our training (31%) was similar to the percentage of zebrafish reaching the learning criterion in other perceptual–cognitive tasks [36,59]. This suggests that, rather than assuming that our training procedure was largely ineffective in this species, the cognitive skills of this important animal model could barely be shaped by extensive training, compared with other fish species (e.g., guppies [60], redtail splitfins [61], and angelfish [62]).

In conclusion, we found that the behavior exhibited in a test measuring brain lateralization seems to be predictive of the side bias exhibited by zebrafish in binary choices. Lateralized individuals tend to turn to a preferred side of the experimental tank regardless of extensive training, a fact that makes it difficult to understand whether these individuals have the cognitive abilities to solve the task.

Author Contributions: Conceptualization, M.E.M.P. and C.A.; Data curation, A.P.; Funding acquisition, M.E.M.P.; Investigation, M.D; Methodology, A.P.; Writing—original draft, M.E.M.P., A.P., M.D. and C.A. All authors have read and agreed to the published version of the manuscript.

Acknowledgments: We performed the present work within the scope of the research grant Dipartimenti di Eccellenza entitled "Innovative methods or technologies for assessment, intervention, or enhancement of psychological functions (cognitive, emotional or behavioral)".

References

1. Parrish, A.E.; Beran, M.J. When less is more: Like humans, chimpanzees (*Pan troglodytes*) misperceive food amounts based on plate size. *Anim. Cogn.* **2014**, *17*, 427–434. [CrossRef]

2. Lucon-Xiccato, T.; Miletto Petrazzini, M.E.; Agrillo, C.; Bisazza, A. Guppies discriminate between two quantities of food items but prioritize item size over total amount. *Anim. Behav.* **2015**, *107*, 183–191. [CrossRef]
3. Santacà, M.; Agrillo, C. Perception of the Müller—Lyer illusion in guppies. *Curr. Zool.* **2020**, *66*, 205–213. [CrossRef] [PubMed]
4. Cantlon, J.; Brannon, E. Basic math in monkeys and collegestudents. *PLoS Biol.* **2007**, *5*, e328. [CrossRef] [PubMed]
5. Sovrano, V.A.; Bisazza, A.; Vallortigara, G. Modularity as a fish (*Xenotoca eiseni*) views it: Conjoining geometric and nongeometric information for spatial reorientation. *J. Exp. Psych. Anim. Behav. Proc.* **2003**, *29*, 199–210. [CrossRef] [PubMed]
6. Robins, A.; Rogers, L.J. Complementary and lateralized forms of processing in *Bufo marinus* for novel and familiar prey. *Neurobiol. Learn. Mem.* **2006**, *86*, 214–227. [CrossRef] [PubMed]
7. Giljov, A.N.; Karenina, K.A.; Malashichev, Y.B. An eye for a worm: Lateralisation of feeding behaviour in aquatic anamniotes. *Laterality* **2009**, *14*, 273–286. [CrossRef]
8. Peirce, J.W.; Leigh, A.E.; Kendrick, K.M. Configurational coding, familiarity and the right hemisphere advantage for face recognition in sheep. *Neuropsychologia* **2000**, *38*, 475–483. [CrossRef]
9. Bortot, M.; Agrillo, C.; Avarguès-Weber, A.; Bisazza, A.; Miletto Petrazzini, M.E.; Giurfa, M. Honeybees use absolute rather than relative numerosity in number discrimination. *Biol. Lett.* **2019**, *15*, 20190138. [CrossRef]
10. Adámková, J.; Svoboda, J.; Benediktová, K.; Martini, S.; Nováková, P.; Tůma, D.; Burda, H. Directional preference in dogs: Laterality and "pull of the north". *PLoS ONE* **2017**, *12*, e0185243. [CrossRef]
11. Bisazza, A.; De Santi, A.; Bonso, S.; Sovrano, V.A. Frogs and toads in front of a mirror: Lateralisation of response to social stimuli in tadpoles of five anuran species. *Behav. Brain Res.* **2002**, *134*, 417–424. [CrossRef]
12. Santacà, M.; Agrillo, C. Two halves are less than the whole: Evidence of a length bisection bias in fish (*Poecilia reticulata*). *PLoS ONE* **2020**, *15*, e0233157. [CrossRef]
13. Gierszewski, S.; Bleckmann, H.; Schluessel, V. Cognitive abilities in Malawi cichlids (*Pseudotropheus* sp.): Matching-to-sample and image/mirror-image discriminations. *PLoS ONE* **2013**, *8*, e57363. [CrossRef] [PubMed]
14. Kuba, M.J.; Byrne, R.A.; Burghardt, G.M. A new method for studying problem solving and tool use in stingrays (*Potamotrygon castexi*). *Anim. Cogn.* **2010**, *13*, 507–513. [CrossRef] [PubMed]
15. Lebovich, L.; Darshan, R.; Lavi, Y.; Hansel, D.; Loewenstein, Y. Idiosyncratic choice bias naturally emerges from intrinsic stochasticity in neuronal dynamics. *Nat. Hum. Behav.* **2019**, *3*, 1190–1202. [CrossRef]
16. Andrade, C.; Alwarshetty, M.; Sudha, S.J.; Suresh Chandra, J. Effect of innate direction bias on T-maze learning in rats: Implications for research. *J. Neurosci. Methods* **2001**, *110*, 31–35. [CrossRef]
17. Danisman, E.; Bshary, R.; Bergmüller, R. Do cleaner fish learn to feed against their preference in a reverse reward contingency task? *Anim. Cogn.* **2010**, *13*, 41–49. [CrossRef] [PubMed]
18. Agrillo, C.; Parrish, A.E.; Beran, M.J. Do primates see the solitaire illusion differently? A comparative assessment of humans (*Homo sapiens*), chimpanzees (*Pan troglodytes*), rhesus mon-keys (*Macaca mulatta*), and capuchin monkeys (*Cebus apella*). *J. Comp. Psychol.* **2014**, *128*, 402–413. [CrossRef]
19. Alves, C.; Chichery, R.; Boal, J.G.; Dickel, L. Orientation in the cuttlefish *Sepia officinalis*: Response versus place learning. *Anim. Cogn.* **2007**, *10*, 29–36. [CrossRef]
20. Miletto Petrazzini, M.E.; Wynne, C.D. What counts for dogs (*Canis lupus familiaris*) in a quantity discrimination task? *Behav. Proc.* **2016**, *122*, 90–97. [CrossRef]
21. Miletto Petrazzini, M.E.; Mantese, F.; Prato Previde, E. Food quantity discrimination in puppies (*Canis lupus familiaris*). *Anim. Cogn.* **2020**, *23*, 703–710. [CrossRef] [PubMed]
22. Collins, R.L. When left-handed mice live in right-handed world. *Science* **1975**, *187*, 181–184. [CrossRef] [PubMed]
23. Ayroles, J.F.; Buchanan, S.M.; O'Leary, C.; Skutt-Kakaria, K.; Grenier, J.K.; Clark, A.G.; Hartl, D.L.; de Bivort, B.L. Behavioral idiosyncrasy reveals genetic control of phenotypic variability. *Proc. Natl. Acad. Sci. USA* **2015**, *112*, 6706–6711. [CrossRef] [PubMed]
24. Iigaya, K.; Ahmadian, Y.; Sugrue, L.P.; Corrado, G.S.; Loewenstein, Y.; Newsome, W.T.; Fusi, S. Deviation from the matching law reflects an optimal strategy involving learning over multiple timescales. *Nat. Commun.* **2019**, *10*, 1466. [CrossRef]

25. Frasnelli, E.; Ponte, G.; Vallortigara, G.; Fiorito, G. Visual lateralization in the cephalopod mollusk *Octopus vulgaris*. *Symmetry* **2019**, *11*, 1121. [CrossRef]
26. Regaiolli, B.; Spiezo, C.; Hopkins, W.D. Asymmetries in mother-infant behaviour in Barbary macaques (*Macaca sylvanus*). *PeerJ* **2018**, *6*, e4736. [CrossRef]
27. Dadda, M.; Agrillo, C.; Bisazza, A.; Brown, C. Laterality enhances numerical skills in the guppy, *Poecilia reticulata*. *Front. Behav. Neurosci.* **2015**, *9*, 285. [CrossRef]
28. Bisazza, A.; Rogers, L.J.; Vallortigara, G. The origins of cerebral asymmetry: A review of evidence of behavioural and brain lateralization in fishes, reptiles and amphibians. *Neurosci. Biobehav. Rev.* **1998**, *22*, 411–426. [CrossRef]
29. Güntürkün, O.; Ströckens, F.; Ocklenburg, S. Brain lateralization: A comparative perspective. *Physiol. Rev.* **2020**, *100*, 1019–1063. [CrossRef]
30. Ströckens, F.; Güntürkün, O.; Ocklenburg, S. Limb preferences in non-human vertebrates. *Laterality* **2013**, *18*, 536–575. [CrossRef]
31. Versace, E.; Caffini, M.; Werkhoven, Z.; de Bivort, B. Individual, but not population asymmetries, are modulated by social environment and genotype in *Drosophila melanogaster*. *Sci. Rep.* **2020**, *10*, 4480. [CrossRef] [PubMed]
32. Miletto Petrazzini, M.E.; Sovrano, V.; Vallortigara, G.; Messina, A. Brain and behavioral asymmetry: A lesson from fish. *Front. Neuroanat.* **2020**, *14*, 11. [CrossRef] [PubMed]
33. Dadda, M.; Zandonà, E.; Agrillo, C.; Bisazza, A. The costs of hemispheric specialization in a fish. *Proc. R. Soc. B Biol. Sci.* **2009**, *276*, 4399–4407. [CrossRef] [PubMed]
34. Bandmann, O.; Burton, E.A. Genetic zebrafish models of neurodege-nerative diseases. *Neurobiol. Dis.* **2010**, *40*, 58–65. [CrossRef] [PubMed]
35. Langenau, D.M.; Zon, L.I. The zebrafish: A new model of T-cell and thymic development. *Nat. Rev.* **2005**, *5*, 307–317. [CrossRef] [PubMed]
36. Agrillo, C.; Miletto Petrazzini, M.E.; Tagliapietra, C.; Bisazza, A. Inter-specific differences in numerical abilities among teleost fish. *Front. Psychol.* **2012**, *3*, 483. [CrossRef]
37. Potrich, D.; Sovrano, V.A.; Stancher, G.; Vallortigara, G. Quantity discrimination by zebrafish (*Danio rerio*). *J. Comp. Psychol.* **2015**, *129*, 388–393. [CrossRef]
38. Potrich, D.; Rugani, R.; Sovrano, V.A.; Regolin, L.; Vallortigara, G. Use of numerical and spatial information in ordinal counting by zebrafish. *Sci. Rep.* **2019**, *9*, 18323. [CrossRef]
39. Baratti, G.; Potrich, D.; Sovrano, V.A. The environmental geometry in spatial learning by zebrafish (*Danio rerio*). *Zebrafish* **2020**, *17*, 131–138. [CrossRef]
40. Gori, S.; Agrillo, C.; Dadda, M.; Bisazza, A. Do fish perceive illusory motion. *Sci. Rep.* **2014**, *4*, 6443. [CrossRef]
41. Santacà, M.; Lucon-Xiccato, T.; Agrillo, C. The Delboeuf illusion's bias in food choice of teleost fishes: An interspecific study. *Anim. Behav.* **2020**, *164*, 105–112. [CrossRef]
42. Facchin, L.; Burgess, H.A.; Siddiqi, M.; Granato, M.; Halpern, M.E. Determining the function of zebrafish epithalamic asymmetry. *Philos. Trans. R. Soc. B Biol. Sci.* **2009**, *364*, 1021–1032. [CrossRef] [PubMed]
43. Stennett, C.R.; Strauss, R.E. Behavioural lateralization in zebrafish and four related species of minnows (Osteichthyes: *Cyprinidae*). *Anim. Behav.* **2010**, *79*, 1339–1342. [CrossRef]
44. Hata, H.; Hori, M. Inheritance patterns of morphological laterality in mouth opening of zebrafish, *Danio rerio*. *Laterality* **2001**, *17*, 741–754. [CrossRef]
45. Brown, C.; Western, J.; Braithwaite, V.A. The influence of early experience on, and inheritance of cerebral lateralization. *Anim. Behav.* **2007**, *74*, 231–238. [CrossRef]
46. Domenici, P.; Allan, B.; McCormick, M.I.; Munday, P.L. Elevated carbon dioxide affects behavioural lateralization in a coral reef fish. *Biol. Lett.* **2012**, *8*, 78–81. [CrossRef]
47. Sovrano, V.A.; Bisazza, A.; Vallortigara, G. Modularity and spatial reorientation in a simple mind: Encoding of geometric and nongeometric properties of a spatial environment by fish. *Cognition* **2002**, *85*, B51–B59. [CrossRef]
48. Agrillo, C.; Miletto Petrazzini, M.E.; Bisazza, A. Numerical abilities in fish: A methodological review. *Behav. Proc.* **2007**, *141*, 161–171. [CrossRef]
49. Oliveira, J.; Silveira, M.; Chacon, D.; Luchiari, A. The zebrafish world of colors and shapes: Preference and discrimination. *Zebrafish* **2015**, *12*, 166–173. [CrossRef]

50. Savage, A.; Dronzek, L.A.; Snowden, C.T. Color discrimination by the cotton-top tamarin (*Saguinus oedipus oedipus*) and its relation to fruit coloration. *Folia Primatol.* **1987**, *49*, 57–69. [CrossRef]
51. Giurfa, M. Conditioning procedure and color discrimination in the honeybee *Apis mellifera*. *Naturwissenschaften* **2004**, *91*, 228–231. [CrossRef] [PubMed]
52. Dunn, T.W.; Fitzgerald, J.E. Correcting for physical distortions in visual stimuli improves reproducibility in zebrafish neuroscience. *eLife* **2020**, *9*, e53684. [CrossRef] [PubMed]
53. Uller, C.; Lewis, J. Horses (*Equus caballus*) select the greater of two quantities in small numerical contrasts. *Anim. Cogn.* **2009**, *12*, 733–738. [CrossRef] [PubMed]
54. Bánszegi, O.; Urrutia, A.; Szenczi, P.; Hudson, R. More or less: Spontaneous quantity discrimination in the domestic cat. *Anim. Cogn.* **2016**, *19*, 879–888. [CrossRef] [PubMed]
55. Uller, C.; Jaeger, R.; Guidry, G.; Martin, C. Salamanders (*Plethodon cinereus*) go for more: Rudiments of number in an amphibian. *Anim. Cogn.* **2003**, *6*, 105–112. [CrossRef]
56. Pritchard, V.L.; Lawrence, J.; Butlin, R.K.; Krause, J. Shoal size in zebrafish, *Danio rerio*: The influence of shoal size and activity. *Anim. Behav.* **2001**, *62*, 1085–1088. [CrossRef]
57. Dadda, M.; Bisazza, A. Does brain asymmetry allow efficient performance of two simultaneous tasks? *Anim. Behav.* **2006**, *72*, 523–529. [CrossRef]
58. Gatto, E.; Agrillo, C.; Brown, C.; Dadda, M. Individual differences in numerical skills are influenced by brain lateralization in guppies (*Poecilia reticulata*). *Intelligence* **2019**, *74*, 12–17. [CrossRef]
59. Gatto, E.; Lucon-Xiccato, T.; Bisazza, A.; Manabe, K.; Dadda, M. The devil is in the detail: Zebrafish learn to discriminate visual stimuli only if salient. *Behav. Proc.*. under review.
60. Bisazza, A.; Agrillo, C.; Lucon-Xiccato, T. Extensive training extends numerical abilities of guppies. *Anim. Cogn.* **2014**, *7*, 1413–1419. [CrossRef]
61. Sovrano, V.A.; Bisazza, A. Perception of subjective contours in fish. *Perception* **2009**, *38*, 579–590. [CrossRef] [PubMed]
62. Miletto Petrazzini, M.E.; Agrillo, C.; Izard, V.; Bisazza, A. Do humans (*Homo sapiens*) and fish (*Pterophyllum scalare*) make similar numerosity judgments? *J. Comp. Psychol.* **2016**, *130*, 380–390. [CrossRef] [PubMed]

10

Effects of Handedness and Viewpoint on the Imitation of Origami-Making

Natalie Uomini [1] and Rebecca Lawson [2,*]

1 Department of Linguistic and Cultural Evolution, Max Planck Institute for the Science of Human History, Kahlaische Strasse 10, 07745 Jena, Germany; traduck@gmail.com
2 School of Psychology, University of Liverpool, Eleanor Rathbone Building, Bedford Street South, Liverpool L69 7ZA, UK
* Correspondence: rlawson@liv.ac.uk

Abstract: The evolutionary origins of the human bias for 85% right-handedness are obscure. The Apprenticeship Complexity Theory states that the increasing difficulty of acquiring stone tool-making and other manual skills in the Pleistocene favoured learners whose hand preference matched that of their teachers. Furthermore, learning from a viewing position opposite, rather than beside, the demonstrator might be harder because it requires more mental transformation. We varied handedness and viewpoint in a bimanual learning task. Thirty-two participants reproduced folding asymmetric origami figures as demonstrated by a videotaped teacher in four conditions (left-handed teacher opposite the learner, left-handed beside, right-handed opposite, or right-handed beside). Learning performance was measured by time to complete each figure, number of video pauses and rewinds, and similarity of copies to the target shape. There was no effect of handedness or viewpoint on imitation learning. However, participants preferred to produce figures with the same asymmetry as demonstrated, indicating they imitate the teacher's hand preference. We speculate that learning by imitation involves internalising motor representations and that, to facilitate learning by imitation, many motor actions can be flexibly executed using the demonstrated hand configuration. We conclude that matching hand preferences evolved due to socially learning moderately complex bimanual skills.

Keywords: social learning; imitation; handedness; laterality; origami; evolution

1. Introduction

Handedness is a behavioural lateralization, defined as a species-level bias to use a certain hand configuration for most tasks. It is expressed in *Homo sapiens* as a species-universal behavioural bias (70–90%) towards using the right hand for fine manipulations and the left hand for stabilising actions [1–3]. Among vertebrates, 61 species (out of 119 measured) show population-level limb preferences, of which 25 species are mammals, 30 birds, and 6 amphibians, reptiles, and fish [4]. Some other animal species also have behavioural hand biases up to 90% at the species level [5–8], and many other species have individually stable hand preferences [9,10]. However, within our evolutionary clade, humans are the only great ape that shows strong, species-universal biases towards one direction of handedness. Non-human great ape hand preferences are characterized by high variability in their direction and a low magnitude of expression [4,11]. In particular, humans have much higher ratios of the dominant to non-dominant hand preference, compared to other apes [4,11,12]. Among the other great apes there are groups of individuals with a majority of right-handers, but there are also groups with a majority of left-handers [13]. In contrast, despite much cross-cultural research, no human group has been found with more than 30% left-handers [14]. The origins of handedness probably lie in brain lateralization [7]. The advantages to having lateralized brain functions, not only in the direction of laterality, but also in the strength of laterality, are ubiquitous in vertebrates [4,15]. In that case, we should ask why other ape species who engage in bimanual manipulations do not show a universal bias to either right- or left-handedness.

The obvious question concerning this bias to right-handedness is why most humans are lateralized in the same direction. Our recent ancestors had a similar majority of right-handers as today, judging by the proportion of right and left handprints and hand stencils in cave art [16,17]. Data on older, prehistoric handedness, from asymmetries in fossil brain endocasts, arm bones, and tooth cut-marks, show that 67–69% of hominins between 3 million and 30,000 years ago were right-handed with only 5–11% left-handed [18–20]. Interestingly, the same data also show a rate of 12% mixed-handedness in Neanderthals (a parallel species with whom we share a common ancestral species around 600,000 years ago). In contrast, present-day estimates for our species are around 4% mixed-handers [21,22]. Thus, *Homo sapiens* is characterised by a reduction of mixed-handers, and an equivalent increase in right-handers, compared to the Neanderthals.

A possible evolutionary driver of this directional bias in *Homo sapiens* is given by the Apprenticeship Complexity Theory [13,23,24]. This emphasizes the importance of the social learning environment of prehistoric hominins as they acquired complex tool manipulations [25]. It [26,27] proposes that group-level handedness biases in humans evolved to facilitate faster learning through imitation of complex tool manufacture. Stone tool-making changed over time towards requiring longer sequences and more subgoals, from the pre-Oldowan to the Late Acheulean [24,28,29]. Throughout the Pleistocene, as stone crafts and other essential survival tasks increased in difficulty, so did the pressure on children to learn those skills [24]. According to the Apprenticeship Complexity Theory, selective pressure for learning efficiently (i.e., quickly and accurately) favoured learners whose hand preference matched that of their teachers. This pressure was probably a factor for all individuals given that, for example, the archaeological evidence suggests that, for most of hominin prehistory, functional stone knapping skills were learned by all individuals in a group; the emergence of craft specialisation was a very recent invention linked to artistic production, reduced mobility, and complexification of human societies from the Mesolithic and Neolithic onward [30–35].

The nature of the social learning environment can also affect the efficiency of skill transmission. There is a broad spectrum of social learning strategies across human cultures and across animal species, ranging from unsupervised observation to interactive teaching [36–41]. Prehistoric hominins could have used any of these learning strategies [28,42–44]. Before the emergence of teaching, hominin children would have engaged in social learning through observation. Imitation is a form of observational learning that does not involve any teacher input, where the learner copies the actions of others.

Imitation is often seen as a goal-directed process involving knowledge and understanding on the part of the learner, rather than merely copying of a sequence of actions. Imitation requires learners to form an internal representation of the teacher's action sequence in order to reproduce it [45,46]. This action representation involves the mirror neuron system in Broca's area [47,48]. Imitation also relies on the learners' ability to adopt the visual perspective of others, in order to understand their actions [49–51]. Children's learning by imitation in various human societies has a wide range of forms [52] such as helping with daily tasks [53] or third-party observation [40]. The learner's position with respect to the demonstrator(s) will vary in different situations. For example, for participatory tasks, such as hunting, the child is most likely to be behind, or alongside, the demonstrator. In contrast, during observatory tasks, such as basket weaving, the child is more likely to be opposite, facing the demonstrator.

Viewing position during imitation tasks has attracted particular focus due to the transformation of visual perspective required to map between the reference frame of the imitator and the demonstrator [46]. When positioned beside a demonstrator (egocentric viewpoint), the observer's viewpoint matches that of the demonstrator. In this case no mental transformation is needed to interpret the demonstrated action. However, when positioned opposite a demonstrator (allocentric viewpoint), the observer must compensate for the discrepancy between their viewpoint and that of the demonstrator. In this case a mental transformation of the input may be necessary, regardless of hand preferences. The brain processes actions differently depending on whether they are observed from beside, versus opposite, the viewer, with greater activation in the contralateral hemisphere in the former case but the ipsilateral hemisphere in the latter case [54], and with greater activity in the sensory-motor system in the former than the latter case [55]. In addition, visual object recognition is affected by the object's orientation [56,57]. People are better at action prediction for images of tools viewed from the perspective that they would see when using them [58]. Furthermore, in haptic (active touch) tasks, recognition is easier when objects are explored from the orientation typically used to manipulate them ([59], but see [60]). However, none of the previous studies on viewpoint also tested the interaction with handedness. In sum, there is some evidence showing that imitation is harder if there is a discrepancy in viewpoint that needs to be compensated for (though such viewpoint effects have not always been observed; for example, as described below, Reference [61] found no difference in an observer's ability to reproduce knot-tying dependent on their viewpoint). Furthermore, it is not known how handedness might affect the mental transformation required to process different viewpoints.

The Apprenticeship Complexity Theory predicts that the transmission of complex tasks is more efficient when the demonstrator and learner have the same hand preference. We define "complexity" here as motoric and conceptual difficulty, reflected in the learning time needed to acquire the skill [62]. In this sense, higher complexity is found in tasks with long learning times, narrow error tolerances, many components, and/or many steps in a sequence [63–65]. In particular, complementary bimanual tasks with asynchronous digit use rank high on the manipulative complexity scale [66] and thus are excellent models for testing the interplay of handedness and learning. We expected that folding origami, as used in the present study, would be a good example of such a task.

Previous research on handedness and skill learning is very limited. Two studies found that a congruent hand preference between the demonstrator and observer resulted in more efficient learning than incongruent hand preferences. Reference [27] taught knot-tying to groups of right-handed and left-handed observers, with right- and left-handed demonstrators. They showed faster learning from same-handed demonstrators in both groups. Similarly, Reference [67] showed that same-hand demonstrations result in higher accuracy and speed for targeted hand movements than opposite-hand demonstrations (in right-handed observers). In early child development, imitation of the demonstrators' hand configuration is apparent. Infants are heavily influenced by the demonstrator's hand used when manipulating objects. When tested experimentally, although most infants showed right-hand preferences when first grasping an object, an action demonstrated by a left-handed researcher led all infants to subsequently use their left hand [68]. However, object recognition in the haptic modality is not affected by the hand used to explore the object, which suggests a constancy in object representations that generalises across the hands [60]. Thus, more work is needed to determine how learning and handedness are related.

Few studies have tested the effect of viewpoint on imitation. Reference [69] showed that imitation of body movements is easier when standing behind a teacher rather than opposite a teacher. Reference [70] found more accurate mirror imitation of body movements when the teacher faced the observer. Two other studies used a knot-tying task where participants reproduced knots after viewing demonstrations from different visual angles. Consistent with the body movement studies, Reference [71] showed that knots demonstrated in videos were learned more effectively if the teacher was shown from a position beside, rather than opposite to, the learner. Another study [61] used live knot-tying demonstrations from three different viewpoints (beside, opposite, and at right angles to the demonstrator) and found no difference in the mean number of trials to successfully replicate each knot. Reference [61] did, though, find that participants preferred to reduce the discrepancy in viewing angles by sitting beside the demonstrator when given the choice. These conflicting results mean that more work is needed to determine when viewpoint affects the learning of complex bimanual skills.

In order to disentangle the variables of hand preference and viewpoint on the acquisition of manual skills, we conducted a bimanual learning study involving making origami. We chose origami folding because it is a complex task that has been used in previous studies of learning [41,72,73]. Origami has several important advantages over "live" stone tool-making experiments: (1) the starting raw materials can be perfectly controlled so that all participants receive identical blank origami papers; (2) people already possess the motor skill to fold paper, so they can concentrate on learning the folding sequence, which was the focus of our experiment; (3) folding origami is clean and safe and does not require special equipment; (4) our experiment is reproducible by any scientist, not just the few who have access to specialist flint knapping resources. Following the method of [74], we showed participants demonstration videos of a teacher making nine different origami figures ranging from easy to hard. Learners were required to reproduce each figure by imitating the demonstrated actions. We manipulated the videos to show left-handed and right-handed teachers, and for the teachers to have either the same perspective as the participant (beside view) or a 180-degree rotated perspective (opposite view). We predicted that demonstrations of the origami figures would be harder to imitate if they showed an incongruent hand configuration, and if they showed the teacher opposite, rather than beside, the learner.

2. Materials and Methods

2.1. Participants

We recruited thirty-two participants (9 male) aged between 18 and 22 years. Participants were University of Liverpool undergraduate students, with no restriction on hand preference. All subjects gave their informed consent before they participated in the study. The study was conducted in accordance with the Declaration of Helsinki, and the protocol was approved by the Ethics Committee of the University of Liverpool (Project identification code PSYC-1011-075).

2.2. Stimuli

Videos were created demonstrating nine asymmetric origami figures being folded. A right-handed teacher folded all of the origami figures using a 21 cm^2 piece of orange paper. The teacher was video recorded from above, at a height of 42 cm from the desk (see Supplementary Video S1 for full videos). Four versions of each of these nine videos were created varying the hand configuration and viewpoint. Following [74], we rotated each video 180 degrees in the picture plane to create the alternate viewing positions and mirror-flipped the video to create a left-handed version in both viewpoints (Figure 1). The camera was placed directly above the teacher's hands to ensure both that the same visual information was available for the two viewing positions and that both viewing positions could occur in actual viewing (this would not be the case if an angled camera angle had been used).

The first video shown to participants was an easy practice stimulus and it was the only one that required the use of scissors. Each participant created all eight origami figures once. They created two figures in each of the four viewpoint conditions (Left-Handed Opposite, Left-Handed Beside, Right-Handed Opposite, and Right-Handed Beside), so that each participant received all conditions. The assignment of the two figures to each condition, and the order of presentation of conditions, was counterbalanced using a Latin Square procedure to reduce order effects. Two participants were assigned to each of the 16 counterbalancing conditions.

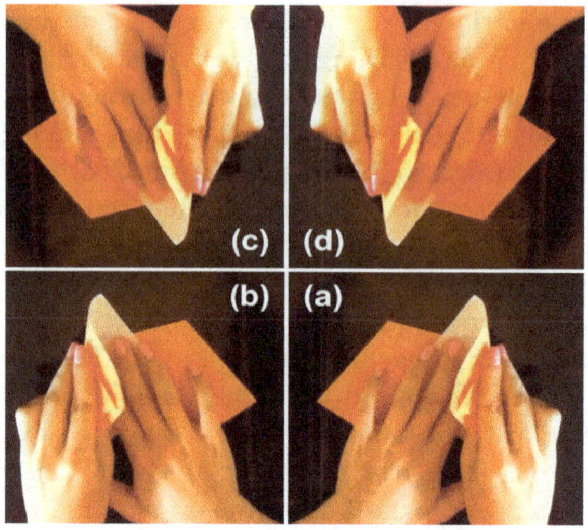

Figure 1. Still images from each of the four conditions created for the "Fish" video showing (**a**) right-handed beside; (**b**) left-handed beside; (**c**) left-handed opposite; and (**d**) right-handed opposite teachers.

2.3. Procedure

Participants initially read an information sheet that stressed that they had to reproduce the origami figures as similarly as possible to the example shown in the video. They were not informed about the different experimental conditions. Participants were given nine 21 cm^2 pieces of paper (one was orange for the practice trial; with two red, yellow, purple, and green papers each assigned to each experimental condition). The demonstration videos were presented to participants on an Apple MacBook Pro 13" using QuickTime player. Participants were free to interact with the video while they reproduced the figures, by pausing with the pause button, and rewinding by dragging the progress bar backwards.

Participants were first shown the practice demonstration video. After the practice reproduction, any queries were resolved before the experiment began. Participants then did the eight experimental trials. While participants were watching the demonstration videos, the experimenter discreetly recorded the number of times the video was paused and was rewound, and also recorded the time taken to complete the figure, using a stopwatch.

After all nine figures were completed, participants were asked a series of questions:

1. Do you know what the experiment is testing?
2. Did you notice anything about the position of the hands in the videos?
3. Did you notice anything about the hands themselves in the videos?
4. Did you find any of the trials particularly hard?

Participants then completed a Short Form Edinburgh Handedness Inventory [75].

2.4. Analyses

Performance at origami folding was coded with respect to preferred hand dominance. For left-handed participants, left-handed demonstrations were coded as congruent and right-handed demonstrations as incongruent. The reverse coding was used for right-handed and mixed-handed participants. We included mixed-handers in the right-handed category because they all had positive scores (range +25 to +62.5) on the Short Form Edinburgh Handedness Inventory (left-handers had scores ranging from −50 to −100). Since human hand performance is not categorical but rather on a continuum [76], we focus here on hand preference, that is, the categorical choice of hand dominance when doing a task.

The efficiency of reproducing origami figures was measured in two ways: first, the time taken to complete the figure divided by the length of the demonstration video; second, the total number of pauses and rewinds for each video.

The accuracy of reproducing origami figures was also measured in two ways. First, subjective ratings were made of the completed origami figures. Two naïve raters who did not take part in the experiment independently rated the similarity of the produced origami figures to the originals. As training, the two raters were initially shown all 32 practice figures and were asked to rate these using the full scale from 1 for figures which looked 'unlike the original' to 10 for figures which looked 'exactly like the original'. Zero was given to incomplete figures. Raters were required to assign at least three figures to each number on the scale to ensure that they used the full scale. Raters then rated each set of eight experimental figures created by each participant using the same scale. The eight demonstration figures were laid out in front of them together with the set of eight figures from one participant. After completing ratings for all 32 participants, the figures from the first two participants that they had rated were re-presented (without informing the raters) for rating to check for the stability of ratings. The raters completed their ratings of participants in reverse orders with respect to each other.

Second, the experimenter recorded the symmetry of all eight figures produced by each of the 32 subjects in turn. Each figure was categorised as having matching asymmetry to the original (MA), having the opposite asymmetry to the original (OA), as being incorrectly folded to be symmetrical rather asymmetrical (IS), or as being uncodeable due to the poor quality of the reproduction.

3. Results

The Short Form Edinburgh Handedness Inventory scores revealed three left-handed participants (scores -100 to -50), five mixed-handers (scores +25 to +62.5), and 24 right-handed participants (scores +75 to +100). Our sample was similar to the usual human distribution of hand dominance with 9% left-handed, 16% mixed and 75% right-handed participants.

Participants were asked questions prior to debrief in order to assess whether they were aware of the aims of the experiment. None of the 32 participants reported the correct overall aims of the experiment. When prompted, only two participants had noticed that the hand configurations in the video changed in some way, and only three noticed that the viewpoint of demonstrations changed.

For the subjective ratings of figures' similarity to originals, inter-rater reliability between the two raters revealed a fair agreement between the two raters, k = 0.35 ($p < 0.001$), 95% CI (0.414, 0.284), as well as moderate agreement within rater 1, k = 0.56, ($p < 0.001$), and substantial agreement within rater 2, k = 0.64, ($p < 0.001$).

3.1. Effect of Viewpoint and Handedness of Demonstrator on the Efficiency of Making Origami Figures

The data were analysed using an ANOVA with two within-subjects variables, viewpoint (Beside or Opposite) and handedness of demonstrator relative to the participant (Congruent, where, for example, a right-handed participant watched a right-handed demonstrator; or Incongruent, where, for example, a left-handed participant watched a right-handed demonstrator) and reaction time as the dependent variable. There was no effect of viewpoint, $F(1,31) = 0.06$, $p = 0.8$, partial $\eta^2 = 0.002$, with similar time to complete figures for Beside (Mean = 231 s, SD = 10.9) and Opposite (Mean = 225 s, SD = 10.2) videos. There was also no effect of handedness, $F(1,31) = 1.16$, $p = 0.3$, partial $\eta^2 = 0.04$, with similar time for Congruent handedness (Mean = 227 s, SD = 10.9) and Incongruent handedness (Mean = 229 s, SD = 11.66) videos. Finally, there was no interaction between viewpoint and handedness, $F(1,31) = 0.35$, $p = 0.6$, partial $\eta^2 = 0.01$.

Repeating this ANOVA using the sum of pauses and rewinds as the dependent variable revealed the same pattern of results. Again, there was no effect of viewpoint, $F(1,31) = 0.07$, $p = 0.8$, partial $\eta^2 = 0.002$, with a similar number of pauses and rewinds for Beside (Mean = 7.9, SD = 0.53) and Opposite (Mean = 7.8, SD = 0.66) videos. There was also no effect of handedness, $F(1,31) = 0.40$, $p = 0.5$, partial $\eta^2 = 0.01$, with a similar number of pauses and rewinds for Congruent handedness

(Mean = 7.7, SD = 0.59) and Incongruent handedness (Mean = 8.1, SD = 0.67) videos. Finally, there was no interaction between viewpoint and handedness, $F(1,31) = 0.03$, $p = 0.9$, partial $\eta^2 = 0.001$.

3.2. *Effect of Viewpoint and Handedness of Demonstrator on the Accuracy of Making Origami Figures*

The ANOVA was repeated with ratings of accuracy of reproduction of the origami figure as the dependent variable. Here, there was no effect of viewpoint, $F(1,31) = 3.06$, $p = 0.09$, partial $\eta^2 = 0.09$, with similar ratings for figures produced from Beside (Mean = 6.2, SD = 0.37) and Opposite (Mean = 5.8, SD = 0.44) videos. There was also no effect of handedness, $F(1,31) = 1.46$, $p = 0.2$, partial $\eta^2 = 0.05$, with similar ratings for figures in the Congruent handedness (Mean = 6.2, SD = 0.42) and Incongruent handedness (Mean = 5.8, SD = 0.42) conditions. Finally, there was no interaction between viewpoint and handedness, $F(1,31) = 0.002$, $p = 0.9$, partial $\eta^2 = 0.00$.

3.3. *Check That Results Were Not Influenced by the Inclusion of Participants Who Were Not Right-Handed*

In order to ascertain that the results reported above were not contaminated by the inclusion of the three left-handed participants and five mixed-handed participants, these three ANOVAs were repeated but only including the 24 right-handed participants. These ANOVAs produced the same pattern of results, with no signficant main effects of viewpoint or of handedness congruency and no significant interactions between these two factors.

3.4. *Analysis of Symmetry of Reproduced Origami Figures*

Participants produced similar numbers of figures with matching asymmetry to the original (MA; 90 figures, 35%), as figures with the reverse asymmetry to the original (RA; 76 figures, 30%). The remainder of figures were incorrectly reproduced as symmetrical (IS; 30 figures, 12%) or were too poorly reproduced to be coded (60 figures, 23%). The IS and uncodeable responses occurred at similar rates across the four conditions (5–10/condition for IS; 13–17/condition for uncodeable).

Of primary interest was the proportion of figures produced with matching (MA) versus reverse (RA) asymmetry across the four conditions. Considering only these two types of responses, for the Beside viewpoint, when handedness was congruent, as expected most figures had matching asymmetry (MA = 38/46 responses, 83%). Critically, when handedness was incongruent, most figures continued to have matching asymmetry (MA = 29/40 responses; 73%). Thus participants continued to fold using the same hand configuration as the teacher even when the teacher had the opposite handedness as them. A similar, but weaker, pattern occurred for the Opposite viewpoint. Here, when handedness was congruent most figures had, as expected, matching asymmetry (MA = 26/39 responses, 67%). Crucially, when handedness was incongruent most figures again continued to have matching asymmetry (MA = 26/41 responses; 63%). Thus people usually used the same hand configuration to fold as shown by the teacher, whether or not the teacher had the same hand preference as them, with this preference being rather weaker for demonstrations shown from the Opposite viewpoint.

4. Discussion

Contrary to our predictions, there was no effect on performance of either viewing position of the participant relative to the teacher or of handedness of the participant relative to the teacher. Performance was assessed in terms of efficiency of reproduction of each figure, as measured both by the amount of time taken to complete the figures and by the number of pauses and rewinds of the demonstration videos needed to finish the figures. Performance was also assessed in terms of the quality of reproduction of each figure using subjective ratings of the figures' similarity to the originals and coding of the asymmetry of each figure relative to that of the original.

Our experiment provides no evidence for an effect of viewing position on performance, with no difference between viewing demonstration videos from the same visual perspective as the demonstrator, or from a 180 degree rotated viewpoint. This result is in line with [61] who found that a change in viewing position did not perturb imitation performance. It goes against [56], that visual object recognition is faster for objects viewed from a beside orientation. One possible explanation is that our participants were able to interpret the opposite viewpoints by mentally rotating their body relative to the object, rather than by mentally rotating the origami figures themselves. Mental object rotation is more difficult than mental body rotation [77] and is more sensitive to angle of rotation. Therefore, it is possible that people imitate origami folding using the easier strategy of copying the hand movements, rather than by trying to reproduce the shape of the origami figures directly. Future work could test this by investigating whether viewpoint affects performance in the visual recognition of origami figures. In addition, for our video stimuli we elected to use the overhead view, rather than the angled views that would be more characteristic of live demonstrations, in order to better control for visual differences across the four conditions. It is possible that an angled view would give learners a stronger cue to the differences in hand configurations, as most of our participants did not notice any change in the hands between conditions. Again, this possibility could be tested in future studies.

Our results also show that participants were no more efficient at completing the task when observing the folding demonstration by the congruent-handed teacher compared to the incongruent-handed teacher. This contradicts previous studies by [27,67] which both showed improved learning with congruent handedness. Our study is, instead, consistent with the results of [58] that handedness congruence had no effect on performance in a tool action prediction task. Our findings are also in line with [60], who suggest that handedness does not affect object representations. Further support for this conclusion comes from the analysis of the asymmetry of the figures produced. This indicated that participants preferred to fold using the hand configuration demonstrated by the teacher whether or not the teacher had the same hand preference as them. We do not know if participants achieved matching symmetry in origami figures by imitating the teacher's hand configuration itself, or by imitating the direction of folding only. Future work could test this directly by video-recording the participants to see exactly how their hands move during the task. Follow-up studies should also recruit more left-handed and mixed-handed participants in order to test a balanced sample of groups with a range of hand dominances.

We interpret our findings as indicative that learning by imitation involves internalising observed motor representations in order to execute them, as [78] found in their study of brain activation during imitation of Mousterian stone knapping actions. An earlier study [73], presented origami folding instructions as a sequence of written instructions with pictures of the folding shown from the Beside viewpoint. They found that when people learn to fold origami from such pictorial-verbal instructions, they creatively interpret the instructions by reformulating them into spatial terms and adding information. Hand configurations were not specified in this study, but the direction of folding was (e.g., "fold the tip diagonally to the left"). They measured folding success by subjective ratings of figure similarity, and found that people who read fewer instructions aloud were more successful [73]. This result suggests that internalising visual representations is a key process in action imitation [78], and that verbal instructions can actually hinder learning. During learning by imitation alone, as in the present study, no explicit teaching occurred and there were no verbal instructions, so the learner was not instructed to use a particular hand configuration. In this case, the internalised motor representations allowed the learner to use any hand configuration. Our results suggest that these motor representations are hand-independent, consistent with what has previously been found by [60]. This enabled learners to flexibly match their hand preference to that used by the demonstrator.

Our finding that incongruent handedness between demonstrator and learner did not affect performance, was thus, we argue, because learners effectively preferred to remove the handedness incongruence by adopting the hand configuration of the demonstrator. Support for this claim comes from our finding that learners preferentially produced origami figures that matched the direction of asymmetry demonstrated by incongruent-handed teachers. The conflicting results found in previous studies could be explained by participants finding it harder to reproduce stimuli created by incongruent-handed teachers, but being able to compensate for this by changing their handedness to be congruent with that of the teacher.

If, as we have suggested, the preferred configuration of hand use is flexible when people learn a complex bimanual task, this indicates that social learning by imitation can be a powerful determinant of handedness. Despite having established hand preferences, our adult participants behaved the same as the infants in [68] who imitated the hand configuration of the demonstrator. We speculate that an ability to facilitate learning by rapidly and temporarily adopting a demonstrator's hand configuration evolved due to the pressure for efficient social learning of complex tasks. Similarly, [79] proposed that hominins were the only species who engaged in sufficiently complex manual tasks to trigger the expression of a handedness bias.

Our evolutionary scenario is as follows: prior to the evolution of complex tool manufacture, hand preferences were evenly distributed among human populations, as is the case in other species of living apes, which we take to reflect the ancestral condition. Thus, some groups would have had a left-hand bias, some groups a right-hand bias, and other groups no bias. During social learning of simple skills such as many foraging tasks like picking fruit or pounding nuts, there was no need to conform to any particular hand configuration. This was because the tasks were simple enough to allow easy mental transformations so that each individual could use their preferred hand. This situation still exists among non-human apes. We propose that human imitation of manual skills began to require congruent handedness only once a certain level of tool complexity was reached. At this stage, learners found it beneficial to flexibly adopt the hand configuration of their teachers, in order to minimise the difficulties of mental transformation for such tasks.

Importantly, if, as we have argued, learners can efficiently imitate their teacher's hand preference, then we would have no reason to expect a drive for dominance of any particular hand preference. Thus, our species-level directional bias towards right-handedness still needs to be explained. We suggest that a combination of, first, functional brain laterality and, second, task expertise effects could be the evolutionary driver for the dominance of right-handedness in *Homo sapiens*.

First, regarding brain laterality, the two brain hemispheres have specialised, complementary roles in controlling the contralateral hand and arm [2]. Evidence from vertebrate lateralization indicates an evolutionarily ancient hemispheric specialisation was already in place before the hominin lineage emerged [5,79,80]. We believe the persistence of 10% left-handers in humans today is due to both a minority advantage in combat (Fighting Hypothesis) [20] and to atypical functional brain lateralization patterns which occur naturally in the population [81].

Second, this hemispheric specialisation could be critical when undertaking a highly complex bimanual task such as stone tool-making. Specifically, the brain's motor control specialisations mean that typically the dominant (right) arm controls movement direction and shape, while the non-dominant (left) arm maintains a stable position [2,82,83]. During direct, hand-held percussion for stone tool-making, these are precisely the bimanual complementary roles required of the two hands [13,17]. The non-dominant hand firmly holds the stone core at an appropriate angle while the dominant hand strikes the core with a fast, accurate, aimed motion. In this task, the hand role differentiation is extreme. In contrast, our origami task required quite similar and sometimes overlapping roles for the two hands. It is likely that the behavioural asymmetries were not salient in this task, as evidenced by the fact that most participants did not notice the change in conditions. Furthermore, the differentiation in difficulty between the motor skill required to, for example, hold the paper flat on the table (typical for the non-dominant hand) while folding one corner (typical for the dominant hand) was much less than for stone tool-making. In addition, task learning is much faster, in part because there is ongoing visual feedback and the error tolerances are much wider than in stone knapping. We suggest that the relative difficulty of the movements required by the two hands during origami-making is likely not enough to cause differential activation of the brain's hemispheric specialisations, as previously proposed by [7]. In contrast, given that the acquisition of stone tool-making skills was both essential for survival and very difficult, we speculate that the most efficient learning strategy used the brain's existing hemispheric specialisations. For example, archaeological evidence from Neanderthals living 80,000 years ago, at the site of Buhlen in Germany, suggests that they experienced childhood pressure to become right-handed through social learning of extremely difficult "Keilmesser" stone tool manufacturing techniques [84].

We thus argue that the level and nature of manual expertise required to master a task may be crucial in determining whether the handedness of a demonstrator influences task performance. In experimental psychology, origami-folding and knot-tying are considered complex tasks. Indeed, 23% of origami figures produced by our participants were poorly formed, indicating that the task was challenging. However, humans can learn to reproduce a particular knot or origami figure in about an hour. For this type of task, flexible imitation of incongruent handers may be sufficient to support successful performance. In contrast, proficient Oldowan stone knapping needs weeks of practice and most stone tool types take years to master [85–87]. While the basic gestures and concepts of stone tool production can be learned in an hour with active teaching ([42], N. Uomini pers. obs.), learning this task by imitation alone is much less efficient [28]. The non-verbal social learning of stone knapping skills requires close attention to fine details of hand postures, stone core geometry, selection of where to strike, and striking direction and speed. It is likely that these essential details are easier to perceive and to reproduce when watching a congruent hander. This prediction could be tested by measuring the frequency of handedness congruence between masters and their apprentices learning modern-day crafts such as stone carving (we are not aware of any published data).

Our experimental findings are consistent with the evolution of concordant hand preferences due to social learning by imitation of complex bimanual skills such as stone tool manufacture. In our study, learners flexibly adapted their hand configuration to match that of the demonstrator, resulting in no decrease of performance for the incongruent-handedness conditions or from viewpoints requiring mental transformation. This result partly supports the Apprenticeship Complexity Theory, at least for origami imitation. We suggest that our origami task was not sufficiently challenging to cause obligate use of the brain's preferred right/left hand specialisations. As a consequence, using an incongruent hand configuration did not disrupt learning. Future work should focus on acquiring difficult craft skills that require extended learning periods and precise motor control. This would allow a check of whether there is a cost to incongruent-handedness and viewpoint on more complex and ecologically valid tasks. More work is also needed to establish how objects are represented during tool creation tasks that require mental transformation, particularly for difficult sequential bimanual actions such as stone knapping.

Acknowledgments: We thank Gabriella Strazzanti for testing the participants reported in this study. This research was supported by the University of Liverpool School of Psychology and the Department of Linguistic and Cultural Evolution, Max Planck Institute for the Science of Human History, Jena. We thank 3 anonymous reviewers for constructive comments on previous drafts, and Bill McGrew and Nele Zickert for discussions. We are grateful to Lesley Rogers for ideas and the invitation to participate in this special issue. Open access publication fees paid by the Max Planck Society.

Author Contributions: R.L. conceived and designed the study and analyzed the data; N.U. and R.L. wrote the paper based on a report by Gabriella Strazzanti.

References

1. Cavanagh, T.; Berbesque, J.C.; Wood, B.; Marlowe, F. Hadza handedness: Lateralized behaviors in a contemporary hunter–gatherer population. *Evolut. Hum. Behav.* **2016**, *37*, 202–209. [CrossRef]
2. Mutha, P.K.; Haaland, K.Y.; Sainburg, R.L. Rethinking motor lateralization: Specialized but complementary mechanisms for motor control of each arm. *PLoS ONE* **2013**, *8*, e58582. [CrossRef] [PubMed]
3. Uomini, N.T. Paleoneurology and behaviour. In *Human Paleoneurology*; Bruner, E., Ed.; Springer: Berlin, Germany, 2014; pp. 121–144.

4. Ströckens, F.; Güntürkün, O.; Ocklenburg, S. Limb preferences in non-human vertebrates. *Laterality* **2013**, *18*, 536–575. [CrossRef] [PubMed]
5. Rogers, L.J.; Andrew, R.J. *Comparative Vertebrate Lateralization*; Cambridge University Press: Cambridge, UK, 2002.
6. Rogers, L.J.; Zucca, P.; Vallortigara, G. Advantages of having a lateralized brain. *Proc. R. Soc. B* **2004**, *271*, S420–S422. [CrossRef] [PubMed]
7. Rogers, L.J. Hand and paw preferences in relation to the lateralized brain. *Philos. Trans. R. Soc. Lond. B* **2009**, *364*, 943–954. [CrossRef] [PubMed]
8. MacNeilage, P.F. Evolution of the strongest vertebrate rightward action asymmetries: Marine mammal sidedness and human handedness. *Psychol. Bull.* **2014**, *140*, 587–609. [CrossRef] [PubMed]
9. Versace, E.; Vallortigara, G. Forelimb preferences in human beings and other species: Multiple models for testing hypotheses on lateralization. *Front. Psychol.* **2015**, *6*, 233. [CrossRef] [PubMed]
10. Karenina, K.; Giljov, A.; Ingram, J.; Rowntree, V.J.; Malashichev, Y. Lateralization of mother-infant interactions in a diverse range of mammal species. *Nat. Ecol. Evolut.* **2017**, *1*, 0030. [CrossRef] [PubMed]
11. Hopkins, W.D.; Phillips, K.A.; Bania, A.; Calcutt, S.E.; Gardner, M.; Russell, J.; Schaeffer, J.; Lonsdorf, E.V.; Ross, S.R.; Schapiro, S.J. Hand preferences for coordinated bimanual actions in 777 great apes: Implications for the evolution of handedness in hominins. *J. Hum. Evolut.* **2011**, *60*, 605–611. [CrossRef] [PubMed]
12. Neufuss, J.; Humle, T.; Cremaschi, A.; Kivell, T.L. Nut-cracking behaviour in wild-born, rehabilitated bonobos (*Pan paniscus*): A comprehensive study of hand-preference, hand grips and efficiency. *Am. J. Primatol.* **2017**, *79*, 1–16. [CrossRef] [PubMed]
13. Uomini, N.T. The prehistory of handedness: Archaeological data and comparative ethology. *J. Hum. Evolut.* **2009**, *57*, 411–419. [CrossRef] [PubMed]
14. Raymond, M.; Pontier, D. Is there geographical variation in human handedness? *Laterality* **2004**, *9*, 35–51. [CrossRef] [PubMed]
15. Rogers, L.J. A matter of degree: Strength of brain asymmetry and behaviour. *Symmetry* **2017**, *9*, 57. [CrossRef]
16. Faurie, C.; Raymond, M. Handedness frequency over more than ten thousand years. *Proc. R. Soc. Lond. B* **2004**, *271*, S43–S45. [CrossRef] [PubMed]
17. Steele, J.; Uomini, N. Humans, tools and handedness. In *Stone knapping: The Necessary Conditions for a Uniquely Hominid Behaviour*; Roux, V., Bril, B., Eds.; McDonald Institute for Archaeological Research: Cambridge, UK, 2005; pp. 217–239.
18. Faurie, C.; Uomini, N.; Raymond, M. Origins, development and persistence of laterality in humans. In *Laterality in Sports: Theories and Applications*; Hagemann, N., Strauss, B., MacMahon, C., Loffing, F., Eds.; Elsevier: San Diego, CA, USA, 2016; pp. 11–30.
19. Frayer, D.W.; Clarke, R.J.; Fiore, I.; Blumenschine, R.J.; Pérez-Pérez, A.; Martinez, L.M.; Estebaranz, F.; Holloway, R.; Bondioli, L. OH-65: The earliest evidence for right-handedness in the fossil record. *J. Hum. Evolut.* **2016**, *100*, 65–72. [CrossRef] [PubMed]
20. Lozano, M.; Bermúdez de Castro, J.M.; Arsuaga, J.L.; Carbonell, E. Diachronic analysis of cultural dental wear at the Atapuerca sites (Spain). *Quat. Int.* **2017**, *433*, 243–250. [CrossRef]
21. McManus, I.C. The history and geography of human handedness. In *Language Lateralization and Psychosis*; Sommer, I.E.C., Kahn, R.S., Eds.; Cambridge University Press: Cambridge, UK, 2009; pp. 37–57.
22. Vuoksimaa, E.; Koskenvuoa, M.; Rosea, R.J.; Kaprioa, J. Origins of handedness: A nationwide study of 30,161 adults. *Neuropsychologia* **2009**, *47*, 1294–1301. [CrossRef] [PubMed]
23. Uomini, N.T. Prehistoric left-handers and prehistoric language. In *The Emergence of Cognitive Abilities: The Contribution of Neuropsychology to Archaeology*; de Beaune, S.A., Coolidge, F.L., Eds.; Cambridge University Press: Cambridge, UK, 2009; pp. 37–55.
24. Högberg, A.; Gärdenfors, P.; Larsson, L. Knowing, learning and teaching—How *Homo* became *Docens*. *Camb. Archaeol. J.* **2015**, *25*, 847–858. [CrossRef]
25. Legare, C.H.; Nielsen, M. Imitation and innovation: The dual engines of cultural learning. *Trends Cogn. Sci.* **2015**, *19*, 688–699. [CrossRef] [PubMed]
26. Bradshaw, J.L.; Nettleton, N.C. Language lateralization to the dominant hemisphere: Tool use, gesture and language in hominid evolution. *Curr. Psychol.* **1982**, *2*, 171–192. [CrossRef]
27. Michel, G.F.; Harkins, D.A. Concordance of handedness between teacher and student facilitates learning manual skills. *J. Hum. Evolut.* **1985**, *14*, 597–601. [CrossRef]

28. Bamforth, D.B.; Finlay, N. Archaeological approaches to lithic production skill and craft learning. *J. Archaeol. Method Theory* **2008**, *15*, 1–27. [CrossRef]
29. Eigeland, L. No man is an island. *Lithic Technol.* **2011**, *36*, 127–140. [CrossRef]
30. Hurcombe, L. Time, skill and craft specialization as gender relations. In *Gender and Material Culture in Archaeological Perspective*; Donald, M., Hurcombe, L., Eds.; Palgrave Macmillan: Basingstoke, UK, 2000; pp. 88–109.
31. Olausson, D.J. Different strokes for different folks: Possible reasons for variation in quality of knapping. *Lithic Technol.* **1998**, *23*, 90–115. [CrossRef]
32. Olausson, D.J. Does practice make perfect? Craft expertise as a factor in aggrandizer strategies. *J. Archaeol. Method Theory* **2008**, *15*, 28–50. [CrossRef]
33. Sternke, F. Stuck between a rock and hard place. *Lithic Technol.* **2011**, *36*, 221–236. [CrossRef]
34. Morgan, T.J.H.; Uomini, N.T.; Rendell, L.E.; Chouinard-Thuly, L.; Street, S.E.; Lewis, H.M.; Cross, C.P.; Evans, C.; Kearney, R.; de la Torre, I.; et al. Experimental evidence for the co-evolution of hominin tool-making teaching and language. *Nat. Commun.* **2015**, *6*, 6029. [CrossRef] [PubMed]
35. Pelegrin, J.; Roche, H. L'humanisation au prisme des pierres taillées. *Comptes Rendus Palevol* **2017**, *16*, 175–181. [CrossRef]
36. Byrne, R.W.; Rapaport, L.G. What are we learning from teaching? *Anim. Behav.* **2011**, *82*, 1207–1211. [CrossRef]
37. Fryling, M.J.; Johnston, C.; Hayes, L.J. Understanding observational learning: An interbehavioural approach. *Anal. Verbal Behav.* **2011**, *27*, 191–203. [CrossRef] [PubMed]
38. Garfield, Z.H.; Garfield, M.J.; Hewlett, B.S. A cross-cultural analysis of hunter-gatherer social learning. In *Social Learning and Innovation in Contemporary Hunter-Gatherers*; Terashima, H., Hewlett, B.S., Eds.; Springer: Tokyo, Japan, 2016; pp. 19–34.
39. Hewlett, B.S.; Roulette, C.J. Teaching in hunter–gatherer infancy. *R. Soc. Open Sci.* **2016**, *3*, 150403. [CrossRef] [PubMed]
40. Legare, C.H.; Harris, P.L. The ontogeny of cultural learning. *Child Dev.* **2016**, *87*, 633–642. [CrossRef] [PubMed]
41. Mejía-Arauz, R.; Rogoff, B.; Paradise, R. Cultural variation in children's observation during a demonstration. *Int. J. Behav. Dev.* **2005**, *29*, 282–291. [CrossRef]
42. Ohnuma, K.; Aoki, K.; Akazawa, T. Transmission of tool-making through verbal and non-verbal communication—Preliminary experiments in Levallois flake production. *Anthropol. Sci.* **1997**, *105*, 159–168. [CrossRef]
43. Putt, S.S.; Woods, A.D.; Franciscus, R.G. The role of verbal interaction during experimental bifacial stone tool manufacture. *Lithic Technol.* **2014**, *39*, 96–112. [CrossRef]
44. Putt, S.S.; Wijeakumar, S.; Franciscus, R.G.; Spencer, J.P. The functional brain networks that underlie Early Stone Age tool manufacture. *Nat. Hum. Behav.* **2017**, *1*, 0102. [CrossRef]
45. Nishitani, N.; Avikainen, S.; Hari, R. Abnormal imitation-related cortical activation sequences in asperger's syndrome. *Am. Neurol. Assoc.* **2004**, *55*, 558–562. [CrossRef] [PubMed]
46. Whiten, A.; Ham, R. On the nature and evolution of imitation in the animal kingdom: Reappraisal of a century of research. In *Advances in the Study of Behaviour*; Slater, P.J.B., Rosenblatt, J.S., Beer, C., Milinski, M., Eds.; Academic Press: San Diego, CA, USA, 1992; pp. 239–283.
47. Heiser, M.; Lacoboni, M.; Maeda, F.; Marcus, J.; Mazziotta, C. The essential role of Broca's area in imitation. *Eur. J. Neurosci.* **2003**, *17*, 1123–1128. [CrossRef] [PubMed]
48. Liepelt, R.; Cramon, D.; Yves, V.; Brass, M. What is matched in direct matching? Intention attribution modulates motor priming. *J. Exp. Psychol.* **2008**, *34*, 587–591. [CrossRef] [PubMed]
49. Bellagamba, F.; Camaioni, L.; Colonnesi, C. Change in children's understanding of others' intentional actions. *Dev. Sci.* **2006**, *9*, 182–188. [CrossRef] [PubMed]
50. Byrne, R.W. *The Thinking Ape*; Oxford University Press: Oxford, UK, 1995.
51. Huang, C.; Heyes, C.; Charman, T. Preschoolers' behavioural reenactment of "failed attempts": The roles of intention-reading, emulation and mimicry. *Cogn. Dev.* **2006**, *21*, 36–45. [CrossRef]
52. Rogoff, B. *The Cultural Nature of Human Development*; Oxford University Press: New York, NY, USA, 2003.
53. Paradise, R.; Rogoff, B. Side by side: Learning by observing and pitching in. *Ethos* **2009**, *37*, 102–138. [CrossRef]

54. Shmuelof, L.; Zohary, E. Mirror-image representation of action in the anterior parietal cortex. *Nat. Neurosci.* **2008**, *11*, 1267–1269. [CrossRef] [PubMed]
55. Campanella, F.; Sandini, G.; Morrone, M.C. Visual information gleaned by observing grasping movement in allocentric and egocentric perspectives. *Proc. R. Soc. Lond. B* **2011**, *278*, 2142–2149. [CrossRef] [PubMed]
56. Lawson, R. Achieving visual object constancy over plane rotation and depth rotation. *Acta Psychol.* **1999**, *102*, 221–245. [CrossRef]
57. Lawson, R. A comparison of the effects of depth rotation on visual and haptic three- dimensional object recognition. *J. Exp. Psychol.* **2009**, *35*, 911–930. [CrossRef] [PubMed]
58. Kelly, R.L.; Wheaton, L.A. Differential mechanisms of action understanding in left and right-handed subjects: The role of perspective and handedness. *Front. Psychol.* **2013**, *4*, 957. [CrossRef] [PubMed]
59. Lawson, R.; Ajvani, H.; Cecchetto, S. Effects of line separation and exploration on the visual and haptic detection of symmetry and repetition. *Exp. Psychol.* **2016**, *63*, 197–214. [CrossRef] [PubMed]
60. Craddock, M.; Lawson, R. Do left and right matter for haptic recognition of familiar objects? *Perception* **2009**, *38*, 1355–1376. [CrossRef] [PubMed]
61. Sambrook, T.D. Does visual perspective matter in imitation? *Perception* **1998**, *27*, 1461–1473. [CrossRef] [PubMed]
62. Sinclair, A. All in a day's work? Early conflicts in expertise, life history and time management. In *Settlement, Society and Cognition in Human Evolution*; Coward, F., Hosfield, R., Pope, M., Wenban-Smith, F., Eds.; Cambridge University Press: Cambridge, UK, 2015; pp. 94–116.
63. Byrne, R.W.; Byrne, J.M. Hand preferences in the skilled gathering tasks of mountain gorillas (*Gorilla g. berengei*). *Cortex* **1991**, *27*, 521–546. [CrossRef]
64. Rugg, G. Quantifying technological innovation. *Palaeonthropology* **2011**, 154–165.
65. Sambrook, T.; Whiten, A. On the nature of complexity in cognitive and behavioural science. *Theory Psychol.* **1997**, *7*, 191–213. [CrossRef]
66. Heldstab, S.A.; Kosonen, Z.K.; Koski, S.E.; Burkart, J.M.; van Schaik, C.P.; Isler, K. Manipulation complexity in primates coevolved with brain size and terrestriality. *Sci. Rep.* **2016**, *6*, 24528. [CrossRef] [PubMed]
67. Rohbanfard, H.; Proteau, L. Effects of the model's handedness and observer's viewpoint on observational learning. *Exp. Brain Res.* **2011**, *214*, 567–576. [CrossRef] [PubMed]
68. Fagard, J.; Lemoine, C. The role of imitation in the stabilization of handedness during infancy. *J. Integr. Neurosci.* **2006**, *5*, 519–533. [CrossRef] [PubMed]
69. Ishikura, T.; Inomata, K. Effects of angle of model-demonstration on learning motor skill. *Percept. Motor Skills* **1995**, *80*, 651–658. [CrossRef] [PubMed]
70. Press, C.; Ray, E.; Heyes, C. Imitation of lateralised body movements: Doing it the hard way. *Laterality* **2009**, *14*, 515–527. [CrossRef] [PubMed]
71. Roshal, S.M. Film-mediated learning with varying representation of the task: Viewing angle, portrayal of demonstration, motion, and student participation. In *Student Response in Programmed Instruction*; Lumsdaine, A.A., Ed.; National Academy of Sciences—National Research Council: Washington, DC, USA, 1961; pp. 107–128.
72. Andreass, B. Origami art as a means of facilitating learning. *Procedia Soc. Behav. Sci.* **2011**, *11*, 32–36. [CrossRef]
73. Tenbrink, T.; Taylor, H.A. Conceptual transformation and cognitive processes in origami paper folding. *J. Probl. Solving* **2015**, *8*, 1. [CrossRef]
74. Zickert, N.; Riedstra, B.; Groothuis, T. Imitational learning and right-handedness bias in humans. In Proceedings of the Tarragona Laterality Conference (TLC), Tarragona, Spain, 11–13 February 2013.
75. Veale, J.F. Edinburgh Handedness Inventory—Short Form: A revised version based on confirmatory factor analysis. *Laterality* **2014**, *19*, 164–177. [CrossRef] [PubMed]
76. Annett, M. The distribution of manual asymmetry. *Br. J. Psychol.* **1972**, *63*, 343–358. [CrossRef] [PubMed]
77. Jola, C.; Mast, F.W. Mental object rotation and egocentric body transformation: Two dissociable processes? *Spat. Cogn. Comput.* **2005**, *5*, 217–237.
78. Miura, N.; Nagai, K.; Yamazaki, M.; Yoshida, Y.; Tanabe, H.C.; Akazawa, T.; Sadato, N. Brain activation related to the imitative learning of bodily actions observed during the construction of a Mousterian stone tool: A functional magnetic resonance imaging study. In *Dynamics of Learning in Neanderthals and Modern*

Humans Volume 2: Cognitive and Physical Perspectives; Akazawa, T., Ogihara, N., Tanabe, H.C., Terashima, H., Eds.; Springer: Tokyo, Japan, 2015; pp. 221–232.

79. Corballis, M.C. Evolution of language and laterality: A gradual descent? *Cah. Psychol. Cogn.* **1998**, *17*, 1148–1155.
80. Bradshaw, J.L. The evolution of human lateral asymmetries: New evidence and second thoughts. *J. Hum. Evolut.* **1988**, *17*, 615–637. [CrossRef]
81. Cai, Q.; Van der Haegen, L. What can atypical language hemispheric specialization tell us about cognitive functions? *Neurosci. Bull.* **2015**, *31*, 220–226. [CrossRef] [PubMed]
82. Ocklenburg, S.; Güntürkün, O. Hemispheric asymmetries: The comparative view. *Front. Psychol.* **2012**, *3*, 5. [CrossRef] [PubMed]
83. Guiard, Y. Asymmetric division of labor in human skilled bimanual action: The kinematic chain as a model. *J. Motor Behav.* **1987**, *19*, 486–517. [CrossRef]
84. Sainburg, R.L. Convergent models of handedness and brain lateralization. *Front. Psychol.* **2014**, *5*, 1092. [CrossRef] [PubMed]
85. Jöris, O.; Uomini, N. Evidence for Neanderthal hand-preferences from the late Middle Palaeolithic site of Buhlen, Germany: Insights into Neanderthal learning behaviour. In *Learning Strategies during the Palaeolithic*; (Replacement of Neanderthals by Modern Humans Series); Nishiaki, Y., Jöris, O., Eds.; Springer: Tokyo, Japan. (In Press)
86. Stout, D. Skill and cognition in stone tool production: An ethnnographic case study from Irian Jaya. *Curr. Anthropol.* **2002**, *43*, 693–722. [CrossRef]
87. Ruck, L. Manual praxis in stone tool manufacture: Implications for language evolution. *Brain Lang.* **2014**, *139*, 68–83. [CrossRef] [PubMed]

11

Distribution of Antennal Olfactory and Non-Olfactory Sensilla in Different Species of Bees

Elisa Frasnelli * and Giorgio Vallortigara

Center for Mind/Brain Sciences, University of Trento, Piazza della Manifattura 1, I-38068 Rovereto, Italy; giorgio.vallortigara@unitn.it

* Correspondence: elisa.frasnelli@gmail.com

Academic Editor: Lesley Rogers

Abstract: Several species of social bees exhibit population-level lateralization in learning odors and recalling olfactory memories. Honeybees *Apis mellifera* and Australian social stingless bees *Trigona carbonaria* and *Austroplebeia australis* are better able to recall short- and long-term memory through the right and left antenna respectively, whereas non-social mason bees *Osmia rufa* are not lateralized in this way. In honeybees, this asymmetry may be partially explained by a morphological asymmetry at the peripheral level—the right antenna has 5% more olfactory sensilla than the left antenna. Here we looked at the possible correlation between the number of the antennal sensilla and the behavioral asymmetry in the recall of olfactory memories in *A. australis* and *O. rufa*. We found no population-level asymmetry in the antennal sensilla distribution in either species examined. This suggests that the behavioral asymmetry present in the stingless bees *A. australis* may not depend on lateral differences in antennal receptor numbers.

Keywords: lateralization; asymmetry; bees; antennal sensilla; olfaction

---

1. Introduction

The different functional specialization of the right and left sides of the nervous system (lateralization) is a feature shared by many vertebrates and also invertebrate species (see [1,2]). Lateralization manifests itself in a substantial range of behaviors and cognitive tasks, and mediates distinct sensory, motor and cognitive processes. In several species, behavioral asymmetries such as, for example, a side-bias in turning in one direction or a preferential use of one eye, ear or nostril to respond to specific stimuli, have been associated with corresponding asymmetries in the anatomical substrates of the nervous system (see [1]). These anatomical differences can be present at different levels: (i) in macroscopic anatomy, such as, for example, the Sylvian fissure of the lateral sulcus in humans that, in most people, is longer in the left hemisphere [3]; (ii) in the different size of the fibers that connect sensory reception and motor afference, such as the Mauthner cells responsible for the lateralization in the C-start bending reaction to danger in fishes [4]; or (iii) at the cellular level, such as in the different arrangement of synapses for specific neurotransmitters between the right and the left side of specific cerebral structures (e.g., the glutamate *N*-methyl-D-aspartate (NMDA) receptor, implied in learning and memory, in the left and right hippocampus of rodents [5]).

Several species of social bees exhibit population-level lateralization in learning odors and recalling olfactory memories. The first evidence comes from a study by Letzkus and colleagues [6], showing that honeybees *Apis mellifera* trained with only one antenna in use to associate an odor with a sugar reward in the proboscis extension reflex (PER) paradigm performed better in a recall test 5–6 h after training when they used their right antenna. Letzkus et al. [6] also looked at the distribution of one type of olfactory sensilla (the *sensilla placodea*) on the antennae and found that the right antenna had more *sensilla placodea* compared to the left antenna, and they linked this result with the better performance of the bees in the PER. Since the bees were both trained and tested with only one antenna in use, it is very difficult to establish whether the behavioral asymmetry observed related to the learning phase or to the recall of the olfactory memory.

Access to unilaterally acquired memories for odors is transferred to the other side of the brain in honeybees [7] and this transfer seems to occur from the right to the left side of the brain. Specifically, Rogers and Vallortigara [8] showed that there is a time-dependence in the behavioral asymmetry in the PER. Specifically, when honeybees are trained in a PER paradigm with both antennae in use, they are better at recalling the olfactory memory 1–2 h after training using their right antenna, and 8–12 h after training using their left antenna [8,9]. The same pattern of lateralization in the recall of short- and long-term olfactory memories has been found in the Australian social stingless bees *Trigona carbonaria*, *Trigona hockingsi* and *Austroplebeia australis*—the three species are better able to recall short- and long-term memories through the right and left antenna respectively [10]. It is important to underline that the results of the study conducted by Rogers and Vallortigara [8] and those of the following studies [9–13] investigated asymmetry in the recall of olfactory memories and not in the learning phase as the bees were trained with both antennae in use. Recent evidence has confirmed that in honeybees trained with only one antenna in use during olfactory learning, the left hemisphere is more responsible for long-term memory and the right hemisphere is more responsible for the learning and short-term memory [14]. Moreover, the gene expression in the brain of these honeybees was also asymmetric, with more genes having higher expression in the right hemisphere than the left hemisphere [14].

Interestingly, the non-social mason bees *Osmia rufa* are not lateralized in this way for the recall of short-term memory since they can retrieve it both through the circuits of the right and left antenna [11]. However, when tested for electroantennographic (EAG) responsivity to different odors, most mason bees showed individual lateralization (seven and eight individuals out of 21 showed significantly stronger responses respectively with the right and the left antenna), whereas honeybees show population-level lateralization with higher EAG responses on the right than on the left antenna [11].

Bumble bees *Bombus terrestris* trained on the PER paradigm with only one antenna in use and tested one hour after training show the same asymmetrical performance favoring the right antenna as do honeybees and the three species of Australian stingless bees. However, in bumble bees EAG responsivity is not lateralized at the population level, as it is in honeybees. In fact, as with mason bees, most bumble bees show individual lateralization (nine and three individuals out of 20 showed significantly stronger responses respectively with the right and the left antenna) [12].

In honeybees, the population-level asymmetry in the recall of olfactory memories may be partially explained by a morphological asymmetry at the peripheral level—the right antenna has about 5% more olfactory sensilla than the left antenna [6,13]. However, this does not exclude that the right antenna may also have a more important role than the left antenna in learning the association between an odor and a sugar reward in the PER paradigm [6]. As a consequence, it is possible that the morphological asymmetry observed in the number of olfactory sensilla influences the learning process and not the recall of the olfactory memory.

Moreover, honeybees with only the right antenna in use are better at discriminating a target from a background odorant in a cross-adaptation experiment (i.e., when a target odor is superimposed on the same or a different background odor), and this behavioral performance is not due to different discrimination of changes in odor concentration, nor to different learning abilities during odor discrimination [15]. Indeed, Rigosi et al. [15] showed that odor representations in the projection neurons of the right and left antennal lobes (ALs) are different with higher Euclidian distances between activity patterns in the right AL compared to the left. Interestingly, it is the odor representation in the right and the left ALs that is different. In fact, the functional activity patterns elicited by stimulation with different odors (both pheromones and environmental odors) in the right and the left AL of the same honeybee are bilaterally symmetrical [16]. In addition, at 14 days post-emergence the levels of neuroligin-1 expression, a protein involved in learning and memory, are higher in honeybees with only their right antenna compared to honeybees with only the left or both antenna [17].

In bumble bees *Bombus terrestris*, morphological counting of the olfactory and non-olfactory sensilla show a predominance in the number of only one type of olfactory sensilla, the *s. trichodea type A*, in the right antenna [12]. In the Australian stingless bee *T. carbonaria*, the right and the left antenna present the same number of olfactory and non-olfactory sensilla [18].

The antennae of female wasps *Anastatus japonicus* Ashmead (Hymenoptera: Eupelmidae), a non-social parasitoid, present more *s. placodea* on the right antenna than on the left antenna. Interestingly, in this species the distribution of *s. trichodea* and *s. basiconica* is asymmetrical between the antennae, but it depends on the segment. In fact, these sensilla are more abundant on the third flagellum antennomere of the right antenna than on the corresponding flagellum of the left antenna—the reverse results were observed for *s. trichodea* on the scape, pedicle, and fourth to fifth flagellum antennomeres, and for *s. basiconica* on the seventh flagellum antennomere and the third clava antennomere— suggesting that the asymmetry between the antennae can vary depending on the segment [19].

Here we looked at the possible correlation between the distribution of antennal sensilla in those species mentioned above that have been previously studied for behavioral asymmetry in the recall of olfactory memories, specifically the social Australian stingless bee *Austroplebeia australis* and the non-social mason bee *Osmia rufa*.

2. Materials and Methods

2.1. Subjects

Female adult mason bees *Osmia rufa* were obtained as they emerged from over-wintering cocoons collected at Crevalcore (Bologna, Italy) during spring 2011. Australian stingless *A. australis* foragers ($N = 14$) of unknown age were caught as they exited a well-established hive located in Valla, NSW, Australia within the natural range of the species in summer 2014.

2.2. Types of Sensilla

The different types of sensilla were identified on the basis of previous studies conducted on other Apoidea species [11,12,15]. For both species, we distinguished three types of putative olfactory sensilla (Figure 1)—*s. placodea*, *s. trichodea type A* (thick), and *s. coeloconica*—and two types of non-olfactory sensilla (Figure 1)—*s. trichodea type B* (thin) and *s. ampullacea* (Figure 2a)—clearly distinguishable from the putative olfactory *s. coeloconica* (Figure 2b) as they are smaller in size. Interestingly, the antennae of *A. australis* also present two more types of sensilla which we could clearly recognize, the non-olfactory *s. coelocapitulum* (Figure 1) and the putative olfactory *s. basiconica* (Figures 1 and 2c), exactly as with honeybees [13] and *T. carbonaria* [18]. Bumble bees *B. terrestris* also possess *s. basiconica*, but not *s. coelocapitulum* [12].

We also observed other types of sensilla in *O. rufa*, the *s. basiconica thick* (Figure 2d)—which is bigger than the standard *s. basiconica* (Figure 2c) and presents only lateral pores—and the *s. trichodea type C* (Figure 2e)—characterized by lateral pores, rifling, and an apical pore, which may have a double taste (because of the apical pore) and olfactory (because of the lateral pores) function. Finally, in *A. australis* we saw another type of *s. trichodea type D* (Figure 2f), with no pores (and thus probably non-olfactory), which given the lack of curvature could be easily recognized and distinguished from the olfactory *s. trichodea type A* (Figure 2f). We decided not to count these three new types of sensilla (i.e., *s. basiconica thick*, *s. trichodea type C* and *s. trichodea type D*) since we were not sure of their function. Thus, we limited our analyses to the sensilla we had already observed in other Apoidea species and which we could clearly distinguish based on previous studies.

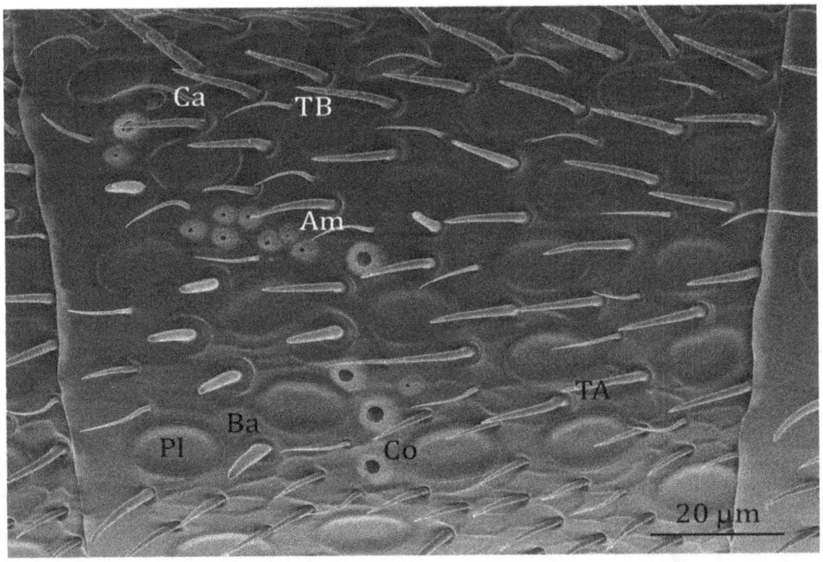

Figure 1. Scanning electron micrograph of the 9th segment of the left antenna of an *A. australis* forager (left view, i.e., imaging of the left antenna side). In black the putative olfactory *s. placodea* (Pl), *s. trichodea type A* (TA), *s. coeloconica* (Co) and *s. basiconica* (Ba); in white the non-olfactory *s. trichodea type B* (TB), *s. ampullacea* (Am) and *s. coelocapitulum* (Co). All the sensilla mentioned above are also present in *O. rufa* females apart from *s. basiconica* and *s. coelocapitulum*.

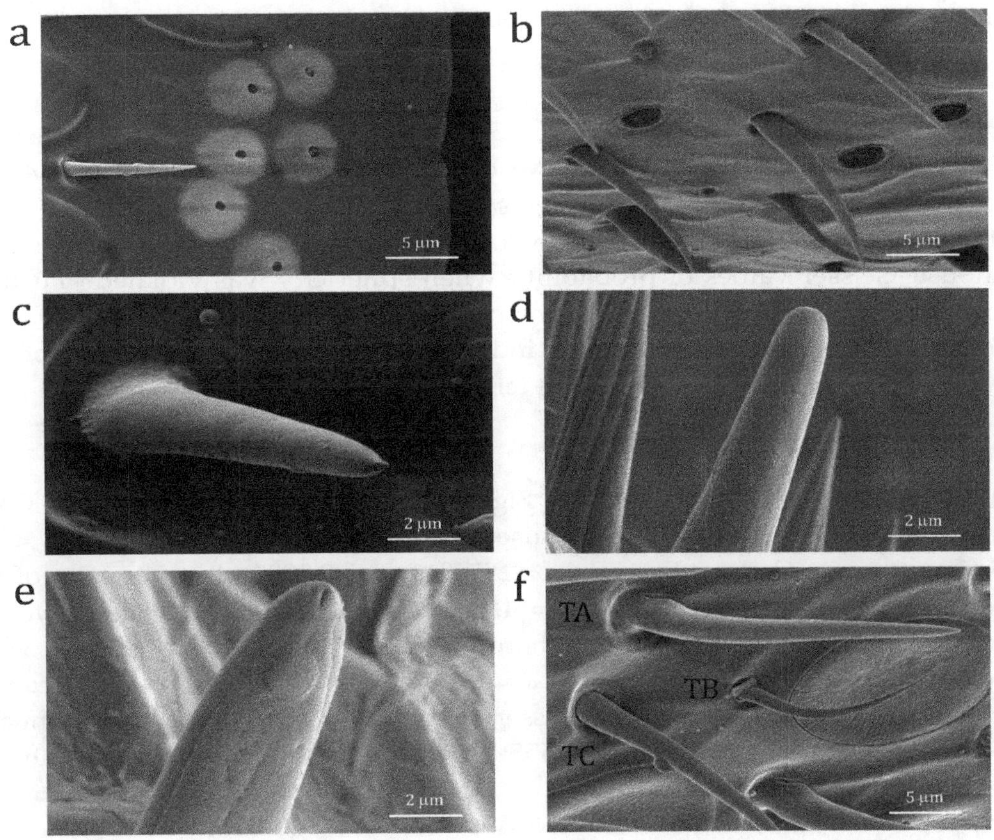

Figure 2. Scanning electron micrographs of details of (**a**) *s. ampullacea* (Am) in *A. australis*; (**b**) *s. coeloconica* (Co) in *A. australis*; (**c**) standard *s. basiconica* (Ba) in *A. australis*; (**d**) *s. basiconica thick* in *O. rufa*; (**e**) *s. trichodea type C* in *O. rufa*; and (**f**) *s. trichodea type D* (TD), *s. trichodea type A* (TA), *s. trichodea type* B (TB) in *A. australis*.

2.3. Scanning Electron Microscopy (SEM)

The mason bees *O. rufa* were preserved in a freezer in Trento before being taken to the Department of Medicine Laboratory, Azienda Provinciale per i Servizi Sanitari (APSS), Trento, Italy for preparation and imaging of the sample. There the antennae of the bees were removed and cleaned using ultrasound in a bath of acetone. The right and left antenna of each bee were then attached to a circular stub by double-sided conductive tape (TAAB Laboratories Equipment Ltd., Aldermaston, UK) and gold-coated to guarantee electrical conductivity during imaging with a XL 30, field emission environmental scanning electron microscope (FEI-Philips, Eindhoven, The Netherlands). Each antenna was imaged from four different viewpoints—ventral view (sample positioned at 0°), right view (sample tilted at −75°, imaging of the right antenna side), left view (sample tilted at +75°, imaging of the left antenna side), and dorsal view (following removal of the antenna from the stub and placing it upside down)—as done previously for honeybees [13], bumblebees [12] and *T. carbonaria* [18].

The same procedure was adopted for the *A. australis* bees with the difference that these bees were preserved in a freezer in Australia before being transported to the Department of Medicine Laboratory in Trento, Italy. Since *A. australis* bees are much smaller in size that mason bees, the whole heads of the bees rather than just the antennae were removed, as previously done for *T. carbonaria* [18]. Then, they underwent the same sample preparation and imaging as mason bees. As there are no olfactory receptors on the first two segments of the mason bee flagellum, only the third to tenth segments were scanned. Each segment from the third to ninth was scanned longitudinally at a magnification of 600 times. A magnification of 800 times was used for the tenth smallest segment (apex). For the same reason, only the second to tenth segments were scanned for *A. australis*. Given that the antennae of this species are smaller than the antennae of mason bees, each segment was scanned longitudinally at a larger magnification of 1000 times rather than 600 times.

2.4. Sensilla Counting and Statistical Analyses

Each sensilla was tagged and counted in all acquired images using ImageJ software (U.S. National Institutes of Health, Bethesda, MD, USA). We conducted analysis of variance (ANOVA) with the antennae (two levels), segments (eight levels for *O. rufa* and nine levels for *A. australis*), and type of sensilla (five and seven levels respectively for *O. rufa* and *A. australis*) as within-subjects factors, using Greenhouse–Geisser values of probability when sphericity was violated. Further analyses were conducted by grouping and separating the putative olfactory from the non-olfactory sensilla. Two-tailed binomial tests were used to evaluate individual differences in the number of olfactory and non-olfactory sensilla between the right and the left antennae.

3. Results

The results for both species are shown in Figure 3. For *O. rufa*, the overall ANOVA revealed significant main effects of segment (Greenhouse–Geisser, $F_{2.841,36.930} = 734.905$, $p < 0.0001$) and sensilla type (Greenhouse–Geisser, $F_{1.416,18.410} = 976.911$, $p < 0.0001$), but no effect of the antenna (left versus right) (sphericity assumed, $F_{1,13} = 4.217$, $p = 0.061$), although there was a tendency towards more sensilla on the left antenna. There was a significant interaction between segment × sensilla type (Greenhouse–Geisser, $F_{3.877,50.399} = 261.403$, $p < 0.0001$) but no significant interaction with antenna (antenna × type, Greenhouse–Geisser, $F_{2.154,28.006} = 2.031$, $p = 0.147$; antenna × segment, Greenhouse–Geisser, $F_{2.005,26.066} = 0.602$, $p = 0.555$; antenna × type × segment, Greenhouse–Geisser, $F_{3.734,48.538} = 1.269$, $p = 0.296$).

Similarly, for *A. australis*, the overall ANOVA revealed significant main effects of segment (Greenhouse–Geisser, $F_{2.002,26.027} = 458.141$, $p < 0.0001$) and sensilla type (Greenhouse–Geisser, $F_{1.545,20.091} = 1982.535$, $p < 0.0001$), but no effect of the antenna (left versus right) (sphericity assumed, $F_{1,13} = 0.045$, $p = 0.835$). There was a significant interaction between segment × sensilla type (Greenhouse–Geisser, $F_{4.941,64.230} = 244.914$, $p < 0.0001$) but no significant interactions with antenna (antenna × type, Greenhouse–Geisser, $F_{1.324,17.206} = 1.380$, $p = 0.267$; antenna × segment, Greenhouse–Geisser, $F_{3.480,45.243} = 1.405$, $p = 0.251$; antenna × type × segment, Greenhouse–Geisser, $F_{5.609,72.911} = 0.917$, $p = 0.483$).

We then summed up all the olfactory sensilla and all the non-olfactory sensilla, and conducted separate ANOVAs with sensilla type (olfactory vs. non-olfactory—two levels) as within-subjects factors to see whether there was any significant antenna × sensilla type interaction. For *O. rufa* (Figure 3a) we found a significant main effect of segment (Greenhouse–Geisser, $F_{2.841,36.930} = 734.905$, $p < 0.0001$) and sensilla type (sphericity assumed, $F_{1,13} = 6102.170$, $p < 0.0001$), but no effect although a tendency of the antenna (sphericity assumed, $F_{1,13} = 4.217$, $p = 0.061$). Again, there was a significant interaction between segment × sensilla type (Greenhouse–Geisser, $F_{2.835,36.855} = 533.080$, $p < 0.0001$) but no significant interaction with antenna (antenna × type, sphericity assumed, $F_{1,13} = 3.337$, $p = 0.091$; antenna × segment, Greenhouse–Geisser, $F_{2.005,26.066} = 0.602$, $p = 0.555$; antenna × type × segment, Greenhouse–Geisser, $F_{2.499,32.488} = 1.040$, $p = 0.378$). Likewise, ANOVA of the data for olfactory vs. non-olfactory sensilla for *A. australis* (Figure 3b) revealed significant main effects of segment (Greenhouse–Geisser, $F_{2.002,26.027} = 458.141$, $p < 0.0001$) and sensilla type (sphericity assumed, $F_{1,13} = 2269.510$, $p < 0.0001$), but no effect of the antenna (sphericity assumed, $F_{1,13} = 0.045$, $p = 0.835$). There was a significant interaction between segment × sensilla type (Greenhouse–Geisser, $F_{3.160,41.079} = 98.505$, $p < 0.0001$) but no significant interactions with antenna (antenna × type, sphericity assumed, $F_{1,13} = 1.893$, $p = 0.192$; antenna × segment, Greenhouse–Geisser, $F_{3.480,45.243} = 1.405$, $p = 0.251$; antenna × type × segment, Greenhouse–Geisser, $F_{3.086,40.112} = 1.029$, $p = 0.391$).

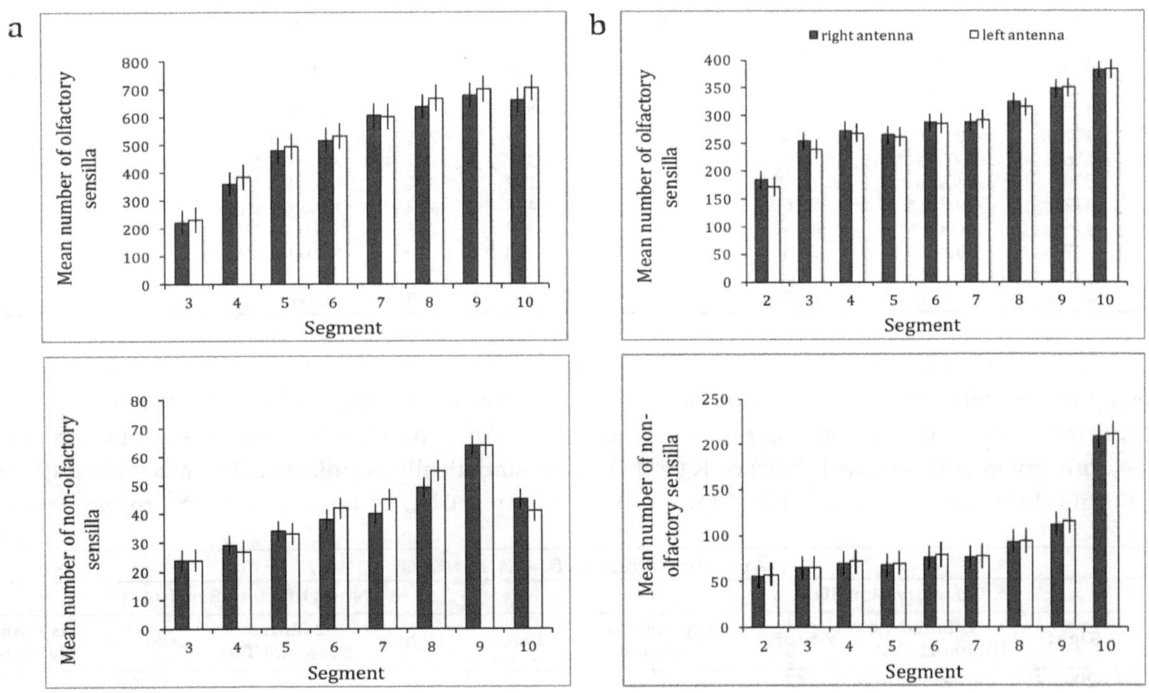

Figure 3. The mean number of olfactory and non-olfactory sensilla with the respective standard error (SE) in function of the segment number for the right antenna (dark grey bars) and for the left antenna (white bars) of (**a**) *O. rufa* females ($N = 14$) and (**b**) *A. australis* foragers ($N = 14$).

We also looked at possible differences between the right and the left antenna when the segment was not considered as a factor. For *O. rufa*, there was no significant effect of antenna (sphericity assumed, $F_{1,13} = 4.217$, $p = 0.061$) nor the antenna × type interaction (Greenhouse–Geisser, $F_{2.154,28.006} = 2.031$, $p = 0.147$), but only the effect of the sensilla type was significant (Greenhouse–Geisser, $F_{1.416,18.410} = 976.911$, $p < 0.0001$). For *A. australis*, the differences between the left and right antennae were not significant (sphericity assumed, $F_{1,13} = 0.045$, $p = 0.835$) nor the antenna × type interaction (Greenhouse–Geisser, $F_{1.324,17.206} = 1.380$, $p = 0.267$), but only the effect of the sensilla type was significant (Greenhouse–Geisser, $F_{1.545,20.091} = 1982.535$, $p < 0.0001$).

Interestingly, when we looked at possible individual differences between the number of olfactory and non-olfactory sensilla on the two antennae, we found that most individuals of both species showed individual-level asymmetry (Tables 1 and 2). Ten out of 14 individual *O. rufa* showed a significantly higher number of olfactory sensilla (estimated by the two-tailed binomial test, $p < 0.05$) either on the right (two individuals) or the left (eight individuals) antenna (Table 1). Nine of 14 mason bees, six of which were the same individuals that showed individual asymmetry for the olfactory sensilla, had more non-olfactory sensilla either on the right (four individuals) or the left (five individuals) antenna (Table 1).

Table 1. Individual-level lateralization in *O. rufa*. The number of olfactory and non-olfactory sensilla on the left and right antennae of individual mason bees *O. rufa* ($N = 14$) is reported with the corresponding p-values and z-scores of two-tailed binomial tests. The direction of asymmetry is indicated as L (left) or R (right) when statistically significant. The asterisks indicate significant difference: n.s. for $p > 0.05$; * for $p \leq 0.05$; ** for $p \leq 0.01$; *** for $p \leq 0.001$; **** for $p \leq 0.0001$.

Mason Bees *O. rufa*									
Olfactory Sensilla					Non-Olfactory Sensilla				
Left	Right	2-Tailed Binomial Test	z-Score	Asymmetry Direction	Left	Right	2-Tailed Binomial Test	z-Score	Asymmetry Direction
4559	3715	<0.0001 ****	9.27	L	372	433	0.035 *	−2.11	R
3833	4139	0.0006 ***	−3.42	R	260	371	<0.0001 ****	−4.38	R
4364	4144	0.013 *	2.48	L	316	324	0.779 n.s.	−0.28	
4647	4548	0.307 n.s.	1.02		407	323	0.0021 **	3.07	L
4517	4219	0.0014 **	3.18	L	403	397	0.857 n.s.	0.18	
4473	4077	<0.0001 ****	4.27	L	298	312	0.596 n.s.	−0.53	
4227	4014	0.019 *	2.34	L	329	231	<0.0001 ****	4.10	L
4506	4183	0.00056 ***	3.45	L	337	225	<0.0001 ****	4.68	L
3958	3966	0.936 n.s.	−0.08		172	304	<0.0001 ****	−6.00	R
4335	4126	0.024 *	2.26	L	408	402	0.857 n.s.	0.18	
3839	4164	0.0003 ***	−3.62	R	350	223	<0.0001 ****	5.26	L
4672	4477	0.042 *	2.03	L	390	270	<0.0001 ****	4.63	L
4071	4104	0.726 n.s.	−0.35		327	333	0.849 n.s.	−0.19	
4378	4291	0.357 n.s.	0.92		266	360	0.0002 ***	−3.72	R

Table 2. Individual-level lateralization in *A. australis*. The number of olfactory and non-olfactory sensilla on the left and right antennae of individual Australian stingless bees *A. australis* ($N = 14$) is reported with the corresponding p-values and z-scores of two-tailed binomial tests. The direction of asymmetry is indicated as L (left) or R (right) when statistically significant. The asterisks indicate significant difference: n.s. for $p > 0.05$; * for $p \leq 0.05$; ** for $p \leq 0.01$; *** for $p \leq 0.001$; **** for $p \leq 0.0001$.

Australian Stingless Bees *A. australis*									
Olfactory Sensilla					Non-Olfactory Sensilla				
Left	Right	2-Tailed Binomial Test	z-Score	Asymmetry Direction	Left	Right	2-Tailed Binomial Test	z-Score	Asymmetry Direction
2199	2090	0.099 n.s.	1.65		683	680	0.960 n.s.	0.05	
2639	2662	0.764 n.s.	−0.30		855	826	0.497 n.s.	0.68	
2648	2639	0.912 n.s.	0.11		846	868	0.610 n.s.	−0.51	
2601	2677	0.303 n.s.	−1.03		823	875	0.215 n.s.	−1.24	
2531	2510	0.779 n.s.	0.28		805	818	0.764 n.s.	−0.30	
2674	2576	0.180 n.s.	1.34		819	764	0.174 n.s.	1.36	
2712	2840	0.089 n.s.	−1.70		904	930	0.562 n.s.	−0.58	
2673	2787	0.126 n.s.	−1.53		937	917	0.659 n.s.	0.44	
2524	2756	0.0015 **	−3.18	R	892	910	0.689 n.s.	−0.40	
2831	2394	<0.0001 ****	6.03	L	874	676	<0.0001 ****	5.00	L
2080	2373	<0.0001 ****	−4.38	R	703	711	0.849 n.s.	−0.19	
2765	2523	0.0009 ***	3.31	L	1000	812	0.0001 ****	4.39	L
2406	2711	<0.0001 ****	−4.25	R	876	893	0.704 n.s.	−0.38	
2715	2972	0.0007 ***	−3.39	R	808	856	0.250 n.s.	−1.15	

Six out of 14 individual *A. australis* showed a significantly higher number of olfactory sensilla (estimated by two-tailed binomial test, $p < 0.05$) either on the right (four individuals) or the left (two individuals) antenna (Table 2). The same two individuals that had more olfactory sensilla on the left antenna, also had significantly more non-olfactory sensilla on the left antenna (Table 2).

4. Discussion

We showed that both *O. rufa* and *A. australis* do not show differences at the population level in the number of olfactory and non-olfactory sensilla on the right and the left antennae. However, about half of the individuals of both species presented individual-level asymmetry—some bees had more olfactory (and/or non-olfactory) sensilla on the right antenna and others had more sensilla on the left antenna.

Our results seem to be partially in line with previous findings. In fact, although previous studies found that the right antenna presents on average (i.e., at the population level) a higher number of at least one type of olfactory sensilla compared to the left antenna in the species *A. mellifera* [13], *B. terrestris* [12] and *A. japonicas* Ashmead [19], no significant differences in the number of either olfactory or non-olfactory sensilla between the left and the right antennae were found in *T. carbonaria* [16].

As both *T. carbonaria* and *A. australis* show population level lateralized behavior in the recall of olfactory memories [10], as do honeybees [8], we are tempted to conclude that this behavioral asymmetry cannot be explained by a different number of sensilla on the right compared to the left antenna. Indeed, for honeybees the difference between the number of olfactory receptors between the right and the left antenna is only 5% [13]. It is likely that behavioral asymmetry in the learning and recall of olfactory memories through the circuits of the right and left antenna is due to other functional asymmetries in the way these memories are represented and processed in the brain, as shown in the antennal lobe of *A. mellifera* [15]. Moreover, lateralized behavior may be due to asymmetries in the expression of specific neurotransmitters between the two sides on the nervous system, as suggested by a study by Biswas and colleagues [17], showing that levels of neuroligin-1 expression are higher in honeybees with only their right antenna compared to honeybees with only the left or both antennae [17].

It is also important to consider that the asymmetrical processing of odors may be advantageous to the single individual as this would allow, for example, the learning of new odors with one hemisphere and the keeping of memories of old odors in the other hemisphere [9]; this does not necessarily imply that all the individuals should be aligned in the same direction. Indeed, in our study we showed that about half of the individuals in the population (depending on the species considered) are lateralized at the individual level. The individual asymmetry that we observed in the current study of *O. rufa* matches well with previous findings of individual-level lateralization in the EAG responses [11]. In fact, 15 individuals out of 21 (71%) were found to have significantly stronger responses with either the right (seven individuals) or the left antenna (eight individuals) [11]. Here, 10 out of 14 (71%—exactly the same proportion) of mason bees showed significant asymmetry in the number of olfactory sensilla, and nine out of 14 individuals in the non-olfactory sensilla, regardless of the direction.

An alignment of lateralization within the population has been suggested to be a consequence of social pressure [20] and to arise as an evolutionarily stable strategy when individually asymmetrical organisms must coordinate their behavior with that of other individually asymmetrical organisms within the same species [21,22]. Recently, evidence has started to emerge suggesting that also so-called "non-social" species of insects are lateralized at the population level when biases in social interactions are considered. This is the case for *O. rufa*, a species that does not show behavioral asymmetry in the recall of short-term olfactory memory, but shows population-level lateralization in aggressive displays [23], similarly to eusocial honeybees [24] and social stingless bees *T. carbonaria* [18]. Thus, it is plausible that *A. australis* would also exhibit population-level biases in competitive and/or cooperative interactions with other individuals.

Clearly, it is the possibility of being engaged in interactions with other individuals rather than the way in which the species nests (socially or not) that may affect lateralization. Nonetheless the reason why some species show individual-level or population-level lateralization at the peripheral level, i.e., in the antenna, and what, if any, is the functional significance of this remains at present unexplained. It is possible that morphological asymmetry in the number of olfactory sensilla on the antennae influences the learning process of odors rather than the recall of the memories associated with these odors. Likewise, an asymmetrical distribution of non-olfactory sensilla may influence other sensory processes and allow parallel processing of different kinds of information in the two sides of the brain.

Acknowledgments: This research was supported by Caritro Foundation to G.V. A special acknowledgement to Lesley J. Rogers for providing the Australian specimens and for inviting us to contribute to this special issue, to Federico Piccoli, Department of Medicine Laboratory, APSS, Trento for the technical support with the scanning electron microscopy, and to Gianfranco Anfora, IASMA Research and Innovation Center, Fondazione E. Mach, for his help in identifying the sensilla types.

Author Contributions: E.F. and G.V. conceived and designed the experiments; E.F. performed the experiments; E.F. analyzed the data; E.F and G.V. wrote the paper.

References

1. Rogers, L.J.; Vallortigara, G.; Andrew, R. *Divided Brains: The Biology and Behaviour of Brain Asymmetries*, 1st ed.; Cambridge UP: Cambridge, UK, 2013.
2. Frasnelli, E.; Vallortigara, G.; Rogers, L.J. Left-right asymmetries of behavioural and nervous system in invertebrates. *Neurosci. Biobehav. Rev.* **2012**, *36*, 1273–1291. [CrossRef] [PubMed]
3. Rubens, A.B.; Mahowald, M.W.; Hutton, J.T. Asymmetry of the lateral (sylvian) fissures in man. *Neurology* **1976**, *26*, 620–624. [CrossRef] [PubMed]
4. Heuts, B.A. Lateralization of trunk muscle volume, and lateralization of swimming turns of fish responding to external stimuli. *Behav. Process* **1999**, *47*, 113–124. [CrossRef]
5. Kawakami, R.; Shinohara, Y.; Kato, Y.; Sugiyama, H.; Shigemoto, R.; Ito, I. Asymmetric allocation of NMDA receptor ε2 subunits in hippocampal circuitry. *Science* **2003**, *300*, 990–994. [CrossRef] [PubMed]
6. Letzkus, P.; Ribi, W.A.; Wood, J.T.; Zhu, H.; Zhang, S.-W.; Srinivasan, M.V. Lateralization of olfaction in the Honeybee *Apis mellifera*. *Curr. Biol.* **2006**, *16*, 1471–1476. [CrossRef] [PubMed]
7. Sandoz, J.C.; Menzel, R. Side-specificity of olfactory learning in the honeybee: Generalization between odours and sides. *Learn. Mem.* **2001**, *8*, 286–294. [CrossRef] [PubMed]
8. Rogers, L.J.; Vallortigara, G. From antenna to antenna: Lateral shift of olfactory memory recall by honeybees. *PLoS ONE* **2008**, *3*, e2340. [CrossRef] [PubMed]
9. Frasnelli, E.; Vallortigara, G.; Rogers, L.J. Response competition associated with right-left antennal asymmetries of new and old olfactory memory traces in honeybees. *Behav. Brain Res.* **2010**, *209*, 36–41. [CrossRef] [PubMed]
10. Frasnelli, E.; Vallortigara, G.; Rogers, L.J. Right-left antennal asymmetry of odour memory recall in three species of Australian stingless bees. *Behav. Brain Res.* **2011**, *224*, 121–127. [CrossRef] [PubMed]
11. Anfora, G.; Frasnelli, E.; Maccagnani, B.; Rogers, L.J.; Vallortigara, G. Behavioural and electrophysiological lateralization in a social (*Apis mellifera*) but not in a non-social (*Osmia cornuta*) species of bee. *Behav. Brain Res.* **2010**, *206*, 236–239. [CrossRef] [PubMed]
12. Anfora, G.; Rigosi, E.; Frasnelli, E.; Ruga, V.; Trona, F.; Vallortigara, G. Lateralization in the invertebrate brain: Left-right asymmetry of olfaction in Bumble bee, *Bombus terrestris*. *PLoS ONE* **2011**, *6*, e18903. [CrossRef] [PubMed]
13. Frasnelli, E.; Anfora, G.; Trona, F.; Tessarolo, F.; Vallortigara, G. Morpho-functional asymmetry of the olfactory receptors of the honeybee (*Apis mellifera*). *Behav. Brain Res.* **2010**, *209*, 221–225. [CrossRef] [PubMed]
14. Guo, Y.; Wang, Z.; Li, Y.; Wei, G.; Yuan, J.; Sun, Y.; Wang, H.; Qin, Q.; Zeng, Z.; Zhang, S.; et al. Lateralization of gene expression in the honeybee brain during olfactory learning. *Sci. Rep.* **2016**, *6*, 34727. [CrossRef] [PubMed]
15. Rigosi, E.; Haase, A.; Rath, L.; Anfora, G.; Vallortigara, G.; Szyszka, P. Asymmetric neural coding revealed by in vivo calcium imaging in the honey bee brain. *Proc. R. Soc. B* **2015**, *282*, 20142571. [CrossRef] [PubMed]

16. Galizia, C.G.; Nägler, K.; Hölldobler, B.; Menzel, R. Odour coding is bilaterally symmetrical in the antennal lobes of honey bees (*Apis mellifera*). *Eur. J. Neurosci.* **1998**, *10*, 2964–2974. [CrossRef] [PubMed]
17. Biswas, S.; Reinhard, J.; Oakeshott, J.; Russell, R.; Srinivasan, M.V.; Claudianos, C. Sensory regulation of neuroligins and neurexin I in the honeybee brain. *PLoS ONE* **2010**, *5*, e9133. [CrossRef] [PubMed]
18. Rogers, L.J.; Frasnelli, E. Antennal asymmetry in social behavior of the Australian stingless bee, *Tetragonula carbonaria*. *J. Insect Behav.* **2016**, *29*, 491–499. [CrossRef]
19. Meng, Z.J.; Yan, S.C.; Yang, C.P.; Ruan, C.C. Asymmetrical distribution of antennal sensilla in the female *Anastatus japonicus* Ashmead (Hymenoptera: Eupelmidae). *Microsc. Res. Tech.* **2012**, *75*, 1066–1075. [CrossRef] [PubMed]
20. Vallortigara, G.; Rogers, L.J. Survival with an asymmetrical brain: Advantages and disadvantages of cerebral lateralization. *Behav. Brain Sci.* **2005**, *28*, 575–633. [CrossRef] [PubMed]
21. Ghirlanda, S.; Vallortigara, G. The evolution of brain lateralization: A game theoretical analysis of population structure. *Proc. R. Soc. Lond. B* **2004**, *271*, 853–857. [CrossRef] [PubMed]
22. Ghirlanda, S.; Frasnelli, E.; Vallortigara, G. Intraspecific competition and coordination in the evolution of lateralization. *Philos. Trans. R. Soc. Lond. B* **2009**, *364*, 861–866. [CrossRef] [PubMed]
23. Rogers, L.J.; Frasnelli, E.; Versace, E. Lateralized antennal control of aggression and sex differences in red mason bees, *Osmia bicornis*. *Sci. Rep.* **2016**, *6*, 29411. [CrossRef] [PubMed]
24. Rogers, L.J.; Rigosi, E.; Frasnelli, E.; Vallortigara, G. A right antenna for social behaviour in honeybees. *Sci. Rep.* **2013**, *3*, 2045. [CrossRef] [PubMed]

12

Cerebral Sulcal Asymmetry in Macaque Monkeys

Kazuhiko Sawada

Department of Nutrition, Faculty of Medical and Health Sciences, Tsukuba International University, Tsuchiura, Ibaraki 300-0051, Japan; k-sawada@tius.ac.jp

Abstract: The asymmetry of the cerebral sulcal morphology is particularly obvious in higher primates. The sulcal asymmetry in macaque monkeys, a genus of the Old World monkeys, in our previous studies and others is summarized, and its evolutionary significance is speculated. Cynomolgus macaques displayed fetal sulcation and gyration symmetrically, and the sulcal asymmetry appeared after adolescence. Population-level rightward asymmetry was revealed in the length of arcuate sulcus (ars) and the surface area of superior temporal sulcus (sts) in adult macaques. When compared to other nonhuman primates, the superior postcentral sulcus (spcs) was left-lateralized in chimpanzees, opposite of the direction of asymmetry in the ars, anatomically-identical to the spcs, in macaques. This may be associated with handedness: either right-handedness in chimpanzees or left-handedness/ambidexterity in macaques. The rightward asymmetry in the sts surface area was seen in macaques, and it was similar to humans. However, no left/right side differences were identified in the sts morphology among great apes, which suggests the evolutionary discontinuity of the sts asymmetry. The diversity of the cortical lateralization among primate species suggests that the sulcal asymmetry reflects the species-related specialization of the cortical morphology and function, which is facilitated by evolutionary expansion in higher primates.

Keywords: non-human primate; Old World monkey; evolution; evolutionary expansion; gyrification

1. Introduction

Brain lateralization has been reported in many species including vertebrates and invertebrates [1]. The gyrencephalic surface morphology is a distinctive feature of the cerebral cortex seen in some mammalian species including humans [2], nonhuman primates [3–5], carnivores [3,6–9], artiodactyla [3,10] and cetaceans [11,12]. The cerebral sulcal morphology in primates is largely influenced by genetic factors that manifest during the second-trimester equivalent [13,14], and is modified under the influences of developmental and environmental factors during the third-trimester equivalent to form adult features [15,16]. In particular, the cortical expansion, known as one of the developmental factors, is closely correlated with gyrification across primate species [17,18] and is involved in species-related patterns of sexual dimorphism and/or individual variability of the sulcal morphology [19,20].

Cerebral sulci are highly lateralized in humans. Leftward sulcal asymmetry reported in the central sulcus (cs) is associated with handedness [21,22]. Additionally, leftward sulcal asymmetry in the paracingulate sulcus has been linked with cognition [23,24], while rightward sulcal asymmetry in the superior temporal sulcus (sts) is relevant to fMRI-defined right-lateralized voice selective responses [25,26]. Cortical lateralization, along with sulcal asymmetry, has been classically considered to be a unique characteristic in humans [27]. However, sulcal asymmetry has been observed in nonhuman primates such as great apes [28,29] and macaque monkeys [29]. This report summarizes the results of our studies and other findings regarding the laterality of sulcal infolding in the cerebral cortices of macaque monkeys—a genus of the Old World monkeys. The pattern of sulcal asymmetry in macaques to other primates was compared to speculate on the evolutionary significance of the sulcal asymmetry in primates. The sulcal asymmetry of the macaque brain and its related characteristics are summarized in Figure 1 in comparison to other primate species.

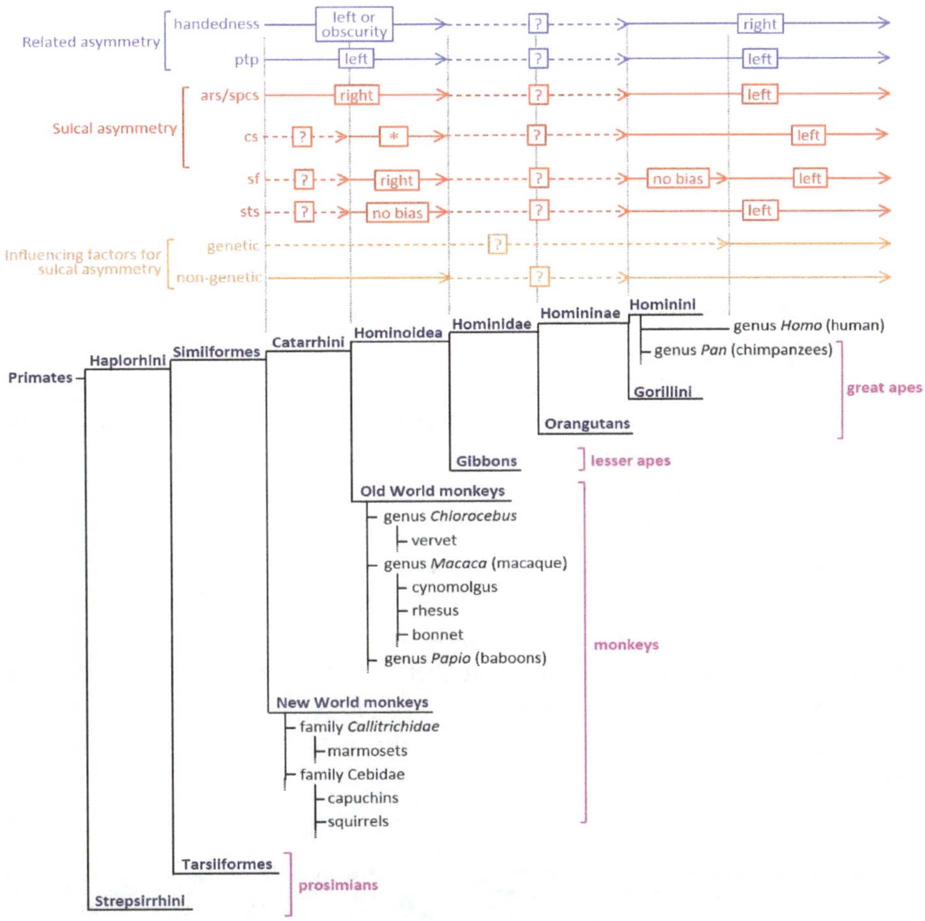

Figure 1. The evolution of sulcal asymmetry and its related asymmetrical characteristics among primate species. The sulcal asymmetry, its related asymmetrical characteristics, and influencing factors for sulcal asymmetry are summarized in reference to previous reports [4,5,13,20,28–47]. An asterisk (*) indicates that the cs symmetry is inconsistent in the Old World monkeys. The presence or absence and the direction of cs asymmetry vary depending on the species. ars, arcuate sulcus; cs, central sulcus; ptp, planum temporale; sf, Sylvian fissure; spcs, superior prefrontal sulcus; sts, superior temporal sulcus.

2. Asymmetrical Development of Cerebral Sulci

Sulcal morphology is influenced by genetic, developmental, and environmental factors [15,30]. In humans, the cs and sts emerge earlier on the right side compared to the left side during fetal development [2,31], which suggests a large influence of genetic factors on the asymmetric sulcal emergence. On the other hand, the sulcal length and depth were variable after birth in the baboon, a genus of the Old World monkeys [13]. Furthermore, sulcal infolding in multimodal association cortices was highly correlated with cortical expansion in cynomolgus macaques [16]. These findings suggest the possibility that the sulcal morphology in the Old World monkeys is modified after birth under the influences of developmental and environmental factors. Cynomolgus macaques experienced fetal sulcation and gyration symmetrically [4,32] and showed the sex-related appearance of sulcal asymmetry after adolescence [20,33]. Thus, sulcal asymmetry in the Old World monkeys may be largely attributed to environmental and developmental factors rather than genetic factors.

Although the New World monkeys are secondarily lissencephalic with reductions in body and brain sizes compared to their gyrencephalic ancestors [48], several primary sulci are sustained [5].

The cs, sts, and the parietooccipital sulcus emerged in adult common marmosets as small indentations, separately, on the left and right sides [5]. The incidence of each sulcus emerging was not biased between the left and light cerebral hemispheres [5], thus suggesting the individual variability of the emergence of asymmetric sulci. Therefore, the shift of nongenetic factor-related sulcal asymmetry from individual to population-level variabilities may appear before the split between the New World monkeys and Old World monkeys. Furthermore, the genetic factor-related sulcal asymmetry may occur after the split between the Old World monkeys and humans.

3. Sulcal Asymmetry in Macaques

The sulcal length asymmetry in macaques has been reported for more than three decades [49–53]. However, these studies failed to obtain consistent results. One possible reason for these discrepancies is that several of these studies used mixed-sex and/or -species samples for measurements of the sulcal lengths. After separating male and female cynomolgus macaques, we measured the sulcal lengths of left and right cerebral hemispheres and found the right-lateralization of the arcuate sulcus (ars) length in males, but not in females [20], following puberty [33]. The AQ values of eight representative primary sulci in our previous report [20] were analyzed using a one-sample *t*-test to determine significant-population level asymmetry of the sulcal lengths in cynomolgus macaques. A significant right-bias of AQ values (0.053 ± 0.069) was only identified after examining the ars length in adult males ($p < 0.05$). A sulcal map of the left and right cerebral hemispheres in cynomolgus macaques is shown in Figure 2. The ars in macaques is infolded in the lateral frontal cortex and identified as the early-emerging sulcal groups, which emerged in cynomolgus macaques between embryonic days 70 to 120 of the 160 day-long gestational period [4,32]. The cs, sts, and cingulate sulcus also appeared during this time [4,32]. However, the ars morphology in the Old World monkeys was greatly influenced by environmental factors rather than genetic factors, unlike the morphologies of other early-emerging sulci [13].

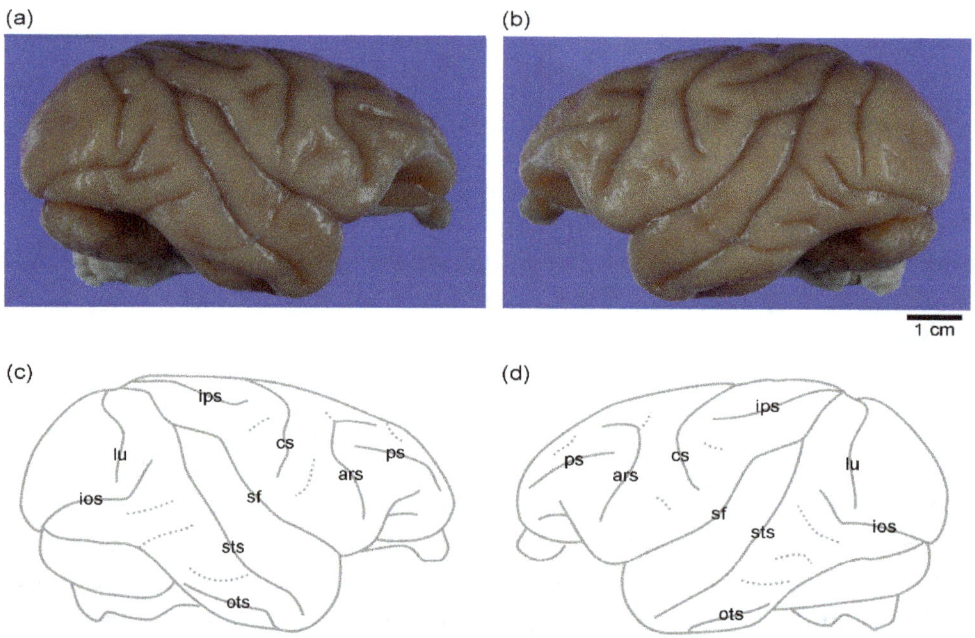

Figure 2. Eternal surface and sulcal map of the left and right cerebral cortex in cynomolgus macaques. (**a**) Photograph of the right hemisphere. (**b**) Photograph of the left hemisphere. (**c**) Sulcal map of the right hemisphere. (**d**) Sulcal map of the left hemisphere. ars, arcuate sulcus; cs, central sulcus; ios, inferior occipital sulcus; ips, intraparietal sulcus; lu, lunate sulcus; ots, occipitotemporal sulcus; ps, principal sulcus; sf, Sylvian fissure; sts, superior temporal sulcus.

One major limitation of our previous study (Imai et al. (2011) [20]) is the use of the "cotton thread" to measure the sulcal length. This method involves placing the cotton thread directly onto the cerebral surface to measure the lengths of each sulcus. However, this method cannot be used to obtain other information besides the sulcal length, e.g., the sulcal depths and surface areas. The sulcal depth, rather than the sulcal length, is known to be a susceptible mediator for evaluating the contributions of environmental factors [13]. Bogart et al. (2012) [29] conducted an MRI-based morphometrical analysis of primary sulci of macaques. This study used combined data from mixed-sex samples of two macaque species (rhesus and bonnet macaques), because no significant main effects or interactions were identified between either sex or species. Significant population-level asymmetries were obtained by the right-side bias in the sts surface area, but not in depths of any primary sulci. On the other hand, a significant individual asymmetry was revealed by the right-lateralization of the ars depth in macaques [29].

The ars in macaques is infolded in the lateral frontal cortex and putatively has cortical connections to premotor areas associated with arm and laryngeal representations, frontal eye fields, and somatomotor/orofacial areas [54]. Although the cerebral cortex continuously expanded after the completion of primary sulcogyrogenesis in cynomolgus macaques [18] and other primates [5,55], the progression of ars infolding correlated with the cortical expansion [16]. This phenomenon was similar to the late-emerging sulcal groups infolded in multimodal association cortices among cynomolgus macaques [16]. Therefore, the right-lateralization of the ars length and depth may be attributed to factors such as androgens, which are predominantly expressed in postpubertal males. This hypothesis is supported by a previous study showing the right-lateralization of androgen receptor levels in the frontal lobe in male rhesus monkeys, but not in female monkeys [56].

The sts is another sulcus that exhibits significant population-level asymmetries among macaques. A significant rightward asymmetry was revealed in the sts surface area [29]. Asymmetric pattern of the sts length may vary regionally among Old World monkeys, which consisted of three species including rhesus macaques: significantly right-lateralized at the lateral portion, but not at the medial and insular portions of the sts [57]. Intriguingly, the rightward sts asymmetry has not been observed in other families of nonhuman primates such as great apes (including chimpanzees) and New World monkeys (including capuchins and squirrels) [57]. In humans, the sts depth exhibited a significant rightward asymmetry that was relevant to fMRI-defined, right-lateralized voice-selective responses [25,26]. Asymmetric aspects of the sts morphology may be comparable between the Old World monkeys and humans. However, no left/right side differences were identified in the sts morphology among great apes, which suggests the evolutionary discontinuity of the sts asymmetry.

4. Comparison to Other Nonhuman Primates

Hopkins and colleagues reported sulcal asymmetry in great apes. They used MRI data from captive chimpanzees (*Pan troglodytes*) of both sexes to analyze the sulcal asymmetry due to the lack of sex differences in either the sulcal surface area or sulcal depth. The sulcal surface areas and/or sulcal depth were significantly left-lateralized in the fronto-orbital sulcus, superior precentral sulcus (spcs), sf, intraparietal sulcus, inferior postcentral sulcus, and the lunate sulcus [29]. The spcs in chimpanzees comprises part of the anterior border of the premotor cortex, and it is anatomically identical to the ars in macaques [34]. Interestingly, the surface areas and depth of the spcs were left-lateralized in chimpanzees—opposite to the direction of the symmetries in ars length and depth in macaques (right-lateralized) [29]. The precentral corticospinal system was associated with handedness in chimpanzees as well as humans [58]. Population-level right-handedness (preference for the right hand) was observed in both wild and captive chimpanzees [35,36,59]. However, the direction of hand use preference in macaques depended on species; while left-handedness predominated in rhesus macaques, ambidexterity predominated in cynomolgus macaques [37].

More than two-thirds of capuchins, which belong to the New World monkeys, showed a preference for left-hand use. The right-lateralized cs depth was obtained in left-handed, but not right-handed capuchins [38,39]. Among baboons, which belong to the genus *Papio* in the Old World monkeys, right-handed and left-handed individuals were equally prevalent. Additionally, the cs depth was lateralized contralaterally to the handedness in baboons [40]. On the other hand, the length and/or surface area of the cs were lateralized contralaterally to the handedness in humans [21,22]. Although handedness may be associated with the lateralization of cerebral sulci demarcating the precentral gyrus, the direction of preferred hands and the affected sides of sulci vary depending on the primate species. The sulcal asymmetry in the precentral cortex may shift from rightward to leftward after the split between the Old World monkeys and great apes, which may be relevant to the acquisition of the right-handedness.

The asymmetry of the sf has reportedly been positively associated with the asymmetry of the planum temporale (ptp) [28]. The ptp, cytoarchitecturally homologous to Brodmann's area 22, was left-lateralized in the surface area and gray matter volume, particularly among right-handed chimpanzees and humans [41]. A positive association between the sf and ptp asymmetries was also revealed in chimpanzees via the population-level leftward asymmetry of the sf depth and surface area [29]. In the Old World monkeys, the ptp volume was left-lateralized in cynomolgus macaques [42] and baboons [43], but not in rhesus macaques, bonnet macaques, and vervet monkeys [44]. However, there were no obvious asymmetries in the sf length in cynomolgus macaques [20] nor the sf depth and surface area in the mixed brain samples from rhesus and bonnet macaques [29]. On the other hand, the handedness, which altered the ptp asymmetry in chimpanzees and humans [41,45], was inconsistent among macaques [37]. While the ptp may have started to lateralize leftward during the evolution of Catarrhini (the common ancestor of the Old World monkeys, great apes, and humans), the sf asymmetry may reflect the enhancement of the ptp left-lateralization by acquiring right-handedness after the evolution of Hominoidea.

5. Possible Mediators for Evaluating Sulcal Asymmetry

One significant strategy for evaluating the sulcal asymmetry is the use of the gyrification index (GI). The GI, which was originally designed by Zilles et al. (1988) [46], is the most commonly used quantitative parameter for evaluating the cortical convolution and better understanding the interspecies differences, ontogeny, sexual dimorphism, and pathological statuses of neurodevelopmental and neurological disorders, as well a linkage with the functional development of particular cortical regions [34]. The GI is defined by the ratio of cortical contours including and excluding sulcal grooves on coronal slices of the cerebrum. Generally, the GI is calculated as the mean value of all coronal slices throughout the cerebral hemisphere. This value is referred to as the "global-GI" in this manuscript. The global-GI is close to 1 in lissencephalic mammals such as rats (1.02) and mice (1.01), while the marked highest value is found in the Pacific pilot whale (5.55). Meanwhile, the global-GI is ~2.56 in humans and between 1.78 and 1.81 in macaques [34]. On the other hand, the sulcal-GI is defined by the ratio of the cortical contours including specific primary sulcus to that excluding other sulcal grooves [9]. The sulcal-GI reflects the length, depth, width, and surface areas of specific sulci as well as the local expansion of particular cortical regions. For example, the sulcal-GI is lower when the sulcal width increases, even if no changes are observed in the sulcal length, depth, and surface area [9]. Furthermore, late-emerging sulcal groups infolded in multimodal association cortices showed significant correlations between sulcal-GIs and cortical volumes in cynomolgus macaques [16]. Further studies will be needed to evaluate the sulcal asymmetry using the sulcal-GI to obtain new insights into the brain lateralization of various species of mammals, including primates.

6. Conclusions

The gyrification of the cortical regions was associated with evolutionary expansion [16] and was higher in humans (global-GI = 2.56) and great apes (global-GI = 2.17–2.31) compared to the Old World monkeys (global GI = 1.64–2.27) [34]. Although the global-GI was correlated with larger brain size within the primate order [18,34,55], the increasing gyrification occurred regionally rather than throughout the entire brain. Particularly, the sulcal infolding has progressed in multimodal association cortices [16]. Therefore, the sulcal asymmetry may reflect the species-related specification of the cortical morphology and function, allowed by the evolutionary expansion in higher primates. On the other hand, morphological and functional lateralization was observed in other brain regions. Several studies have reported on the cerebellar asymmetry in mammalian species such as humans [47], chimpanzees [38], capuchins [38], ferrets [60–62], and dogs [63]. Cerebellar asymmetry is known to involve the large-scale fiber connections, which have a contralateral linkage to the cerebellar hemispheres with the cerebral association cortices [64]. An association between the sulcal asymmetry and the lateralization of other brain regions such as the cerebellum will provide new insights into the evolution of the mammalian brain regarding species-related specialization of the brain morphology and function.

References

1. Rogers, L.J.; Vallortigara, G.; Andrew, R.J. *Divided Brains-The Biology and Behaviour of Brain Asymmetries*; Cambridge Univ. Press: New York, NY, USA, 2013.
2. Chi, J.G.; Dooling, E.C.; Gilles, F.H. Gyral development of the human brain. *Ann. Neurol.* **1977**, *1*, 86–93. [CrossRef]
3. Pillay, P.; Manger, P.R. Order-specific quantitative patterns of cortical gyrification. *Eur. J. Neurosci.* **2007**, *25*, 2705–2712. [CrossRef] [PubMed]
4. Sawada, K.; Fukunishi, K.; Kashima, M.; Imai, N.; Saito, S.; Sakata-Haga, H.; Aoki, I.; Fukui, Y. Neuroanatomic and MRI references for normal development of cerebral sulci of laboratory primate, cynomolgus monkeys (*Macaca fascicularis*). *Congenit. Anom. (Kyoto)* **2012**, *52*, 16–27. [CrossRef] [PubMed]
5. Sawada, K.; Hikishima, K.; Murayama, A.Y.; Okano, H.J.; Sasaki, E.; Okano, H. Fetal sulcation and gyrification in common marmosets (Callithrix jacchus) obtained by ex vivo magnetic resonance imaging. *Neuroscience* **2014**, *257*, 158–174. [CrossRef] [PubMed]
6. Ferrer, I.; Hernández-Martí, M.; Bernet, E.; Galofré, E. Formation and growth of the cerebral convolutions I. Postnatal development of the median-suprasylvian gyrus and adjoining sulci in the cat. *J. Anat.* **1988**, *160*, 89–100.
7. Wosinski, M.; Schleicher, A.; Zilles, K. Quantitative analysis of gyrification of cerebral cortex in dogs. *Neurobiology* **1996**, *4*, 441–468.
8. Sawada, K.; Watanabe, M. Development of cerebral sulci and gyri in ferrets (*Mustela putorius*). *Congenit. Anom. (Kyoto)* **2012**, *52*, 168–175. [CrossRef]
9. Sawada, K.; Aoki, I. Biphasic aspect of sexually dimorphic ontogenetic trajectory of gyrification in the ferret cerebral cortex. *Neuroscience* **2017**, *364*, 71–81. [CrossRef]
10. Louw, G.J. The development of the sulci and gyri of the bovine cerebral hemispheres. *Anat. Histol. Embryol.* **1989**, *18*, 246–264. [CrossRef]
11. Marino, L.; Connor, R.C.; Fordyce, R.E.; Herman, L.M.; Hof, P.R.; Lefebvre, L.; Lusseau, D.; McCowan, B.; Nimchinsky, E.A.; Pack, A.A.; et al. Cetaceans have complex brains for complex cognition. *PLoS Biol.* **2007**, *5*, e139. [CrossRef]
12. Mortensen, H.S.; Pakkenberg, B.; Dam, M.; Dietz, R.; Sonne, C.; Mikkelsen, B.; Eriksen, N. Quantitative relationships in delphinid neocortex. *Front. Neuroanat.* **2014**, *8*, 132. [CrossRef] [PubMed]
13. Kochounov, P.; Castro, C.; Davis, D.; Dudley, D.; Brewer, J.; Zhang, Y.; Kroenke, C.D.; Purdy, D.; Fox, P.T.; Simerly, C.; et al. Mapping primary gyrogenesis during fetal development in primate brains: High-resolution in utero structural MRI of fetal brain development in pregnant baboons. *Front. Neurosci.* **2010**, *4*, 20.
14. Kochounov, P.; Glahn, D.C.; Fox, P.; Lancaster, J.L.; Saleem, K.; Shelledy, W.; Zilles, K.; Thompson, P.M.; Coulon, O.; Mangin, J.F.; et al. Genetics of primary cerebral gyrification: Heritability of length, depth and area of primary sulci in an extended pedigree of baboons. *Neuroimage* **2010**, *53*, 1126–1134. [CrossRef]

15. Clark, G.M.; Mackay, C.E.; Davidson, M.E.; Iversen, S.D.; Collinson, S.L.; James, A.C.; Roberts, N.; Crow, T.J. Paracingulate sulcus asymmetry; sex difference, correlation with semantic fluency and change over time in adolescent onset psychosis. *Psychiatry Res.* **2010**, *184*, 10–15. [CrossRef] [PubMed]
16. Sawada, K.; Fukunishi, K.; Kashima, M.; Imai, N.; Saito, S.; Aoki, I.; Fukui, Y. Regional difference in sulcal infolding progression correlated with cerebral cortical expansion in cynomolgus monkey fetuses. *Congenit. Anom. (Kyoto)* **2017**, *57*, 114–117. [CrossRef] [PubMed]
17. Rogers, J.; Kochunov, P.; Zilles, K.; Shelledy, W.; Lancaster, J.; Thompson, P.; Duggirala, R.; Blangero, J.; Fox, P.T.; Glahn, D.C. On the genetic architecture of cortical folding and brain volume in primates. *Neuroimage* **2010**, *53*, 1103–1108. [CrossRef] [PubMed]
18. Sawada, K.; Sun, X.Z.; Fukunishi, K.; Kashima, M.; Satio, S.; Sakata-Haga, H.; Tokado, H.; Aoki, I.; Fukui, Y. Ontogenetic pattern of gyrification in fetuses of cynomolgus monkeys. *Neuroscience* **2010**, *167*, 735–740. [CrossRef]
19. Liu, T.; Wen, W.; Zhu, W.; Trollor, J.; Reppermund, S.; Crawford, J.; Jin, J.S.; Luo, S.; Brodaty, H.; Sachdev, P. The effects of age and sex on cortical sulci in the elderly. *Neuroimage* **2010**, *51*, 19–27. [CrossRef]
20. Imai, N.; Sawada, K.; Fukunishi, K.; Sakata-Haga, H.; Fukui, Y. Sexual dimorphism of sulcal length asymmetry in cerebrum of adult cynomolgus monkeys (*Macaca fascicularis*). *Congenit. Anom. (Kyoto)* **2011**, *51*, 161–166. [CrossRef]
21. Foundas, A.L.; Hong, K.; Leonard, C.M.; Heilman, K.M. Hand preference and magnetic resonance imaging asymmetries of the central sulcus. *Neuropsychiatry Neuropsychol. Behav. Neurol.* **1998**, *11*, 65–71.
22. Klöppel, S.; Mangin, J.F.; Vongerichten, A.; Frackowiak, R.S.; Siebner, H.R. Nurture versus nature: Long-term impact of forced right-handedness on structure of pericentral cortex and basal ganglia. *J. Neurosci.* **2010**, *30*, 3271–3275. [CrossRef] [PubMed]
23. Fornito, A.; Wood, S.J.; Whittle, S.; Fuller, J.; Adamson, C.; Saling, M.M.; Velakoulis, D.; Pantelis, C.; Yücel, M. Variability of the paracingulate sulcus and morphometry of the medial frontal cortex: Associations with cortical thickness, surface area, volume, and sulcal depth. *Hum. Brain Mapp.* **2008**, *29*, 222–236. [CrossRef] [PubMed]
24. Amiez, C.; Wilson, C.R.E.; Procyk, E. Variations of cingulate sulcal organization and link with cognitive performance. *Sci. Rep.* **2018**, *8*, 1–13. [CrossRef] [PubMed]
25. Bonte, M.; Frost, M.A.; Rutten, S.; Ley, A.; Formisano, E.; Goebel, R. Development from childhood to adulthood increases morphological and functional inter-individual variability in the right superior temporal cortex. *Neuroimage* **2013**, *83*, 739–750. [CrossRef] [PubMed]
26. Bodin, C.; Takerkart, S.; Belin, P.; Coulon, O. Anatomo-functional correspondence in the superior temporal sulcus. *Brain Struct. Funct.* **2018**, *223*, 221–232. [CrossRef] [PubMed]
27. Corballis, M.C. *The Lopsided Brain: Evolution of the Generative Mind*; Oxford University Press: New York, NY, USA, 1992.
28. Cantalupo, C.; Pilcher, D.L.; Hopkins, W.D. Are planum temporale and sylvian fissure asymmetries directly related? A MRI study in great apes. *Neuropsychologia* **2003**, *41*, 1975–1981. [CrossRef]
29. Bogart, S.L.; Mangin, J.F.; Schapiro, S.J.; Reamer, L.; Bennett, A.J.; Pierre, P.J.; Hopkins, W.D. Cortical sulci asymmetries in chimpanzees and macaques: A new look at an old idea. *Neuroimage* **2012**, *61*, 533–541. [CrossRef]
30. Bonan, I.; Argenti, A.M.; Duyme, M.; Hasboun, D.; Dorion, A.; Marsault, C.; Zouaoui, A. Magnetic resonance imaging of cerebral central sulci: A study of monozygotic twins. *Acta Genet. Med. Gemellol. (Roma)* **1998**, *47*, 89–100. [CrossRef]
31. Kasprian, K.; Langs, G.; Brugger, P.C.; Bittner, M.; Weber, M.; Arantes, M.; Prayer, D. The prenatal origin of hemispheric asymmetry: An in utero neuroimaging study. *Cereb. Cortex* **2011**, *21*, 1076–1083. [CrossRef]
32. Sawada, K.; Fukunishi, K.; Kashima, M.; Saito, S.; Sakata-Haga, H.; Aoki, I.; Fukui, Y. Fetal gyrification in cynomolgus monkeys: A concept of developmental stages of gyrification. *Anat. Rec. (Hoboken)* **2012**, *295*, 1065–1074. [CrossRef]
33. Sakamoto, K.; Sawada, K.; Fukunishi, K.; Imai, N.; Sakata-Haga, H.; Fukui, Y. Postnatal change in sulcal length asymmetry in cerebrum of cynomolgus monkeys (*Macaca fascicularis*). *Anat. Rec. (Hoboken)* **2014**, *297*, 200–207. [CrossRef] [PubMed]
34. Zilles, K.; Palomero-Gallagher, N.; Amunts, K. Development of cortical folding during evolution and ontogeny. *Trends Neurosci.* **2013**, *36*, 275–284. [CrossRef] [PubMed]

35. Lonsdorf, E.V.; Hopkins, W.D. Wild chimpanzees show population level handedness for tool use. *Proc. Natl. Acad. Sci. USA* **2005**, *102*, 12634–12638. [CrossRef] [PubMed]
36. Corp, N.; Byrne, R.W. Sex difference in chimpanzee handedness. *Am. J. Phy. Anthropol.* **2004**, *123*, 62–68. [CrossRef] [PubMed]
37. Chatagny, P.; Badoud, S.; Kaeser, M.; Gindrat, A.D.; Savidan, J.; Fregosi, M.; Moret, V.; Roulin, C.; Schmidlin, E.; Rouiller, E.M. Distinction between hand dominance and hand preference in primates: A behavioral investigation of manual dexterity in nonhuman primates (macaques) and human subjects. *Brain Behav.* **2013**, *3*, 575–595. [CrossRef] [PubMed]
38. Phillips, K.; Hopkins, W.D. Exploring the relationship between cerebellar asymmetry and handedness in chimpanzees (*Pan troglodytes*) and capuchins (*Cebus apella*). *Neuropsychologia* **2007**, *45*, 2333–2339. [CrossRef] [PubMed]
39. Phillips, K.A.; Thompson, C.R. Hand preference for tool-use in capuchin monkeys (*Cebus apella*) is associated with asymmetry of the primary motor cortex. *Am. J. Primatol.* **2013**, *75*, 435–440. [CrossRef]
40. Margiotoudi, K.; Marie, D.; Claidière, N.; Coulon, O.; Roth, M.; Nazarian, B.; Lacoste, R.; Hopkins, W.D.; Molesti, S.; Fresnais, P.; et al. Handedness in monkeys reflects hemispheric specialization within the central sulcus. An in vivo MRI study in right- and left-handed olive baboons. *Cortex* **2019**, *118*, 203–211. [CrossRef]
41. Hopkins, W.D.; Nir, T. Planum temporale surface area and grey matter asymmetries in chimpanzees (*Pan troglodytes*): The effect of handedness and comparison within findings in humans. *Behav. Brain Res.* **2010**, *208*, 436–443. [CrossRef]
42. Gannon, P.J.; Holloway, R.L.; Broadfield, D.C.; Braum, A.R. Asymmetry of chimpanzee planum temporale: Humanlike pattern of Wernicke's brain language area homolog. *Science* **1998**, *279*, 220–222. [CrossRef]
43. Marie, D.; Roth, M.; Lacoste, R.; Nazarian, B.; Bertello, A.; Anton, J.L.; Hopkins, W.D.; Margiotoudi, K.; Love, S.A.; Meguerditchian, A. Left brain asymmetry of the planum temporale in a nonhominid primate: Redefining the origin of brain specialization for language. *Cereb. Cortex* **2018**, *28*, 1808–1815. [CrossRef] [PubMed]
44. Lyn, H.L.; Pierre, P.; Bennett, A.J.; Fears, S.C.; Woods, R.P.; Hopkins, W.D. Planum temporale grey matter asymmetries in chimpanzees (*Pan troglodytes*), vervet (*Chlorocebus aethiops sabaeus*), rhesus (*Macaca mulatta*) and bonnet (*Macaca radiata*) monkeys. *Neuropsychologia* **2011**, *49*, 2004–2012. [CrossRef] [PubMed]
45. Hopkins, W.D. Neuroanatomical asymmetries and handedness in chimpanzees (*Pan troglodytes*): A case for continuity in the evolution of hemispheric specialization. *Ann. N. Y. Acad. Sci.* **2013**, *1288*, 17–35. [CrossRef] [PubMed]
46. Zilles, K.; Armstrong, E.; Schleicher, A.; Kretschmann, H.J. The human pattern of gyrification in the cerebral cortex. *Anat. Embryol.* **1988**, *179*, 173–179. [CrossRef] [PubMed]
47. Rosch, R.E.; Ronan, L.; Cherkas, L.; Gurd, J.M. Cerebellar asymmetry in a pair of monozygotic handedness-discordant twins. *J. Anat.* **2010**, *217*, 38–47. [CrossRef]
48. Kelava, I.; Lewitus, E.; Huttner, W.B. The aecondary loss of gyrencephaly as an example of evolutionary phenotypical reversal. *Front. Neuroanat.* **2013**, *7*, 16. [CrossRef]
49. Yeni-Komshian, G.H.; Benson, D.A. Anatomical study of cerebral asymmetry in the temporal lobe of humans, chimpanzees, and rhesus monkeys. *Science* **1976**, *192*, 387–389. [CrossRef]
50. Falk, D.; Cheverud, J.; Vannier, M.W.; Conroy, G.C. Advanced computer graphics technology reveals cortical asymmetry in endocasts of rhesus monkeys. *Folia Primatol.* **1986**, *4*, 98–103. [CrossRef]
51. Falk, D.; Hildebolt, C.; Cheverud, J.; Vannier, M.; Helmkamp, R.C.; Konigsberg, L. Cortical asymmetries in frontal lobes of rhesus monkeys (*Macaca mulatta*). *Brain Res.* **1990**, *512*, 40–45. [CrossRef]
52. Heilbroner, P.L.; Holloway, R.L. Anatomical brain asymmetries in New World and Old World monkeys: Stages of temporal lobe development in primate evolution. *Am. J. Phys. Anthropol.* **1988**, *76*, 39–48. [CrossRef]
53. Heilbroner, P.L.; Holloway, R.L. Anatomical brain asymmetry in monkeys: Frontal, temporoparietal, and limbic cortex in Macaca. *Am. J. Phys. Anthropol.* **1989**, *80*, 203–211. [CrossRef] [PubMed]
54. Goulas, A.; Stiers, P.; Hutchison, R.M.; Everling, S.; Petrides, M.; Margulies, D.S. Intrinsic functional architecture of the macaque dorsal and ventral lateral frontal cortex. *J. Neurophysiol.* **2017**, *117*, 1084–1099. [CrossRef] [PubMed]
55. Armstrong, E.; Schleicher, A.; Omran, H.; Curtis, M.; Zilles, K. The ontogeny of human gyrification. *Cereb. Cortex* **1995**, *5*, 56–63. [CrossRef] [PubMed]

56. Sholl, S.A.; Kim, K.L. Androgen receptors are differentially distributed between right and left cerebral hemispheres of the fetal male rhesus monkey. *Brain Res.* **1990**, *516*, 122–126. [CrossRef]
57. Hopkins, W.D.; Pilcher, D.L.; MacGregor, L. Sylvian fissure asymmetries in nonhuman primates revisited: A comparative MRI study. *Brain Behav. Evol.* **2000**, *56*, 293–299. [CrossRef]
58. Li, L.; Preuss, T.M.; Rilling, J.K.; Hopkins, W.D.; Glasser, M.F.; Kumar, B.; Nana, R.; Zhang, X.; Hu, X. Chimpanzee (*Pan troglodytes*) precentral corticospinal system asymmetry and handedness: A diffusion magnetic resonance imaging study. *PLoS ONE* **2010**, *21*, e12886. [CrossRef]
59. Humle, T.; Matsuzawa, T. Laterality in hand use across four tool use behaviors among the wild chimpanzees of Bossou, Guinea, West Africa. *Am. J. Primatol.* **2009**, *71*, 40–48. [CrossRef]
60. Sawada, K.; Horiuchi-Hirose, M.; Saito, S.; Aoki, I. Male prevalent enhancement of leftward asymmetric development of the cerebellar cortex in ferrets (*Mustela putorius*). *Laterality* **2015**, *20*, 723–737. [CrossRef]
61. Sawada, K.; Aoki, I. Age-dependent sexually-dimorphic asymmetric development of the ferret cerebellar cortex. *Symmetry* **2017**, *9*, 40. [CrossRef]
62. Sawada, K.; Kamiya, S.; Aoki, I. Asymmetry of cerebellar lobular development in ferrets. *Symmetry* **2020**, *12*, 735. [CrossRef]
63. Koyun, N.; Aydinlioğlu, A.; Aslan, K. A morphometric study on dog cerebellum. *Neurol. Res.* **2011**, *33*, 220–224. [CrossRef] [PubMed]
64. Wang, D.; Buckner, R.L.; Liu, H. Cerebellar asymmetry and its relation to cerebral asymmetry estimated by intrinsic functional connectivity. *J. Neurophysiol.* **2013**, *109*, 46–57. [CrossRef] [PubMed]

13

Effects of Emotional Valence on Hemispheric Asymmetries in Response Inhibition

Sebastian Ocklenburg [1,*,†], Jutta Peterburs [2,†], Janet Mertzen [1], Judith Schmitz [1], Onur Güntürkün [1] and Gina M. Grimshaw [3]

1 Institute of Cognitive Neuroscience, Biopsychology, Department of Psychology, Ruhr-University Bochum, 44801 Bochum, Germany; janet.mertzen@rub.de (J.M.); judith.schmitz@rub.de (J.S.); Onur.Guentuerkuen@rub.de (O.G.)
2 Institute of Medical Psychology and Systems Neuroscience, University of Münster, 48149 Münster, Germany; jutta.peterburs@uni-muenster.de
3 Cognitive and Affective Neuroscience Lab, School of Psychology, Victoria University of Wellington, 6140 Wellington, New Zealand; Gina.Grimshaw@vuw.ac.nz
* Correspondence: sebastian.ocklenburg@rub.de
† These authors contributed equally to the manuscript.

Academic Editor: Lesley Rogers

Abstract: Hemispheric asymmetries are a major organizational principle in human emotion processing, but their interaction with prefrontal control processes is not well understood. To this end, we determined whether hemispheric differences in response inhibition depend on the emotional valence of the stimulus being inhibited. Participants completed a lateralised Go/Nogo task, in which Nogo stimuli were neutral or emotional (either positive or negative) images, while Go stimuli were scrambled versions of the same pictures. We recorded the N2 and P3 event-related potential (ERP) components, two common electrophysiological measures of response inhibition processes. Behaviourally, participants were more accurate in withholding responses to emotional than to neutral stimuli. Electrophysiologically, Nogo-P3 responses were greater for emotional than for neutral stimuli, an effect driven primarily by an enhanced response to positive images. Hemispheric asymmetries were also observed, with greater Nogo-P3 following left versus right visual field stimuli. However, the visual field effect did not interact with emotion. We therefore find no evidence that emotion-related asymmetries affect response inhibition processes.

Keywords: emotion; lateralisation; hemispheric asymmetry; executive functions; EEG

---

1. Introduction

Hemispheric asymmetries, i.e., functional and structural differences between the left and the right brain hemisphere, affect behaviour and cognition in all vertebrate classes [1–5]. One of the least well understood asymmetric systems is the one that supports emotion processing [6–8]. First reports that the hemispheres might differ in emotional processing are often attributed to Hughlings-Jackson [9], who noted that aphasic patients (with left hemisphere lesions) often had preserved emotional language. Later patient studies showed that left hemisphere lesions are more commonly associated with depressed or catastrophic reactions, whereas right hemisphere lesions are more likely to trigger inappropriate euphoria [10]. These early studies have since been complemented by research using a range of methodologies, including the testing of patients with unilateral lesions [11], asymmetric EEG activity [12,13], visual half-field and dichotic listening techniques [14,15], and functional imaging [16,17], to show that the hemispheres differ in how they process emotional information, and in the emotional responses they generate.

Two asymmetric systems have been proposed to account for hemispheric differences in emotional processing. The first (described by the "right-hemisphere hypothesis") suggests that the right hemisphere is specialised for the processing of all emotions. The other (described by the "valence" hypothesis) proposes lateralisation as a function of valence, with the left specialised for positive (or approach-related) emotions, and the right for negative (or withdrawal-related) emotions. For decades, researchers have tried to determine which hypothesis better explains emotional asymmetry [18–21]. Rather than pitting these hypotheses against each other, recent research has been based on the premise that both might be correct, and has instead focused on the situations in which emotion-based or valence-based processing might arise [22–24].

There is an emerging consensus that the right hemisphere hypothesis applies largely to emotion perception, regardless of modality, and reflects lateralisation of the right posterior cortex. Such asymmetries may depend largely on the emotional nature of the stimulus, and emerge in a bottom-up fashion. Valence-based processing is more closely tied to emotional experience or expression, and appears to reflect asymmetries in the dorsolateral prefrontal cortex (dlPFC). This asymmetry has been linked to both emotional valence (positive/negative) [25,26] and motivational direction (approach/withdrawal) [27], although valence-related asymmetries are sometimes also reported in perception. Schepman and colleagues have argued that valence effects should emerge when tasks include top-down processing (for example, related to expectancies) that engage frontal emotional processing networks [22,23]. Grimshaw and Carmel [28] have further argued that prefrontal asymmetries in emotional processing may not reflect emotional experience, but the top-down control of emotional information, with the left hemisphere specialised for the inhibition or control of negative information, and the right for inhibition or control of positive emotion. Their rationale is based largely on the fact that prefrontal mechanisms (and particularly those localised to lateral PFC) play a key role in both cognitive and/or attentional control on the one hand, and on emotion regulation on the other [29]. Like Schepman, they argue that valence-based effects are most likely to be observed when tasks involve the use of top-down control mechanisms.

As yet, few experimental studies have directly assessed asymmetries in inhibition or control processes, and so it is unknown whether such control processes show emotional asymmetries, and if so, whether they are in line with either a right hemisphere or valence-based explanation. To address this gap in the literature, we used a lateralized version of the classic Go/Nogo Task in which we manipulated the emotional nature of the stimuli. In this type of task, two categories of stimuli are presented to the subjects: the more frequent Go stimuli to which subjects are asked to respond, e.g., by button press, and the less frequent Nogo stimuli to which participants are asked to withhold responses [30,31]. When Nogo stimuli are rare, participants adopt a prepotent response that must be inhibited when the imperative Nogo signal appears. Poor inhibitory control is indicated by errors of commission on Nogo trials. These behavioural measures are complemented by two neural measures revealed by event-related potentials (ERPs): the Nogo-N2 and the Nogo-P3 [32,33]. These components are assumed to reflect different sub-processes of the response inhibition. The earlier of the two components is the Nogo-N2, a negative component that is thought to reflect either pre-motor inhibition [32] or monitoring of response conflict [34]. The later of the two components is the Nogo-P3, a positive deflection that has been linked to the evaluation of successful inhibition, given that it peaks too late after the response to directly reflect inhibition processes [35–38].

In our version of the task, Go and Nogo stimuli were presented tachistoscopically in the left (LVF) or right visual field (RVF). This ensures that initial visual and emotional processing of the stimulus is lateralized to the contralateral hemisphere [39–42]. To examine emotional processing, we used pictures of emotional and neutral scenes as Nogo stimuli and unidentifiable scrambled versions of the same pictures as Go stimuli. Participants were asked to press a button in response to scrambled stimuli and to refrain from responding whenever intact stimuli were presented. Half of the (intact) Nogo stimuli had a neutral valence, while the other half showed emotional pictures, taken from the International Affective Picture System (IAPS) [43]. We manipulated the valence of the emotional images between subjects; for half of the participants, emotional pictures were negative (mutilations), and for the other half positive (erotic scenes). In this task, the emotional content of the Nogo stimuli was not the imperative aspect for the subjects' responses, but instead served merely as a task-irrelevant distraction; that is, participants withheld their response whenever an intact image appeared, regardless of its content. This is an important aspect of the design, as it allows us to assess the effects of the emotional nature of the stimulus to be controlled, independent of any effects of emotion on the generation or inhibition of the response itself (for example, positive and negative stimuli are associated with approach and avoidance responses, respectively).

To our knowledge, no studies have assessed the effects of lateralised emotional stimuli on Go-Nogo task performance. However, a number of studies have manipulated the emotional nature of imperative stimuli in central vision, while still keeping emotion itself incidental to the task [44–49]. The effect of emotion on behavioural measures is mixed across these studies, with some showing more errors on Nogo trials in emotional contexts [50], but most showing no behavioural effects [44,45,49]. However, more consistent findings are reported in the ERP measures. Most studies show no effect of emotion on the Nogo-N2 [44,45,49,51], although some have reported an attenuation of the N2 for emotional relative to neutral stimuli [46,47]. In contrast, emotional stimuli consistently enhance the Nogo-P3 [46,47,51], with effects sometimes greater for positive than for negative stimuli [44,45]. This enhanced Nogo-P3 is typically interpreted as a more effortful or less efficient inhibitory control in emotional contexts [44,45,48]. Our question concerns the effects of lateralisation of the emotional stimuli on response inhibition processes. Importantly, emotional information can be extracted from peripherally-presented complex scenes, even with very brief stimulus presentations [52,53]. We therefore determined whether emotion affected either behavioural or electrophysiological measures of the response inhibition. Based on the right hemisphere hypothesis, we would expect emotion effects to be stronger for imperative stimuli presented in the LVF. However, because response inhibition depends on top-down control processes, it might be sensitive to emotional valence [22,23,28]. If so, we predict stronger effects of negative stimuli in the LVF, and stronger effects of positive stimuli in the RVF.

It is also possible that our experiment will show that response inhibition processes are affected by asymmetries in stimulus processing that are not specific to emotion. Using verbal stimuli, we previously showed that magnitudes of both Nogo-N2 and Nogo-P3 were affected by hemispheric asymmetries in stimulus processing [54]. When lateralised stimuli were presented tachistoscopically, the Nogo-N2 and related delta frequency band power were stronger when response inhibition was applied to stimuli presented in the LVF, implying greater response conflict generated by stimuli presented to the non-dominant hemisphere. A similar, albeit weaker, effect also reached significance for the P3 [54].

2. Materials and Methods

2.1. Subjects

Forty-two healthy adults (22 women, 20 men) participated in the present study. Subjects were recruited at the Institute of Cognitive Neuroscience, Department of Biopsychology at Ruhr-University Bochum by public advertisement and received course credit or monetary reimbursement (20 €) for participation. The mean age was 24.5 ± 4.3 years (range 18 to 34 years). Exclusion criteria were current or past psychiatric or neurological disorders, current psychotropic medication, colour blindness, mixed- or left-handedness, and ages younger than 18 or older than 35 years. Furthermore, subjects were required to be heterosexual due to the nature of the stimulus material (see below). All subjects were right-handed (mean laterality quotient 86.5 ± 16.1; range 37.5–100), as assessed with the Edinburgh Handedness Inventory [55], had normal or corrected-to normal vision, and were naïve to the study's intent.

Written informed consent was obtained from all subjects prior to participation. The study conforms to the Declaration of Helsinki and has received ethical clearance by the Ethics Board of Faculty of Psychology at Ruhr-University Bochum, Germany.

2.2. Experimental Task

The task was a tachistoscopic adaptation of a classic Go/Nogo task [30,54] that included emotional and neutral pictures as imperative stimuli. Pictures were taken from the International Affective Picture System (IAPS) [43]. Stimulus presentation and timing was controlled by Presentation software (Neurobehavioural Systems, Inc., Berkeley, CA, USA). Figure 1 provides a schematic illustration of the sequence and time course of stimulus presentation. At the beginning of each trial, a fixation cross was presented in the centre of the screen for 1000 ms. Subsequently an imperative stimulus (emotional or neutral; intact or scrambled picture) was presented in the left (LVF) or right visual field (RVF), with the inner edge of the stimulus located at 3 degrees of visual angle from the fixation cross. Stimuli had a width of 4 degrees of visual angle and a height of 3.5 degrees of visual angle. Stimuli were presented for 185 ms. Stimulus presentation was followed by the fixation cross for 525 ms. Trials were separated by inter-trial intervals jittered between 750 ms and 950 ms. There was a short break in fixation between the end of the inter-trial interval and the beginning of the next trial in which the fixation cross disappeared and reappeared again.

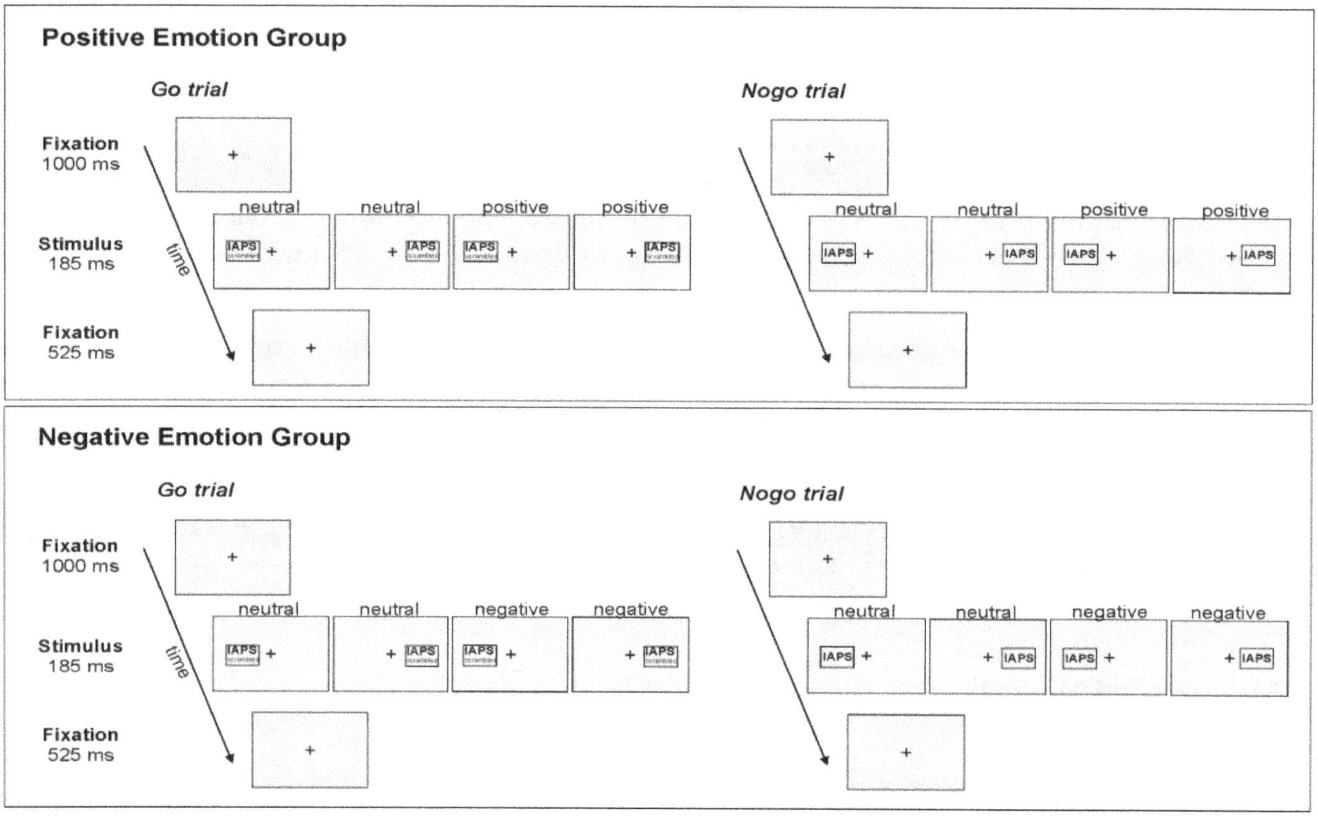

Figure 1. Schematic illustration of the sequence and time course of stimulus presentation. Half of the stimuli for each condition (Go/Nogo) and each valence (positive/neutral or negative/neutral) were presented in the left, the other half in the right visual field. Nogo stimuli were intact IAPS pictures; Go stimuli were scrambled versions of the same IAPS pictures. Trials were separated by inter-trial intervals jittered between 750 ms and 950 ms.

Stimuli were presented on a 17 inch CRT monitor in a dimly lit room, with subjects seated at a viewing distance of 57 cm. Note that at this viewing distance 1 cm on the screen equals 1° of visual angle. Head position was stabilized with a chin rest. Subjects were instructed to keep their gaze on the central fixation cross throughout the entire task, and to press the arrow up key on a key board as fast and as accurately as possible whenever a Go stimulus was presented. Participants responded with their right hand on all trials. Only the right hand was used to respond in order to maximize trial numbers in critical conditions. Although contralateral movement-related potentials can arise prior to the imperative stimulus and potentially affect nogo-ERPs, these do not interact with stimulus lateralization, and should therefore have equivalent effects on left and right visual field stimuli [56,57]. Furthermore, subjects had to withhold their response whenever a Nogo stimulus was presented. Nogo stimuli were intact (i.e., non-scrambled) emotional or neutral pictures, while Go stimuli were scrambled images of the same emotional or neutral pictures (see Figure 1). For half of the subjects, emotional pictures had a negative valence (negative emotion group). There were 12 images in each category. Negative emotional pictures depicted bodily mutilation, injury, or dead bodies. For the other half of the participants, emotional pictures had a positive valence and depicted erotic (heterosexual) couples (positive emotions group). Neutral images all depicted people engaged in common activities. Comparison of normative ratings [8] revealed that positive images were rated as more pleasant and more arousing than neutral images, and negative images were rated as more unpleasant and more arousing than neutral images (all $p < 0.001$). Positive and negative images did not differ in arousal ($p = 0.13$). The same picture sets were used for male and female participants, as men and women rate these images similarly. There were 12 female and 10 male participants in the negative emotion group and 10 female and 10 male participants in the positive emotions group. There were no significant differences in gender composition between the two groups ($p = 0.77$).

In total, the task comprised 672 trials, with 29% (192) Nogo and 71% (480) Go trials. For each trial type (Go/Nogo), half of the stimuli were emotional (Go: 240; Nogo: 96) and half were neutral, and of those, half were presented in the LVF (Go: 120; Nogo: 48) and half in the RVF. Note, however, that because Go stimuli were scrambled images, they were emotional only in that they were derived from emotional images; they had no emotional meaning of their own. Stimulus presentation was randomized. Task completion took approximately 16 minutes. Accuracy (percentages of correct responses), false alarms (that is, responses on Nogo trials), misses (that is, non-responses on Go trials), and mean response times (RTs) for correct responses were assessed.

2.3. Electrophysiological Recordings

EEG was recorded from 64 channels using an actiCAP electrode system with Ag-AgCL electrodes and a standard BrainAmp amplifier, and the corresponding recording BrainVision Recorder software (Brain Products, Gilching, Germany) at a sampling rate of 1000 Hz. Electrodes were arranged according to the International 10-20 system (FCz, FP1, FP2, F7, F3, F4, F8, FC5, FC1, FC2, FC6, T7, C3, Cz, C4, T8, TP9, CP5, CP1, CP2, CP6, TP10, P7, P3, Pz, P4, P8, PO9, O1, Oz, O2, PO10, AF7, AF3, AF4, AF8, F5, F1, F2, F6, FT9, FT7, FC3, FC4, FT8, FT10, C5, C1, C2, C6, TP7, CP3, CPz, CP4, TP8, P5, P1, P2, P6, PO7, PO3, POz, PO4, PO8). Electrode FCz was used as a primary reference. Impedances were kept below 10 kΩ, mostly ranging from 5 to 10 kΩ. Initially, 44 subjects were tested, but in two subjects (1 male, 1 female), not enough electrodes could be recorded throughout the task due to technical problems. Data from these subjects were excluded from all analyses, rendering a sample of N = 42 for the study, as described above.

EEG data were processed off-line using BrainVision Analyzer 2 (Brain Products, Gilching, Germany). Raw data were first down-sampled to 500 Hz and filtered with 0.5 Hz low cutoff and 20 Hz high cutoff (48 dB/oct). The filtered data were visually inspected and all trials containing gross technical artefacts were rejected. Horizontal and vertical eye movements as well as pulse artefacts were then corrected using infomax independent component analysis (ICA), which was applied to the unepoched data. Epoched data were subjected to automatic artefact rejection applying the following rejection criteria: maximum voltage steps of more than 50 μV/ms, maximum value differences of 200 μV in 200 ms intervals, or activity below 0.1 μV. The overall number of trials rejected by this procedure was below 5% of all trials for each condition and channel.

Data analyses (peak and latency quantification) were performed after the calculation of current source density (CSD) of the signal in order to ensure reference-free evaluation [54]. CSD transformation replaces the potential at each electrode with the CSD, thereby eliminating the reference potential. The algorithm applies the spherical Laplace operator to the scalp distribution of the potential. Since this distribution is only known for electrodes that were actually used, spherical spline interpolation is applied to calculate a continuous potential distribution [58].

Data were segmented into 1200 ms epochs starting 200 ms before and ending 1000 ms after onset of Go or Nogo stimuli, respectively. Baseline correction was applied based on the 200 ms directly preceding the stimulus onset. Segments were averaged according to condition (Go/Nogo), emotionality (emotional/neutral), and side (LVF/RVF). Note that only trials with a correct Go or Nogo response were included. Electrodes used for amplitude and latency quantification were chosen based on the typical scalp topographies for the N2 and P3, as well as on careful visual inspection of grand-average ERPs in the present data set. N2 amplitude and latency were measured based on the maximum negative peak occurring in a time window from 190 to 390 ms after stimulus onset at electrode FCz. P3 amplitude and latency were measured based on the maximum positive peak occurring in a time window from 300 to 600 ms after stimulus onset at electrode Pz.

2.4. Statistical Analysis

Statistical analyses were performed using IBM SPSS 23 software (IBM Corporation, Armonk, New York, USA). With regard to behavioural performance and accuracy (percentage of correct responses, that is, button presses in the Go condition, and non-responses in the Nogo condition); RTs for correct responses in the Go condition were also analyzed. The significance level was set to $p < 0.05$. Effect sizes are provided as the proportion of variance accounted for (partial η^2). Mean amplitudes are provided together with the standard error of the mean (SEM as measure of variability).

3. Results

3.1. Behavioural Data

Overall, participants were significantly more accurate when responding to Go stimuli (98.10%) as compared to when withholding their responses to Nogo stimuli (87.75%) ($t_{(41)} = 8.39$; $p < 0.001$). Subsequent analyses were carried out only for Nogo trials (see Figure 2), as the factor emotionality could only be interpreted for these trials because stimuli were scrambled on Go trials. Also, as indicated by very high accuracy on Go trials (>98%), there was possibly a ceiling effect in the Go condition.

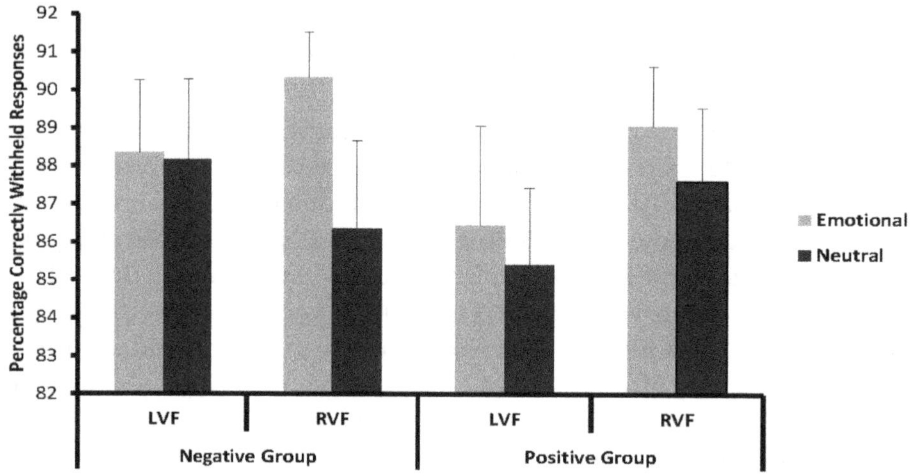

Figure 2. Mean percentage of correctly withheld responses in the Nogo condition for emotional and neutral stimuli in left (LVF) and right (RVF) visual field in the positive and negative emotion groups.

Accuracy data for the Nogo condition was analysed with a 2 × 2 × 2 repeated measures ANOVA with the within-subjects factors side (LVF/RVF) and emotionality (emotional/neutral), and the between-subjects factor valence (positive/negative). Here, the main effect of emotionality showed a strong trend towards significance ($F_{(1,40)} = 3.89$; $p = 0.056$; partial $\eta^2 = 0.09$), indicating that participants were more accurate in withholding their responses to emotional (88.55%), as compared to neutral, pictures (86.89%). All other effects failed to reach significance (all $p > 0.13$).

3.2. EEG Data

3.2.1. N2

N2 Amplitude

For N2 amplitude (see Figure 3), analysis revealed a more negative N2 in the Nogo (−13.82 µV ± 1.28) compared to the Go condition (−9.25 µV ± 0.30), as was to be expected for a Go/Nogo task ($t_{(41)} = 4.47$; $p < 0.001$). Subsequent analyses of emotion effects were carried out within the Nogo trials. N2 amplitudes in the Nogo condition were analysed with a 2 × 2 × 2 repeated measures ANOVA with the within-subjects factors side (LVF/RVF) and emotionality (emotional/neutral), and the between-subjects factor valence (positive/negative). In this analysis, all effects failed to reach significance (all $p > 0.20$).

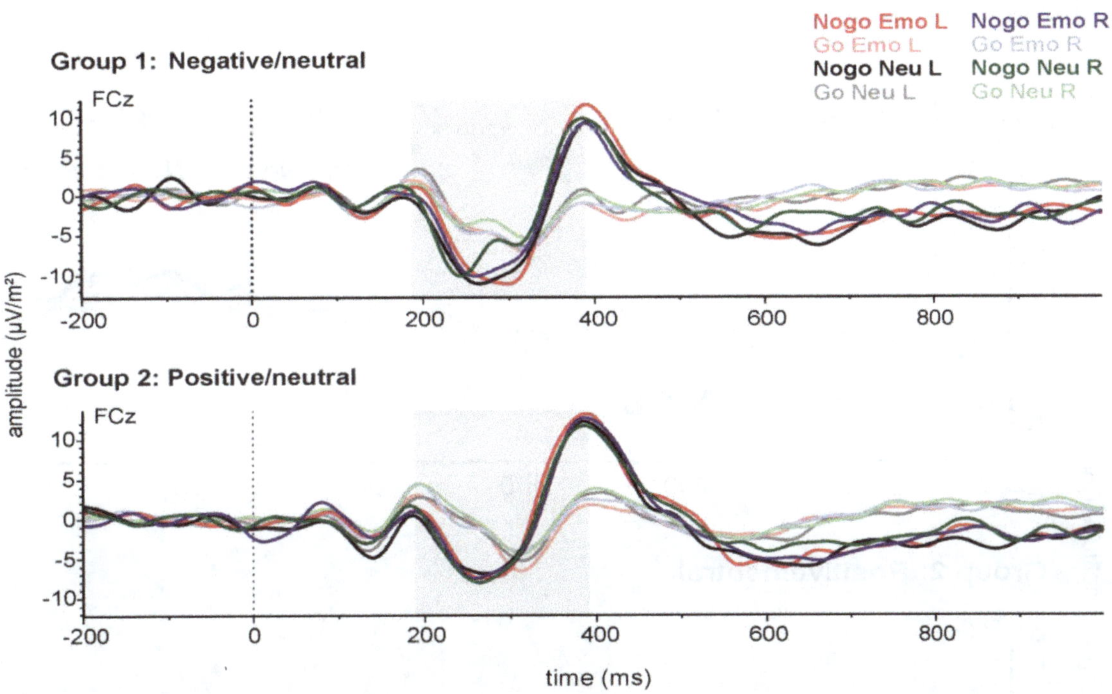

Figure 3. Stimulus-locked grand-average event-related potentials (ERPs) for emotional and neutral Go and Nogo stimuli presented on the left (**L**) or right (**R**) side at electrode FCz. The upper panel shows data from the negative emotion group and the lower panel data from the positive emotion group.

N2 Latency

With regard to latency, the N2 emerged earlier in the Nogo (291.29 ms ± 5.12) than in the Go condition (297.28 ms ± 5.84) ($t_{(41)} = 3.44$; $p < 0.01$). Subsequent analyses of emotion effects were carried out within the Nogo trials. N2 latencies in the Nogo condition were analysed with a 2 × 2 × 2 repeated measures ANOVA with the within-subjects factors side (LVF/RVF), and emotionality (emotional/neutral) and the between-subjects factor valence (positive/negative). In this analysis, all effects failed to reach significance (all $p > 0.18$).

3.2.2. P3

P3 Amplitude

For P3 amplitude (see Figure 4), greater amplitudes were observed in the Go (17.27 μV ± 1.64) as compared to the Nogo condition (12.43 μV ± 1.60) ($t_{(41)} = -5.01$; $p < 0.001$). Subsequent analyses were carried out only for Nogo trials, to evaluate effects of emotion. P3 amplitudes in the Nogo condition were analysed with a 2 × 2 × 2 repeated measures ANOVA with the within-subjects factors side (LVF/RVF) and emotionality (emotional/neutral), and the between-subjects factor valence (positive/negative). Here, the main side effect reached significance ($F_{(1,40)} = 4.12$; $p < 0.05$; partial $\eta^2 = 0.09$), indicating a more positive P3 after stimulus presentation in the LVF (13.31 ± 1.55) as compared to the RVF (11.71 ± 1.53). Moreover, the main effect of emotionality ($F_{(1,40)} = 16.32$; $p < 0.001$; partial $\eta^2 = 0.29$) reached significance, indicating that emotional stimuli lead to a higher P3 (14.01 ± 1.65) than neutral stimuli (11.01 ± 1.41). This effect of emotionality on P3 amplitude was modulated by stimulus valence, as indicated by a significant valence × emotionality interaction ($F_{(1,40)} = 11.28$; $p < 0.01$; partial $\eta^2 = 0.22$). Post-hoc tests revealed no difference between emotional and neutral stimuli in the group of subjects who saw negative emotional images ($p = 0.65$). However, for those who saw positive emotional images, P3 amplitude was greater for emotional stimuli (16.86 ± 2.39) than for neutral stimuli (11.37 ± 2.07) ($p < 0.001$). Importantly for our hypotheses, the effects of side and emotion did not interact.

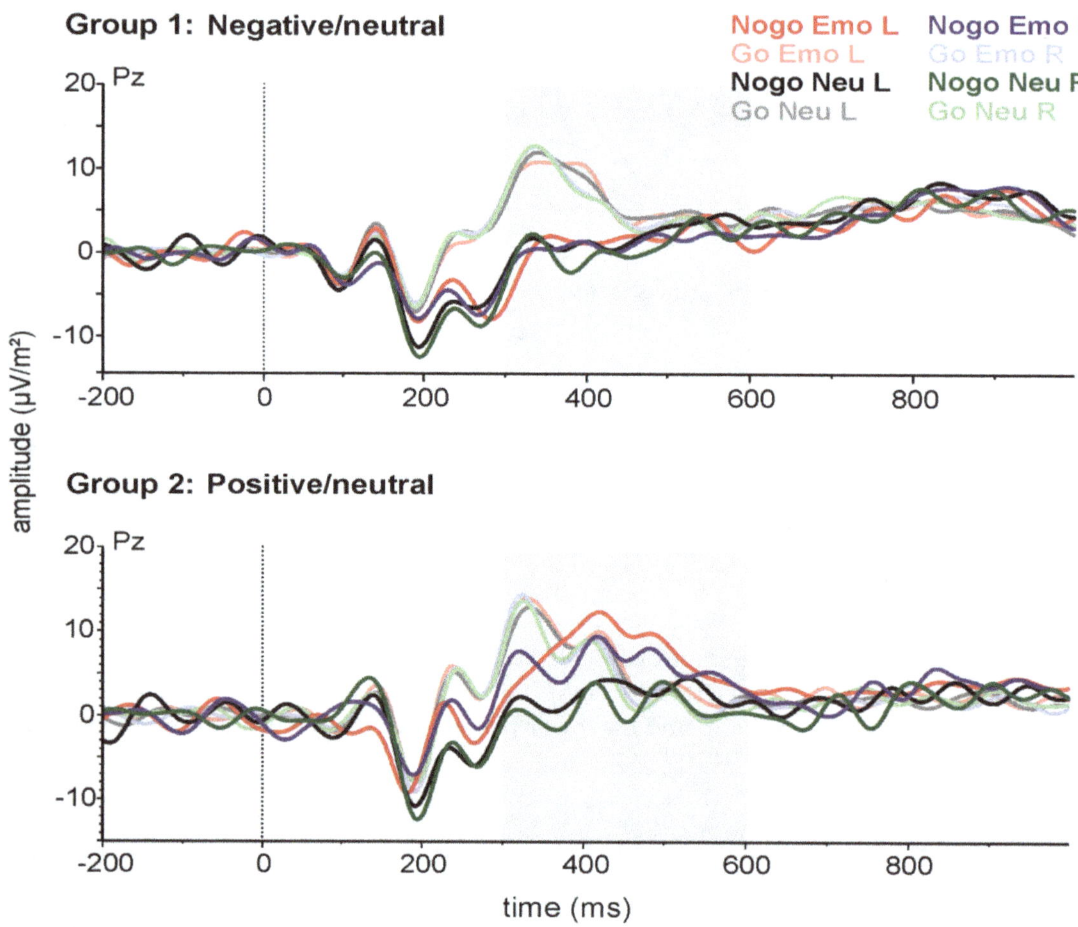

Figure 4. Stimulus-locked grand-average ERPs for emotional and neutral Go and Nogo stimuli presented on the left (**L**) or right (**R**) side at electrode Pz. The upper panel shows data from the negative emotion group and the lower panel data from the positive emotions group.

P3 Latency

For latency, the P3 emerged earlier in the Go (372.53 ms ± 9.00) as compared to the Nogo condition (404.61 ms ± 8.41) ($t_{(41)} = -2.84$; $p < 0.01$). Subsequent analyses were carried out only for Nogo trials, to evaluate emotion-related effects. P3 latencies in the Nogo condition were analysed with a 2 × 2 × 2 repeated measures ANOVA with the within-subjects factors side (LVF/RVF) and emotionality (emotional/neutral), and the between-subjects factor valence (positive/negative). In this analysis, all effects failed to reach significance (all $p > 0.22$).

4. Discussion

Functional hemispheric asymmetries are one of the core organizational principles underlying many cognitive functions in the human brain, including emotion processing [6–8], but their interaction with prefrontal functions, e.g., executive control, is not well understood. The present study was designed to elucidate the neurophysiological basis of this relationship by recording N2 and P3 ERP components during a divided visual field Go/Nogo task with scrambled (Go) or intact (Nogo) pictures with emotional or neutral content that was incidental to the task. Based on right-hemisphere dominance for emotional processing, we would expect emotion effects to be stronger for imperative stimuli presented in the left visual field than in the right. Alternatively, valence-based models lead to the prediction of stronger effects of negative stimuli in the left visual field, and stronger effects of positive stimuli in the right visual field.

We observed expected differences between Go and Nogo trials in the accuracy data, indicating that our task effectively elicited response conflict and response inhibition [30,32]. Additionally, accuracy on both Go and Nogo trials was high (98% and 88%, respectively), showing that participants were able to distinguish intact from scrambled images even though they were presented only briefly in the periphery. High accuracy also meant that sufficient trials were available for analysis of N2 and P3 responses.

We observed effects of emotion that are broadly consistent with those reported in other studies that have manipulated the emotion of imperative stimuli in Go/Nogo tasks. Behaviourally, emotional stimuli were associated with marginally better performance on Nogo trials, consistent with a "freezing" effect of emotion, perhaps driven by attentional prioritisation of emotional stimulus processing [50]. Turning to the ERP measures, we found no effect of emotion on the Nogo-N2, consistent with other studies [44,45]. Collectively, these studies suggest that conflict monitoring processes are not sensitive to emotion. Also consistent with other studies, we observed that Nogo-P3 was enhanced in the presence of positive emotional stimuli [44,45]. The most common interpretation of emotional potentiation of the P3 is that sustained attentional engagement with positive emotional stimuli affects the execution or evaluation of inhibitory processing.

Emotion effects were observed even though stimuli were only briefly presented in peripheral locations, meaning that our experimental paradigm should be sensitive to hemispheric differences in emotional processing if they exist. Nonetheless, neither emotionality nor valence interacted with the visual field on any measure. Our findings therefore do not support either a right hemisphere or valence-based interpretation of emotional processing in the context of response inhibition. This complete lack of asymmetry in emotional processing was unexpected, given robust findings of emotional asymmetry on perceptual processing [6–8]. It is possible that asymmetries were not observed because emotion was incidental to the task, which required participants only to distinguish intact from scrambled stimuli. Many studies that have produced evidence for emotional asymmetries use explicit emotional identification or judgments [6–8], or involve tasks in which emotion is relevant to response [53]. We purposefully made emotion itself task-irrelevant so that we could observe the effects of emotion on control processes independent of any effects on motor execution (e.g., approach and avoidance tendencies that might have been activated by positive and negative stimuli, respectively) [7]. Further studies on the task dimensions that influence emotional asymmetries would be necessary to evaluate this hypothesis.

Although emotion did not interact with visual field, hemispheric differences were still observed, in that the Nogo-P3 was enhanced for the left visual field relative to right visual field stimuli. This finding is partially consistent with our previous study in which both Nogo-N2 and Nogo-P3 were enhanced for verbal stimuli presented in the left visual field [54]. The fact that similar effects have been observed for both verbal and pictorial stimuli suggests that this effect might not be stimulus-specific, and might instead reflect asymmetry in the application of inhibitory control more broadly. Notably, response inhibition mechanisms have been localised to the right hemisphere [59], and specifically to right inferofrontal cortex [60,61].

The use of lateralised stimuli in Go/Nogo task (especially with ERP measures) is not common in the literature, and further studies are needed using a broader range of stimulus modalities before drawing strong conclusions about how hemispheric asymmetries in stimulus processing affect response inhibition processes. For example, in order to render findings on emotional lateralisation in inhibition-related ERPs more comparable to those found for verbal stimuli [54], it would be an interesting follow-up study to use the emotional content of the stimuli not as a distracting task-irrelevant feature but as the Go/Nogo indicator. Here, emotional stimuli with reduced stimulus complexity should be used. While IAPS pictures are widely used and thus constitute a well-validated stimulus set in emotion processing research, they typically are presented for longer intervals than in the present tachistoscopic experiment when participants must make judgments of valence based on stimulus content. This brief presentation may lead to reduced accuracy when using them as Go/Nogo stimuli. Less complex emotional stimuli, e.g., emotional faces, might be better suited for such tasks (see [62] for a tachistoscopic EEG study that successfully used emotional faces as imperative stimuli). Moreover, in the present study, although it was task-irrelevant, emotion was a stimulus property of the Go/Nogo stimuli. To further disentangle stimulus- and distractor-related effects, it would be informative to use a paradigm with central presentation of non-verbal Go/Nogo stimuli without emotional content (e.g., red and green coloured squares). The distractors (IAPS pictures or emotional faces) would then be presented in the LVF or RVF. By comparing distractor trials to trials without distractors, a more fine-tuned assessment of the effects of left- or right-hemispheric stimulus processing on prefrontal inhibition processes would be possible. Moreover, we used a between-subjects design in the present study, with one group of subjects tested with positive and neutral stimuli and the other group with negative and neutral stimuli. A within-subjects design in which each participant is tested in both conditions would have greater statistical power and should be used in future studies addressing ERP-correlates of emotional lateralization. Additionally, the Go/Nogo task is only one of several paradigms that allow investigation of prefrontally mediated inhibition processes. Other paradigms targeting prefrontal functions that involve inhibition, e.g., the stop-signal task [63], stop-change task [64], or the task-switching paradigm [65] could yield further evidence for a relationship between emotional lateralisation and prefrontal inhibition.

5. Conclusions

Emotional asymmetries are commonly observed in perception and in emotional expression and experience. We manipulated the emotional nature of the Nogo stimulus in order to distinguish between right hemisphere and valence-based explanations of emotional asymmetry. P3 amplitudes were enhanced when stimuli were presented in the left visual field, suggesting that evaluative processes involved in response inhibition are sensitive to hemispheric differences in stimulus processing. P3 amplitudes were also potentiated by positive images, showing that the evaluative processes reflected by the P3 are sensitive to emotional content. However, contrary to both right-hemisphere and valence models, we found no evidence that emotional effects depended on the hemisphere to which those stimuli were presented.

Acknowledgments: This work was partially supported by the G.A. Lienert Foundation with a research stipend awarded to Jutta Peterburs. It was also partially supported by a travel grant from the Global Young Faculty to Sebastian Ocklenburg and by grant VUW1307 from the Royal Society of New Zealand Marsden fund to Gina M. Grimshaw.

Author Contributions: Sebastian Ocklenburg, Jutta Peterburs, Onur Güntürkün and Gina M. Grimshaw conceived and designed the experiments; Janet Mertzen and Judith Schmitz performed the experiments; Janet Mertzen and Sebastian Ocklenburg analysed the data; Onur Güntürkün contributed reagents/materials/analysis tools; Sebastian Ocklenburg, Jutta Peterburs, Onur Güntürkün and Gina M. Grimshaw wrote the manuscript.

References

1. Rogers, L.J. Asymmetry of brain and behavior in animals: Its development, function, and human relevance. *Genesis* **2014**, *52*, 555–571. [CrossRef] [PubMed]
2. Rogers, L.J. Development and function of lateralization in the avian brain. *Brain Res. Bull.* **2008**, *76*, 235–244. [CrossRef] [PubMed]
3. Vallortigara, G.; Rogers, L.J. Survival with an asymmetrical brain: Advantages and disadvantages of cerebral lateralization. *Behav. Brain Sci.* **2005**, *28*, 575–589. [CrossRef] [PubMed]
4. Ocklenburg, S.; Ströckens, F.; Güntürkün, O. Lateralisation of conspecific vocalisation in non-human vertebrates. *Laterality* **2013**, *18*, 1–31. [CrossRef] [PubMed]
5. Ströckens, F.; Güntürkün, O.; Ocklenburg, S. Limb preferences in non-human vertebrates. *Laterality* **2013**, *18*, 536–575. [CrossRef] [PubMed]
6. Davidson, R.J. Anterior cerebral asymmetry and the nature of emotion. *Brain Cogn.* **1992**, *20*, 125–151. [CrossRef]
7. Onal-Hartmann, C.; Pauli, P.; Ocklenburg, S.; Güntürkün, O. The motor side of emotions: Investigating the relationship between hemispheres, motor reactions and emotional stimuli. *Psychol. Res.* **2012**, *76*, 311–316. [CrossRef] [PubMed]
8. Thompson, J.K. Right brain, left brain; left face, right face: Hemisphericity and the expression of facial emotion. *Cortex* **1985**, *21*, 281–299. [CrossRef]
9. Hughlings-Jacckson, J. On affections of speech from disease of the brain. *Brain* **1878**, *1*, 304–330. [CrossRef]
10. Gainotti, G. Emotional behavior and hemispheric side of the lesion. *Cortex* **1972**, *8*, 41–55. [CrossRef]
11. Borod, J.C.; Cicero, B.A.; Obler, L.K.; Welkowitz, J.; Erhan, H.M.; Santschi, C.; Grunwald, I.S.; Agosti, R.M.; Whalen, J.R. Right hemisphere emotional perception: Evidence across multiple channels. *Neuropsychology* **1998**, *12*, 446–458. [CrossRef] [PubMed]
12. Coan, J.A.; Allen, J.J.B. Frontal EEG asymmetry as a moderator and mediator of emotion. *Biol. Psychol.* **2004**, *67*, 7–49. [CrossRef] [PubMed]
13. Harmon-Jones, E.; Gable, P.A. On the role of asymmetric frontal cortical activity in approach and withdrawal motivation: An updated review of the evidence. *Psychophysiology* **2017**. [CrossRef] [PubMed]
14. Ley, R.G.; Bryden, M.P. Hemispheric differences in processing emotions and faces. *Brain Lang.* **1979**, *7*, 127–138. [CrossRef]
15. Grimshaw, G.M.; Séguin, J.A.; Godfrey, H.K. Once more with feeling: The effects of emotional prosody on hemispheric specialisation for linguistic processing. *J. Neurol.* **2009**, *22*, 313–326. [CrossRef]
16. Buchanan, T.W.; Lutz, K.; Mirzazade, S.; Specht, K.; Shah, N.J.; Zilles, K.; Jäncke, L. Recognition of emotional prosody and verbal components of spoken language: An fMRI study. *Brain Res. Cogn. Brain Res.* **2000**, *9*, 227–238. [CrossRef]
17. Herrington, J.D.; Heller, W.; Mohanty, A.; Engels, A.S.; Banich, M.T.; Webb, A.G.; Miller, G.A. Localization of asymmetric brain function in emotion and depression. *Psychophysiology* **2010**, *47*, 442–454. [CrossRef] [PubMed]
18. Borod, J.C.; Kent, J.; Koff, E.; Martin, C.; Alpert, M. Facial asymmetry while posing positive and negative emotions: Support for the right hemisphere hypothesis. *Neuropsychologia* **1988**, *26*, 759–764. [CrossRef]
19. Canli, T.; Desmond, J.E.; Zhao, Z.; Glover, G.; Gabrieli, J.D. Hemispheric asymmetry for emotional stimuli detected with fMRI. *Neuroreport* **1998**, *9*, 3233–3239. [CrossRef] [PubMed]

20. Davidson, R.J.; Ekman, P.; Saron, C.D.; Senulis, J.A.; Friesen, W.V. Approach-withdrawal and cerebral asymmetry: Emotional expression and brain physiology. I. *J. Pers. Soc. Psychol.* **1990**, *58*, 330–341. [CrossRef] [PubMed]
21. Silberman, E.K.; Weingartner, H. Hemispheric lateralization of functions related to emotion. *Brain Cogn.* **1986**, *5*, 322–353. [CrossRef]
22. Rodway, P.; Schepman, A. Valence specific laterality effects in prosody: Expectancy account and the effects of morphed prosody and stimulus lead. *Brain Cogn.* **2007**, *63*, 31–41. [CrossRef] [PubMed]
23. Schepman, A.; Rodway, P.; Geddes, P. Valence-specific laterality effects in vocal emotion: Interactions with stimulus type, blocking and sex. *Brain Cogn.* **2012**, *79*, 129–137. [CrossRef] [PubMed]
24. Killgore, W.D.S.; Yurgelun-Todd, D.A. The right-hemisphere and valence hypotheses: Could they both be right (and sometimes left)? *Soc. Cogn. Affect. Neurosci.* **2007**, *2*, 240–250. [CrossRef] [PubMed]
25. Heller, W. Neuropsychological mechanisms of individual differences in emotion, personality, and arousal. *Neuropsychology* **1993**, *7*, 476–489. [CrossRef]
26. Heller, W.; Nitschke, J.B.; Miller, G.A. Lateralization in emotion and emotional disorders. *Curr. Dir. Psychol. Sci.* **1998**, *7*, 26–32. [CrossRef]
27. Harmon-Jones, E.; Gable, P.A.; Peterson, C.K. The role of asymmetric frontal cortical activity in emotion-related phenomena: A review and update. *Biol. Psychol.* **2010**, *84*, 451–462. [CrossRef] [PubMed]
28. Grimshaw, G.M.; Carmel, D. An asymmetric inhibition model of hemispheric differences in emotional processing. *Front. Psychol.* **2014**, *5*, 489. [CrossRef] [PubMed]
29. Kane, M.J.; Engle, R.W. The role of prefrontal cortex in working-memory capacity, executive attention, and general fluid intelligence: An individual-differences perspective. *Psychon. Bull. Rev.* **2002**, *9*, 637–671. [CrossRef] [PubMed]
30. Falkenstein, M. Inhibition, conflict and the Nogo-N2. *Clin. Neurophysiol.* **2006**, *117*, 1638–1640. [CrossRef] [PubMed]
31. Garavan, H.; Ross, T.J.; Murphy, K.; Roche, R.A.P.; Stein, E.A. Dissociable executive functions in the dynamic control of behavior: Inhibition, error detection, and correction. *NeuroImage* **2002**, *17*, 1820–1829. [CrossRef] [PubMed]
32. Falkenstein, M.; Hoormann, J.; Hohnsbein, J. ERP components in Go/Nogo tasks and their relation to inhibition. *Acta Psychol.* **1999**, *101*, 267–291. [CrossRef]
33. Bokura, H.; Yamaguchi, S.; Kobayashi, S. Electrophysiological correlates for response inhibition in a Go/NoGo task. *Clin. Neurophysiol.* **2001**, *112*, 2224–2232. [CrossRef]
34. Nieuwenhuis, S.; Yeung, N.; van den Wildenberg, W.; Ridderinkhof, K.R. Electrophysiological correlates of anterior cingulate function in a go/no-go task: Effects of response conflict and trial type frequency. *Cogn. Affect. Behav. Neurosci.* **2003**, *3*, 17–26. [CrossRef] [PubMed]
35. Band, G.P.; van Boxtel, G.J. Inhibitory motor control in stop paradigms: Review and reinterpretation of neural mechanisms. *Acta Psychol.* **1999**, *101*, 179–211. [CrossRef]
36. Beste, C.; Saft, C.; Andrich, J.; Gold, R.; Falkenstein, M. Response inhibition in Huntington's disease-a study using ERPs and sLORETA. *Neuropsychologia* **2008**, *46*, 1290–1297. [CrossRef] [PubMed]
37. Beste, C.; Dziobek, I.; Hielscher, H.; Willemssen, R.; Falkenstein, M. Effects of stimulus-response compatibility on inhibitory processes in Parkinson's disease. *Eur. J. Neurosci.* **2009**, *29*, 855–860. [CrossRef] [PubMed]
38. Roche, R.A.P.; Garavan, H.; Foxe, J.J.; O'Mara, S.M. Individual differences discriminate event-related potentials but not performance during response inhibition. *Exp.Brain Res.* **2005**, *160*, 60–70. [CrossRef] [PubMed]
39. Liu, L.; Ioannides, A.A. Emotion separation is completed early and it depends on visual field presentation. *PloS ONE* **2010**, *5*, e9790. [CrossRef] [PubMed]
40. Rigoulot, S.; D'Hondt, F.; Honoré, J.; Sequeira, H. Implicit emotional processing in peripheral vision: Behavioral and neural evidence. *Neuropsychologia* **2012**, *50*, 2887–2896. [CrossRef] [PubMed]
41. Rigoulot, S.; Delplanque, S.; Despretz, P.; Defoort-Dhellemmes, S.; Honoré, J.; Sequeira, H. Peripherally presented emotional scenes: A spatiotemporal analysis of early ERP responses. *Brain Topogr.* **2008**, *20*, 216–223. [CrossRef] [PubMed]
42. Ocklenburg, S. Tachistoscopic viewing and dichotic listening. In *Lateralized Brain Functions: Methods in Human and Non-human Species*; Rogers, L.J., Vallortigara, G., Eds.; Humana Press; Springer: New York, NY, USA, 2017; Volume 122.

43. Lang, P.J.; Bradley, M.M.; Cuthbert, B.N. Motivated attention: Affect, activation, and action. In *Attention and Orienting: Sensory and Motivational Processes*; Lang, P.J., Simons, R.F., Balaban, M., Eds.; Lawrence Erlbaum Associates: Mahwah, NJ, USA, 1997; pp. 97–135.
44. Albert, J.; López-Martín, S.; Carretié, L. Emotional context modulates response inhibition: Neural and behavioral data. *NeuroImage* **2010**, *49*, 914–921. [CrossRef] [PubMed]
45. Albert, J.; López-Martín, S.; Tapia, M.; Montoya, D.; Carretié, L. The role of the anterior cingulate cortex in emotional response inhibition. *Hum. Brain Mapp.* **2012**, *33*, 2147–2160. [CrossRef] [PubMed]
46. Buodo, G.; Sarlo, M.; Mento, G.; Messerotti Benvenuti, S.; Palomba, D. Unpleasant stimuli differentially modulate inhibitory processes in an emotional Go/NoGo task: An event-related potential study. *Cogn. Emot.* **2017**, *31*, 127–138. [CrossRef] [PubMed]
47. Chiu, P.H.; Holmes, A.J.; Pizzagalli, D.A. Dissociable recruitment of rostral anterior cingulate and inferior frontal cortex in emotional response inhibition. *NeuroImage* **2008**, *42*, 988–997. [CrossRef] [PubMed]
48. López-Martín, S.; Albert, J.; Fernández-Jaén, A.; Carretié, L. Emotional response inhibition in children with attention-deficit/hyperactivity disorder: Neural and behavioural data. *Psychol. Med.* **2015**, *45*, 2057–2071. [CrossRef] [PubMed]
49. Yu, F.; Yuan, J.; Luo, Y.-J. Auditory-induced emotion modulates processes of response inhibition: An event-related potential study. *Neuroreport* **2009**, *20*, 25–30. [CrossRef] [PubMed]
50. De Houwer, J.; Tibboel, H. Stop what you are not doing! Emotional pictures interfere with the task not to respond. *Psychon. Bull. Rev.* **2010**, *17*, 699–703. [CrossRef] [PubMed]
51. Zhang, W.; Lu, J. Time course of automatic emotion regulation during a facial Go/Nogo task. *Biol. Psychol.* **2012**, *89*, 444–449. [CrossRef] [PubMed]
52. Grimshaw, G.M.; Kranz, L.S.; Carmel, D.; Moody, R.E.; Devue, C. Contrasting reactive and proactive control of emotional distraction. *Emotion* **2017**. [CrossRef] [PubMed]
53. Calvo, M.G.; Avero, P. Affective priming of emotional pictures in parafoveal vision: Left visual field advantage. *Cogn. Affect. Behav Neurosci* **2008**, *8*, 41–53. [CrossRef] [PubMed]
54. Ocklenburg, S.; Güntürkün, O.; Beste, C. Lateralized neural mechanisms underlying the modulation of response inhibition processes. *NeuroImage* **2011**, *55*, 1771–1778. [CrossRef] [PubMed]
55. Oldfield, R.C. The assessment and analysis of handedness: The Edinburgh inventory. *Neuropsychologia* **1971**, *9*, 97–113. [CrossRef]
56. Wascher, E.; Wauschkuhn, B. The interaction of stimulus- and response-related processes measured by event-related lateralizations of the EEG. *Electroencephalogr. Clin. Neurophysiol.* **1996**, *99*, 149–162. [CrossRef]
57. Miller, J. Contralateral and ipsilateral motor activation in visual simple reaction time: A test of the hemispheric coactivation model. *Exp. Brain Res.* **2007**, *176*, 539–558. [CrossRef] [PubMed]
58. Perrin, F.; Pernier, J.; Bertrand, O.; Echallier, J.F. Spherical splines for scalp potential and current density mapping. *Electroencephalogr. Clin. Neurophysiol.* **1989**, *72*, 184–187. [CrossRef]
59. D'Alberto, N.; Funnell, M.; Potter, A.; Garavan, H. A split-brain case study on the hemispheric lateralization of inhibitory control. *Neuropsychologia* **2017**, *99*, 24–29. [CrossRef] [PubMed]
60. Aron, A.R.; Robbins, T.W.; Poldrack, R.A. Inhibition and the right inferior frontal cortex. *Trends Cogn. Sci.* **2004**, *8*, 170–177. [CrossRef] [PubMed]
61. Aron, A.R.; Robbins, T.W.; Poldrack, R.A. Inhibition and the right inferior frontal cortex: One decade on. *Trends Cogn. Sci.* **2014**, *18*, 177–185. [CrossRef] [PubMed]
62. Ocklenburg, S.; Ness, V.; Güntürkün, O.; Suchan, B.; Beste, C. Response inhibition is modulated by functional cerebral asymmetries for facial expression perception. *Front. Psychol.* **2013**, *4*, 879. [CrossRef] [PubMed]
63. Livesey, E.J.; Livesey, D.J. Validation of a Bayesian Adaptive Estimation Technique in the Stop-Signal Task. *PLoS ONE* **2016**, *11*, e0165525. [CrossRef] [PubMed]
64. Verbruggen, F.; McLaren, R. Effects of reward and punishment on the interaction between going and stopping in a selective stop-change task. *Psychol. Res.* **2016**. [CrossRef] [PubMed]
65. Lange, F.; Seer, C.; Müller, D.; Kopp, B. Cognitive caching promotes flexibility in task switching: Evidence from event-related potentials. *Sci. Rep.* **2015**, *5*, 17502. [CrossRef] [PubMed]

14

A Matter of Degree: Strength of Brain Asymmetry and Behaviour

Lesley J. Rogers

School of Science and Technology, University of New England, Armidale, NSW 2351, Australia; lrogers@une.edu.au; Tel.: +61-266-515-006

Academic Editor: John H. Graham

Abstract: Research on a growing number of vertebrate species has shown that the left and right sides of the brain process information in different ways and that lateralized brain function is expressed in both specific and broad aspects of behaviour. This paper reviews the available evidence relating *strength* of lateralization to behavioural/cognitive performance. It begins by considering the relationship between limb preference and behaviour in humans and primates from the perspectives of direction and strength of lateralization. In birds, eye preference is used as a reflection of brain asymmetry and the strength of this asymmetry is associated with behaviour important for survival (e.g., visual discrimination of food from non-food and performance of two tasks in parallel). The same applies to studies on aquatic species, mainly fish but also tadpoles, in which strength of lateralization has been assessed as eye preferences or turning biases. Overall, the empirical evidence across vertebrate species points to the conclusion that stronger lateralization is advantageous in a wide range of contexts. Brief discussion of interhemispheric communication follows together with discussion of experiments that examined the effects of sectioning pathways connecting the left and right sides of the brain, or of preventing the development of these left-right connections. The conclusion reached is that degree of functional lateralization affects behaviour in quite similar ways across vertebrate species. Although the direction of lateralization is also important, in many situations strength of lateralization matters more. Finally, possible interactions between asymmetry in different sensory modalities is considered.

Keywords: functional asymmetry; strength of lateralization; direction of lateralization; advantages; disadvantages; vertebrate species; limb preference; eye bias

---

1. Introduction

A number of papers have reviewed the evidence for functional asymmetry of the brain, citing research showing that it is present in a growing list of vertebrate species [1–4], as well as more recent research demonstrating its presence in invertebrate species (summarized in [5]). The ubiquity of functional asymmetry suggests that it confers selective advantages [6], and some evidence in support of this deduction has been found by comparing the performance, within a species, of individuals with strongly versus weakly lateralized brains. By summarizing the research on different species, this paper attempts to arrive at a conclusion about the benefits versus deficits of strong versus weak lateralization.

The first obstacle encountered in an attempt to bring the research together is that different measures of the strength of laterality have been used [7]. Strength of paw or hand preference has been used as the axiom of strength of laterality in humans and other primates, although other techniques are now being used. In birds, strong versus weak or no laterality of visual responses has been generated by incubating eggs in the light or in darkness during the final days before hatching [4,8], and a similar method has been used to manipulate strength of lateralization in fish [9].

Although it is recognized that using different measures of the strength of lateralization could lead to different results, at this juncture it is worth taking a broad perspective to see how these disparate measures of laterality may be related to cognitive performance. The hypothesis considered is that cognitive ability is enhanced by having a strongly lateralized brain. That is, general cognitive performance may be enhanced by having a brain that is largely, if not entirely, subdivided to process information differently on the left and right sides (i.e., with distinctly separate computational processes being carried out in the left and right hemispheres [10,11]).

As summarised previously [3,4], in a range of vertebrate species the left hemisphere is specialized to categorize stimuli (e.g., food from inedible objects, general characteristics shared by all conspecifics versus those of other species), to focus attention and attend to specific targets and cues, to control established/learnt patterns of behaviour under relaxed conditions and to sustain responding by inhibiting fleeing and inhibiting attention to extraneous stimuli. The right hemisphere has broad attention, used to monitor the surrounds for the presence of predators and attend to other distracting stimuli, and also to detect novel stimuli. The right hemisphere also attends to social cues and, as part of that, recognizes faces of conspecifics, controls aggressive and sexual behaviour, as well as fear responses, and assesses multiple properties of stimuli. As an example of the right hemisphere's control of social responding, pigeons display more rapid social reactions to members of the flock on their left side, processed by the right hemisphere [12]. Also, as shown in a wide range of vertebrate species, infants are positioned more commonly on their mother's left side [13], thus being monitored by her right hemisphere. The right hemisphere also comes into play when the animal is under stress, and in these circumstances it has a dominant role in controlling responses [4].

Left-analytic encoding versus right-global encoding has been demonstrated clearly in chicks using tests similar to those designed for testing humans [14]. These subdivisions of function have been determined by testing a range of non-human species, primarily but not exclusively domestic chicks [15], pigeons [16], zebra fish [17], sheep [18] and dogs [19]. Observation of some species in the wild has confirmed that these asymmetries are seen not only in laboratory settings but also in natural habitats; for example, in Australian magpies responding to a predator [20] and in cetaceans feeding with a right side bias [21].

Similar or the same left-right specialisations are present in humans. A body of research has shown ([1], for example) that the majority of humans use the left hemisphere when they perform established or routine patterns of behaviour and, when using this hemisphere, their attention is focused. By contrast, the right hemisphere of humans has a broad attention used in detecting and responding to unexpected stimuli and responding to affective stimuli [22]. The right hemisphere of humans is also used to recognize faces, especially their emotional expressions [23], and to process other aspects of social information. Not surprising therefore, the right hemisphere is specialized for expressing anger and hostility and for processing of speech with emotional prosody [24] and it also has a role in depression (see later).

The question addressed in this paper is: does cognitive performance depend on the *degree* of lateralization of all or any of these respective hemispheric specializations present in vertebrate species?

2. Limb Preference and Performance

Not surprisingly, since each limb is controlled by its contralateral hemisphere [25], a good deal of research on humans has investigated associations between hand preference and cognitive performance. In general, left-handed subjects excel in tasks requiring cognitive functioning and behaviour associated with the right hemisphere, such as visuospatial ability [26,27] and arithmetic ability [28], whereas right-handed subjects excel on tasks associated with the left hemisphere, such as verbal tasks [29]. It is noted, however, that the association between handedness and cerebral asymmetry is not strong and, as Badzakova-Trajkov et al. [30] found, there is no correlation between handedness and spatial attention, measured in a line-bisection task and as memory of faces.

A study by Denny [31] conducted on a very large population of people from various European countries found that left-handers were significantly more likely to have depressive symptoms than were right handers. Non-right handers, meaning either ambidextrous or left-handed (also referred to as mixed handedness), are more prone than right-handers to suffer from a range of conditions, including schizophrenia [32,33], psychosis [34] and post-traumatic stress disorder [35]. Also, as found in a large sample of 11-year-old children [36], ambidextrous handedness is associated with poorer verbal, nonverbal, reading and mathematical skills compared to either left- or right-handers. This finding has been supported by the results of follow-up studies conducted on children of various ages and adolescents [37,38].

Many studies have compared right-handed with non-right-handed subjects and not weak handedness with strong handedness; this may not be the best way to categorise subjects. A study by Tsuang et al. [39] classified subjects into three categories (left-, right- and mixed handedness) and reported that schizotypy is associated with mixed handedness only, thus making the point that classification into right- versus non-right handed groups is not sufficient to reveal significant relationships. One study found heightened anxiety in strongly left- and right-handed people compared to mixed-handers [40]. Another study reported higher incidence of health problems, including heart disease, thyroid disorders, allergies and epilepsy, in individuals with inconsistent handedness, or ambidexterity [41]. Along these lines, research linking handedness to the development of dyslexia is now progressing and dyslexia-candidate genes have been discovered to play a role in the biological mechanisms that establish left-right asymmetry of the body and influence handedness [42]. Nevertheless, as Ocklenburg et al. [43] point out, the ontogenetic relationship of handedness to lateralization of language (and, by extrapolation, dyslexia) is multifactorial and complex.

Some studies have calculated hand preference using several tasks for scoring the hand used and then categorized subjects into consistent versus inconsistent left- or right-preferring. For example, using this method Hardie et al. [44] found that social anxiety was highest in the inconsistent left-hand preferring group. This result exemplifies the need for precise measurement of hand preference as a finer approach in future studies.

Using another measure of laterality, Johnson et al. [45] have reported that weak lateralization of auditory perception is more common in humans with dyslexia. Neuroimaging studies can also reveal lateral asymmetries, as for example hypoactivity in the left extrastriate cortex in dyslexic subjects compared to controls [46]. These are just some examples from the quite extensive body of research on functional lateralization and behaviour in humans. Handedness has commonly been used as the proxy measure of lateralization but more recent studies have used more direct measures of cerebral asymmetry [47,48].

In nonhuman primates, as in humans, strength of hand preference has been used as a proxy measure of strength of brain lateralization. An early report of association between strength of hand preference and performance in chimpanzees was made by McGrew and Marchant [49] and it concerned termite fishing. This behaviour involves tool use: the chimpanzee holds a stick in one hand and inserts it into the termite nest. The termites attack, and they remain clinging to the probe as the chimpanzee withdraws it, thus allowing the chimpanzee to consume them, usually after rubbing them off the stick by running it over their other hand or arm. Chimpanzees with a stronger preference to insert the probe repeatedly using the same hand were more successful in gaining termites to consume than were those with weaker hand preferences. Some chimpanzees preferred to use their right hand and some their left hand but direction of hand preference did not determine success in termite fishing. It was the strength of hand preference that counted.

Even though this review is focused on vertebrate species, it is worth mentioning a study of motor performance in desert locusts showing that locusts with strong limb preferences make fewer errors when they cross a gap than do locusts with weak limb preference [50]. To my knowledge, this is the only study, so far, investigating strength of lateralization and performance in invertebrates.

Strength of hand preference is associated with ability to attend to two tasks simultaneously, as shown in common marmosets [51]. The marmosets had to forage for food and at the same time respond to a model predator. First their hand preferences were determined by scoring the hand used to pick up pieces of food and take them to their mouth, scored 100 times per subject over several days. They were also trained to search for mealworms, a favourite food, presented in blue bowls at different locations within a room furnished with branches at various angles and heights and to avoid green bowls, placed next to the blue bowls and not containing mealworms. Hence, they were trained to use a win-shift strategy. On testing they were released into the room to search for mealworms and, once they had commenced searching, one of three model predators was presented. One predator was a taxidermic specimen of a kestrel moved overhead using a fishing line and a system of pulleys. Another was a model snake pulled across the floor. The third was a wooden carving of two frogs, resembling rearing snakes, also moved across the floor, and chosen because previous research had shown that the marmosets mobbed this stimulus consistently [52]. The stronger the hand preference the shorter was the latency to detect/react to the predator and the negative correlation between latency and strength of hand preference was significant for the test using the kestrel and the test using the frog carving. Marmosets utter phee calls when aroused and tsik calls when they mob a predator, and the number of these calls correlated positively with strength of hand preference. In summary, marmosets with stronger hand preferences, regardless of whether their preference was for the left or right hand, detected the predator sooner and reacted to it more strongly. Since in control trials, in which the predator was presented but the marmosets were not required to search for food, no significant relationship was found between hand preference and latency to detect the predator or number of calls, it can be concluded that strength of laterality has an effect only when the two tasks have to be undertaken simultaneously. Given that marmosets with weaker laterality are less able to perform the two tasks simultaneously, one can predict that they would be more vulnerable to predation in the natural environment.

The above results did not depend on whether the left or right hand was preferred by the marmosets. However, a number of other studies on primates have found behavioural differences between left- and right-hand preferring animals. Left-handed marmosets are generally more fearful that right-handed marmosets: they are less likely to touch novel objects [53], less likely to sample novel foods and react more strongly to calls made by a natural predator [54], and they are more likely to have a negative cognitive bias [55]. Left-handed marmosets are less responsive to social group influences than are right-handed ones [56]. Similar left- versus right-hand differences in behaviour have also been reported for chimpanzees [57] and rhesus macaques [58] and at least one study of humans has shown that left-handed subjects are more cautious in a novel problem-solving task than are right-handed ones [59].

A number of studies have examined relationships between paw preference and general performance [60–64]. One measure of paw preference in dogs involves scoring repeated trials in which the dog holds steady a Kong with one paw while it licks inside it to obtain a favourite food. A study using this measure found that dogs with no significant preference to use one paw over the other expressed more fear on hearing the sounds of thunderstorms than did dogs with either a left- or right-paw preference [60]. Other studies have found that dogs without a significant paw preference are more excitable when exposed to novel stimuli or environments [61] and are less aggressive to strangers [62]. Dogs without a significant paw preference also show shorter latency to obtain food from a novel puzzle-box than do either left- or right-pawed dogs [63]. In contrast, Siniscalchi et al. [64] found no association between paw preference and the reactivity of dogs to hearing thunderstorms although the dogs used their right hemisphere to respond to the sounds.

In conclusion, and despite some reported differences in behaviour between subjects with significant left- and right-forelimb preferences, the above studies show that subjects without a preference, or with a relatively weak preference, to use one hand/paw consistently are more fearful and excitable, less able to perform two tasks simultaneously, less responsive to novel stimuli and less responsive to social group influences.

A recent report on wild elk [65] supports some aspects of this conclusion: viz., elk with weaker forelimb preferences were more reactive to predator-like chases by humans than were those with stronger forelimb preferences (cf. similar findings in dogs). Other results obtained in this study (e.g., elk with stronger limb preferences were more likely to migrate) have not yet been matched by similar studies of group behavior in other species.

3. Strength of Lateralization and Performance in Birds

A strong body of experimental data demonstrates the presence of lateralization of visual processing and behaviour in the avian brain (summarized in [66]). Although the focus of this research has been on lateralization in domestic chicks and pigeons, laterality has been reported for visual behaviour in other avian species (e.g., zebra finches [67]; Australian magpies [20]; parrots [68]) and for production and processing of song (e.g., canaries [69]; and see paper by Kaplan in this special issue).

Lateralization of control of visual behaviour in the avian brain was first reported in 1979 [70], but it was not until some twenty years later that the potential function of the strength of lateralization, which varies between individuals, was examined. The first paper was published by Güntürkün et al. [71] and it reported a significant correlation between strength of lateralization in pigeons and success in discriminating grain from inedible grit. Pigeons were tested in three conditions: left-eye covered, right eye covered and both eyes uncovered. A laterality index for each bird was determined by the comparison of left- versus right-eye performance, the absolute value of which gave the strength of asymmetry. This value was then correlated against binocular performance and it revealed that the stronger the asymmetry, the more successful was the binocular performance (better at avoiding pecking at grit). Since most birds performed better on this task when they used the right eye (and left hemisphere) [72], as found previously to be the case in chicks [70] (also summarized in [66]), on this task the right eye is dominant. The authors suggested that asymmetry of the visual system enhances computational speed of object recognition by confining to one hemisphere the particular processing necessary to categorize grain as separate from grit (actually in the left hemisphere) and preventing conflicting information from the other hemisphere.

Experiments using domestic chicks have tested this hypothesis by manipulating conditions during development in order to produce groups of chicks that are lateralized for a range of visual functions and groups not lateralized for these same functions. The two types of chicks were generated by either exposing the developing embryos to light in the final days before hatching or by keeping them in darkness until after hatching (summarized in [66]). As a consequence of embryos being oriented in the egg so that the right eye is next to the shell and the left eye is next to the body and thus occluded, light exposure during this critical period stimulates only the right eye and causes asymmetrical development of the visual pathways [73]. In the absence of light exposure no such asymmetry develops and this difference persists throughout the first few weeks of life. Hence, it is possible to test the advantages of having (or not having) brain asymmetry for visual processing by comparing light- versus dark-incubated chicks, usually during the first and second week of post-hatching life. Clear differences in performance have been found.

Rogers et al. [74] tested the hypothesis that lateralization would enhance performance when two tasks had to be performed simultaneously, one relying on processing by the left hemisphere and the other on processing by the right hemisphere. One task was to search for grains of food scattered on a floor to which pebbles had been adhered: chicks learn to avoid pecking at pebbles using their right eye and left hemisphere [75]. The other task was to detect, and respond to, a model predator (a silhouette of a hawk) moved over the top of the cage, a function of the left eye and right hemisphere [76]. The light-exposed (lateralized) chicks performed well on both tasks, whereas the non-lateralized, dark-incubated chicks performed poorly on both tasks and their performance deteriorated as the task continued. Not only were they unable to avoid pecking at the pebbles, but also they were slow to detect the model predator and, once they had detected it, they became less and less able to peck at grains of food and avoid pebbles. They became very disturbed. This result was confirmed by Dharmaretnam and Rogers [77], who additionally found that the dark-incubated chicks made more distress calls during the dual task than did the light-exposed chicks. This was also confirmed more recently by Archer and Mench [78], who found that the effect extends to at least six weeks post-hatching. Since monitoring for predators while searching for food is a common demand in the natural environment, the results of these experiments demonstrate a survival-relevant function of having a lateralized brain.

Chiandetti et al. [79] compared the performance of chicks exposed to light in ovo during the last three days before hatching and chicks incubated in the dark on a task in which grains of food were given to them in small paper cones with either a striped pattern or a checked pattern. The cones were placed along the walls of a rectangular arena, those with one type of pattern to the chick's right side and those with the other pattern on its left side. First the chicks were trained to expect food only in the cones with one of the patterns. Then they were tested either monocularly or binocularly with the cones, now empty, on the opposite sides (position reversed) and the choice made by the chicks was determined to see whether they chose the cones that they expected to contain food using object-specific cues (pattern) or position-specific cues (place). The dark-incubated (not visually lateralized) chicks chose pattern and largely ignored place: they attended to object-specific cues only. The light-exposed (lateralized) chicks chose either pattern or place, meaning that they attended to both possible cues specifying the location of food. Since the left-hemisphere attends to object-specific cues and the right hemisphere to position [80,81], it appears that the light-exposed chicks were able to use both hemispheres, whereas the dark-incubated ones could use only their left hemisphere. In other words, having a lateralized brain permits use of both hemispheres and thereby allows the chick to take into account more of the cues specifying food.

Later Chiandetti and Vallortigara [82] extended this research to show that, whereas light-exposed chicks could discriminate the left from right side, dark incubated chicks could not do so. The former could discriminate between a bowl of food placed in the corner of a cage with a blue wall on the right side from one placed with the blue wall on the left side. Dark-incubated chicks treated both bowls as the same.

In a study of eight species of Australian parrots, Magat and Brown [68] found that strength of laterality was associated with performance on a task requiring discrimination of pebbles from seed and another task requiring the bird to obtain a food reward suspended from its perch on the end of a string. On the pebble-seed discrimination task, individuals with stronger lateralization (measured as eye preference) scored better than individuals with weak lateralization, and performance of those with strong left-eye preference did not differ from those with strong right-eye preference. However, this relationship did not hold for lateralization measured as foot preference, which was contrary to the prediction made from a later paper by the same researchers showing, in 11 out of 16 species of parrot, that eye and foot preferences were correlated [83]. On the string-pulling task, strength of foot, but not eye, preference was associated with performance and, again, direction of foot preference had no significant association with performance. Overall, this study supports the previous research with chicks and pigeons in that performance is better in more strongly lateralized individuals, although it raises an issue about what behaviour is chosen to measure lateralization.

In birds, therefore, the evidence is clear that strength of lateralization is significantly related to performance.

4. Strength of Lateralization and Performance in Aquatic Vertebrates

In studies of species without limbs, laterality can be measured using eye preferences. One method is to determine the eye preferred by the test animal to view its image in a mirror [84]. Using such a measure of laterality and linking this to a test for "boldness", measured in terms of time to emerge from a dark box into an unfamiliar illuminated environment, Brown and Bilbost [85] found that rainbowfish not displaying an eye preference in the mirror test emerged sooner (were more "bold") than fish with significant eye preferences. Since it is currently impossible to say what cognitive abilities underlie this test, one can only speculate that earlier emergence could depend on attention to fewer cues by the non-lateralized fish and hence the expression of less fear. Other possible explanations for the result were discussed by Brown and Bilbost [85]. For the purpose of this review, it is a question of whether shorter emergence time is advantageous or not, and that would depend on the potential presence of predators. Indeed, it has been shown that strongly lateralized fish respond to predators more rapidly than do non-lateralized fish [86], and exposing fish to higher levels of predation increases the strength of lateralization, irrespective of whether it is to the left or right side [87].

In an experiment designed to replicate that of Rogers et al. [74] but using fish, Dadda and Bisazza [88] tested gathering of prey by weakly versus strongly lateralized fish in the presence of a predator. Similar to the result obtained by testing chicks, the strongly lateralized fish obtained the prey in a shorter time than did the weakly lateralized fish, and they did so by attending to the prey with one eye and the predator with the other eye. Sailfish show a similar advantage of being lateralized, as shown in a recent study [89]. Sailfish attack schools of sardines by slashing with their bill to the left or right side and they have individual side preferences. The study found that prey capture is more successful in fish with strong biases than in those that are weakly biased [89].

Along similar lines, Sovrano et al. [90] found that lateralized fish (assessed by turning preference) displayed superior performance compared to non-lateralized fish on a task requiring them to orient using either geometric or non-geometric spatial cues. Within the lateralized group the direction of lateralization had no effect. Once again, strength but not direction of lateralization has been found to be important.

Lateralized tadpoles (*Lithobates sylvaticus*), determined using a swimming test and scoring clockwise versus anticlockwise rotation, are better at learning to recognize a predator's odour than are non-lateralized ones [91]. In this study, however, there was also a difference within the lateralized group: those with clockwise rotation learnt to recognize the threat associated with a predator's odour, whereas those with anticlockwise rotation were less able to do so. In other words, laterality in one particular direction enhanced predator detection and, in this aspect, these results diverge from the ones discussed immediately above.

Empirical evidence obtained by testing aquatic species indicates that stronger lateralization of the brain has advantages over weaker lateralization but there is some contrary evidence also. Dadda et al. [92] have found that fish (*Girardinus falcatus*) with weaker lateralization (determined from preferred eye used to monitor a predator behind a barrier) perform better than those with stronger lateralization on a task requiring them to enter a tank via a middle door in an array of nine doors: fish with stronger lateralization made more mistakes by swimming through doors to the left or right of the middle door. In addition, when these fish had to choose to join one of two shoals, each seen with a different eye, weakly lateralized fish were more likely to choose the high quality (larger) shoal, whereas strongly lateralized fish choose the shoal seen with the eye dominant for social behaviour regardless of the quality of the shoal.

5. Interhemispheric Communication and Lateralization

Communication between the left and right sides of the brain is essential for a lateralized brain. In humans this is achieved primarily via the large corpus callosum and, in other mammalian species, by a less well-developed corpus callosum. In birds a small anterior commissure connects the hemispheres and the tectal and posterior commissures (TC and PC) connect each side of the midbrain. In addition, the avian brain has a decussation that crosses the midline of the brain to allow left-right sharing of information [93,94]. Known as the supraoptic decussation (SOD), it is comprised of neural projections from the thalamus on one side of the brain to the hyperpallial region of the hemisphere/forebrain on the other side. In the SOD of chicks, more projections cross from left to right than from right to left [93,95]. This structural asymmetry correlates with some functional asymmetries: sectioning the SOD of chicks aged two days post-hatching removes the lateralization of visual search performance normally present in the second week of life [96]. Sham operated control chicks tested monocularly on a search task requiring them to find grain scattered amongst pebbles (for details of the task see [97]) learn to avoid pecking pebbles when tested with a patch over their left eye but they cannot learn if the patch is on their right eye. This asymmetry is weakened or absent in chicks with a sectioned SOD: in these chicks performance is poor when using either the left or the right eye [83]. Furthermore, chicks tested binocularly after sectioning of the SOD are unable to perform the task, compared to excellent learning in the sham-operated controls. This result demonstrates the importance of thalamofugal visual projections that cross the midline of the brain. In the intact brain, and when both eyes are able to see, these midline-crossing projections enable learning by limiting it to the right eye/left hemisphere system.

Birds have two sets of visual projections: one involving the thalamus and SOD, discussed above, and the other involving the optic tecta and projecting to the entopallial region of the forebrain hemispheres. The optic tecta on each side of the brain are linked by a tectal commissure (TC) and crossing the midline right alongside the TC is the PC. Sectioning the TC/PC commissural system of the chick brain, on day two post-hatching, leads to lateralization of one particular type of visual behaviour [98]. When, on day five or six after hatching, the chicks were tested monocularly by presenting them with a small red bead, which stimulates pecking, unoperated chicks and sham-operated chicks pecked at the bead and did so on average only once each time it was presented (for 15 s and on eight times to each eye): no lateralization was apparent. Chicks with their TC/PC sectioned behaved in the same manner when tested using their left eye but, when they were tested using their right eye, they pecked at the bead more and more each time it was presented: the group data showed that there was a linear increase in pecking to over four pecks in 15 s on the eighth presentation. They appeared to find the bead more attractive each time they saw it. Such dishabituation suggests that, in intact chicks, the TC/PC commissure must transmit information from one optic tectum to the other in order to suppress continued and increasing responding to novel and attractive stimuli, such as the red bead. It is likely that this relies on a firm categorical memory of the red bead, which intact chicks tested using the right eye access via the TC/PC. Denied access to this memory the chicks using their right eye and without a TC/PC may be forced to use an imperfect memory, which makes the bead more attractive each time it is seen.

Interhemispheric communication is more effective in strongly lateralized brains, as found by comparing pigeons hatched from eggs that had received exposure to light with pigeons hatched from eggs incubated in the dark [99]. In a task reliant on use of both hemispheres together, Manns and Römling [99] tested pigeons that had been hatched from eggs either incubated in the dark or exposed to light. The task, known as transitive inference, required monocular training in which one eye was presented with red and blue keys, only the red being rewarded, and then blue versus green keys, only the blue being rewarded. This established a hierarchy of red preferred over blue and blue over green. A similar hierarchy was established when the bird could see using the other eye, except that, for this eye, two of the colours were different (green versus yellow, with green rewarded, and yellow versus pink, with yellow rewarded). Then in testing the birds were binocular and they were confronted with pairs of colours that they had not seen previously (e.g., blue versus yellow). Light exposed chicks could combine their training to choose, for example, blue over yellow, showing that they could integrate information stored in both hemispheres. Dark-incubated pigeons were unable to integrate the information from both hemispheres even though they we able to learn the combinations in the monocular condition just as well as could the light-incubated birds. Thus, binocular (normal) performance of tasks requiring integration of information on both sides of the brain, and depending on interhemispheric communication, is not possible in a non-lateralized (or weakly lateralized) brain. Since this research did not extend to investigation of what pathways might be involved in the transfer of information between hemispheres, it is not possible to say whether the communication is indirect via, for example, the TC/PC or, perhaps, occurs at the hemispheric level via the anterior commissure.

Although in its infancy, research on functional lateralization and interhemispheric communication at both the behavioural and neural levels promises to be a fruitful way of progressing our understanding of lateralized brain function.

6. Multiple Modality Laterality and Future Research

So far, lateralization has been discussed as a unitary phenomenon, involving processing of all information in the same way and to the same degree. However, it is possible that brains may be lateralized for processing, say, visual information, and not for processing auditory or olfactory information. We know, for example, that light exposure of chick embryos establishes lateralization for certain sorts of visual processing (discussed above) but this treatment has no effect on lateralization of olfactory processing [100] or on decision making about approach to familiar versus unfamiliar stimuli [101].

What does it mean to be strongly lateralized for some types of processing but weakly lateralized for others? Moreover, is there any concordance of lateralization of the brain and lateralization of the viscera? According to studies on zebra fish, some neural asymmetries are concordant with visceral asymmetry, since they are reversed together in *fsi* mutants, but not all behavioural asymmetries are concordant with visceral asymmetry and this appears to lead to the emergence of new patterns of behaviour [102].

Research examining the relationship of laterality across modalities and how they interact should provide a rich field of study and enhance knowledge of cognitive processing. So far we have very little information on the interaction between lateralization in different sensory modalities but fascinating evidence for the interaction between light exposure and birds' ability to orient using their magnetic compass has been discovered [103], and see the paper by Gehring and colleagues in this Special Issue, showing that monocular light stimulation influences the lateralization of processing magnetic compass information.

This raises another important aspect of lateralization: viz., that it is not fixed but can change in strength over an individual's lifespan. From research on chicks, we know that visual lateralization changes markedly over early, and critical, stages of development (see [4,104], p. 120) and that it can be modulated by steroid hormones [105–107] and environmental stimulation (e.g., light exposure, discussed above). A recent review by Hausmann [108] considers the influence of sex hormones on lateralization in humans and points out the difficulties in drawing conclusions from the research on humans. Future research on non-human species promises to shed light on all of these issues.

To conclude, the evidence indicates that brain lateralization is advantageous because it allows parallel processing in the two hemispheres and it suggest that greater efficiency is achieved by confining the neural circuits used in different types of processing to separate hemispheres, thereby reducing conflict and redundancy.

References

1. MacNeilage, P.; Rogers, L.J.; Vallortigara, G. Origins of the left and right brain. *Sci. Am.* **2009**, *301*, 60–67. [CrossRef] [PubMed]
2. Ocklenburg, S.; Güntürkün, O. Hemispheric asymmetries: the comparative view. *Front. Psychol.* **2012**, *3*, 5. [CrossRef] [PubMed]
3. Rogers, L.J.; Vallortigara, G. When and why did brains break symmetry? *Symmetry* **2015**, *7*, 2181–2194. [CrossRef]
4. Rogers, L.J.; Vallortigara, G.; Andrew, R.J. *Divided Brains: The Biology and Behaviour of Brain Asymmetries*; Cambridge University Press: Cambridge, UK, 2013.
5. Frasnelli, E.; Vallortigara, G.; Rogers, L.J. Left-right asymmetries of behaviour and nervous system in invertebrates. *Neurosci. Biobehav. Rev.* **2012**, *36*, 1273–1291. [CrossRef] [PubMed]

6. Vallortigara, G.; Rogers, L.J. Survival with an asymmetrical brain: Advantages and disadvantages of cerebral lateralization. *Behav. Brain Sci.* **2005**, *28*, 575–633. [CrossRef] [PubMed]
7. *Lateralized Brain Functions: Methods in Human and Non-Human Species*; Rogers, L.J.; Vallortigara, G., Eds.; Neuromethods; Springer Protocols Volume 122; Humana Press: New York, NY, USA, 2017.
8. Rogers, L.J. Light experience and asymmetry of brain function in chickens. *Nature* **1982**, *297*, 223–225. [CrossRef] [PubMed]
9. Budaev, S.; Andrew, R.J. Patterns of early embryonic light exposure determine behavioural asymmetries in zebrafish: A habenular hypothesis. *Behav. Brain Res.* **2009**, *200*, 91–94. [CrossRef] [PubMed]
10. Vallortigara, G. Comparative neuropsychology of the dual brain: A stroll through left and right animals' perceptual worlds. *Brain Lang.* **2000**, *73*, 189–219. [CrossRef] [PubMed]
11. Manns, M.; Güntürkün, O. Dual coding of visual asymmetries in the pigeon brain: The interaction of bottom-up and top-down systems. *Exp. Brain Res.* **2009**, *199*, 323–332. [CrossRef] [PubMed]
12. Nagy, M.; Akos, Z.; Biro, D.; Vicsek, T. Hierarchical group dynamics in pigeon flocks. *Nature* **2010**, *464*, 890–893. [CrossRef] [PubMed]
13. Karenina, K.; Giljov, A.; Ingram, J.; Rowntree, V.J.; Malashichev, Y. Lateralization of mother-infant interactions in a diverse range of mammal species. *Nat. Ecol. Evol.* **2017**, *1*, 30. [CrossRef]
14. Chiandetti, C.; Pecchia, T.; Patt, F.; Vallortigara, G. Visual hierarchical processing and lateralization of cognitive functions through domestic chicks' eyes. *PLoS ONE* **2014**, *9*, e84435. [CrossRef] [PubMed]
15. Rogers, L.J. The two hemispheres of the avian brain: their differing roles in perceptual processing and the expression of behaviour. *J. Ornithol.* **2012**, *153*, S61–S74. [CrossRef]
16. Güntürkün, O. The ontogeny of visual lateralization in pigeons. *Ger. J. Psychol.* **1993**, *17*, 276–287.
17. Sovrano, V.A. Visual lateralization in response to familiar and unfamiliar stimuli in fish. *Behav. Brain Res.* **2004**, *152*, 385–391. [CrossRef] [PubMed]
18. Kendrick, K.M. Brain asymmetries for face recognition and emotion control in sheep. *Cortex* **2006**, *42*, 96–98. [CrossRef]
19. Siniscalchi, M.; Sasso, R.; Pepe, A.M.; Vallortigara, G.; Quaranta, A. Dogs turn left to emotional stimuli. *Behav. Brain. Res.* **2010**, *208*, 516–521. [CrossRef] [PubMed]
20. Koboroff, A.; Kaplan, G.; Rogers, L.J. Hemispheric specialization in Australian magpies (*Gymnorhina. tibicen*) shown as eye preferences during response to a predator. *Brain Res. Bull.* **2008**, *76*, 304–306. [CrossRef] [PubMed]
21. Karenina, K.; Giljov, A.; Ivkovich, T.; Malashichev, Y. Evidence for the perceptual origin of right-sided feeding biases in cetaceans. *Anim. Cogn.* **2016**, *19*, 239–243. [CrossRef] [PubMed]
22. Schepman, A.; Rodway, P.; Pritchard, H. Right-lateralized unconscious, but not conscious, processing of affective environmental sounds. *Laterality* **2016**, *21*, 606–632. [CrossRef] [PubMed]
23. Innes, B.R.; Burt, D.M.; Birch, Y.K.; Hausmann, M. A leftward bias however you look at it: Revisiting the emotional chimeric face task as a tool for measuring emotion lateralization. *Laterality* **2016**, *21*, 643–661. [CrossRef] [PubMed]
24. Godfrey, H.K.; Grimshaw, G.M. Emotional language is all right: Emotional prosody reduces hemispheric asymmetry for linguistic processing. *Laterality* **2016**, *21*, 568–584. [CrossRef] [PubMed]
25. Yousry, T.A.; Schmid, U.; Jassoy, A.G.; Schmidt, D.; Eisner, W.E.; Reulen, H.; Reiser, M.F.; Lissner, J. Topography of the cortical motor hand area: Prospective study with functional MR imaging and direct motor mapping at surgery. *Radiology* **1995**, *195*, 23–29. [CrossRef] [PubMed]
26. Annett, M. Spatial ability in subgroups of left and right-handers. *Br. J. Psychol.* **1992**, *83*, 493–515. [CrossRef] [PubMed]
27. Bishop, D.V.M. *Handedness and Development Disorder*; Lawrence Erlbaum Assoc. Ltd.: Hove, UK, 1995.
28. Annett, M.; Manning, M. Arithmetic and laterality. *Neuropsychologia* **1990**, *28*, 61–69. [CrossRef]
29. Corballis, M.C. *The Lopsided Ape*; Oxford University Press: New York, NY, USA, 1991.
30. Badzakova-Trajkov, G.; Häberling, I.S.; Roberts, R.P.; Corballis, M.C. Cerebral asymmetries: Complementary and independent processes. *PLoS ONE* **2010**, *5*, e9682. [CrossRef] [PubMed]
31. Denny, K. Handedness and depression: evidence from a large population survey. *Laterality* **2009**, *14*, 246–255. [CrossRef] [PubMed]
32. Crow, T.J. Schizophrenia as a failure of hemispheric dominance for language. *TINS* **1997**, *20*, 339–343. [PubMed]

33. Delisi, L.E.; Svetina, C.; Razi, K.; Shields, G.; Wellman, N.; Crow, T.J. Hand preference and hand skill in families with schizophrenia. *Laterality* **2002**, *7*, 321–332. [CrossRef] [PubMed]
34. Chapman, J.P.; Chapman, L.J. Handedness of hypothetically psychosis-prone subjects. *J. Abnorm. Psychol.* **1987**, *96*, 89–93. [CrossRef] [PubMed]
35. Spivak, B.; Segal, M.; Mester, R.; Weizman, A. Lateral preference and post-traumatic stress disorder. *Psychol. Med.* **1998**, *28*, 229–232. [CrossRef] [PubMed]
36. Crow, T.J.; Crow, L.R.; Done, D.J.; Leask, S. Relative hand skill predicts academic ability: Global deficits at the point of hemispheric indecision. *Neuropsychologia* **1998**, *36*, 1275–1282. [CrossRef]
37. Corballis, M.C.; Hattie, J.; Fletcher, R. Handedness and intellectual achievement: An even-handed look. *Neuropsychologia* **2008**, *46*, 374–378. [CrossRef] [PubMed]
38. Rodriguez, A.; Kaakinen, M.; Moilanen, I.; Taanila, A.; McGough, J.J.; Loo, S.; Järvelin, M.-R. Mixed-handedness is linked to mental health problems in children and adolescents. *Pediatrics* **2010**, *125*, e340–e348. [CrossRef] [PubMed]
39. Tsuang, H.-C.; Chen, W.J.; Kuo, S.-Y.; Hsiao, P.-C. The cross-cultural nature of the relationship between schizotypy and mixed-handedness. *Laterality* **2013**, *18*, 476–490. [CrossRef] [PubMed]
40. Weinrich, A.M.; Wells, P.A.; McManus, C. Handedness, anxiety and sex differences. *Br. J. Psychol.* **1982**, *73*, 69–72. [CrossRef]
41. Bryden, P.J.; Bruyn, P.J.; Fletcher, P. Handedness and health: An examination of the association between different handedness classifications and health disorders. *Laterality* **2005**, *10*, 429–440. [CrossRef]
42. Brandler, W.M.; Paracchini, S. The genetic relationship between handedness and neurodevelopmental disorders. *Trends Mol. Med.* **2014**, *20*, 83–90. [CrossRef] [PubMed]
43. Ocklenburg, S.; Beste, C.; Arning, L.; Peterburs, J.; Güntürkün, O. The ontogenesis of language lateralization and its relation to handedness. *Neurosci. Biobehav. Rev.* **2014**, *43*, 191–198. [CrossRef] [PubMed]
44. Hardie, S.M.; Wright, L.; Clark, L. Handedness and social anxiety: Using Bryden's research as a catalyst to explore the influence of familial sinistrality and degree of handedness. *Laterality* **2016**, *21*, 329–347. [CrossRef] [PubMed]
45. Johnson, B.W.; McArthur, G.; Hautus, M.; Reid, M.; Brock, J.; Castles, A.; Crain, S. Lateralized auditory brain function in children with normal reading ability and in children with dyslexia. *Neuropsychologia* **2013**, *51*, 633–641. [CrossRef] [PubMed]
46. Maisog, J.M.; Einbinder, E.R.; Flowers, D.L.; Turkeltaub, P.E.; Eden, G.F. A meta-analysis of functional neuroimaging studies of dyslexia. *Ann. N. Y. Acad. Sci.* **2008**, *1145*, 237–259. [CrossRef] [PubMed]
47. Ocklenburg, S. Tachistposcopic viewing and dichotic listening. In *Lateralized Brain Functions: Methods in Human and Non-human Species*; Rogers, L.J., Vallortigara, G., Eds.; Neuromethods; Springer Protocols; Humana Press: New York, NY, USA, 2017; Volume 122, pp. 3–28.
48. Mazza, V.; Pagno, S. Electroencephalographic asymmetries in human cognition. In *Lateralized Brain Functions: Methods in Human and Non-human Species*; Rogers, L.J., Vallortigara, G., Eds.; Neuromethods; Springer Protocols; Humana Press: New York, NY, USA, 2017; Volume 122, pp. 407–440.
49. McGrew, W.C.; Marchant, L.F. Laterality of hand use pays off in foraging success for wild chimpanzees. *Primates* **1999**, *40*, 509–513. [CrossRef]
50. Bell, A.T.A.; Niven, J.E. Strength of forelimb lateralization predicts motor errors in an insect. *Biol. Lett.* **2016**, *12*, 20160547. [CrossRef] [PubMed]
51. Piddington, T.; Rogers, L.J. Strength of hand preference and dual task performance by common marmosets. *Anim. Cogn.* **2013**, *16*, 127–135. [CrossRef] [PubMed]
52. Clara, E.; Tommasi, L.; Rogers, L.J. Social mobbing calls in common marmosets (*Callithrix. jacchus*): Effects of experience and associated cortisol levels. *Anim. Cogn.* **2008**, *11*, 349–358. [CrossRef] [PubMed]
53. Cameron, R.; Rogers, L.J. Hand preference of the common marmoset, problem solving and responses in a novel setting. *J. Comp. Psychol.* **1999**, *113*, 149–157. [CrossRef]
54. Braccini, S.; Caine, N.G. Hand preference predicts reactions to novel foods and predators in marmosets (*Callithrix. geoffroyi*). *J. Comp. Psychol.* **2009**, *123*, 18–25. [CrossRef] [PubMed]
55. Gordon, D.J.; Rogers, L.J. Cognitive bias, hand preference and welfare of common marmosets. *Behav. Brain Res.* **2015**, *287*, 100–108. [CrossRef] [PubMed]
56. Gordon, D.J.; Rogers, L.J. Differences in social and vocal behavior between left- and right-handed common marmosets (*Callithrix. jaachus*). *J. Comp. Psychol.* **2010**, *124*, 402–411. [CrossRef] [PubMed]

57. Hopkins, W.D.; Bennett, A. Handedness and approach-avoidance behavior in chimpanzees. *J. Exp. Psychol.* **1994**, *20*, 413–418.
58. Westergaard, G.C.; Chavanne, T.J.; Houser, L.; Cleveland, A.; Snoy, P.J.; Suomi, S.J.; Higley, J.D. Biobehavioral correlates of hand preference in free-ranging female primates. *Laterality* **2004**, *9*, 267–285. [PubMed]
59. Wright, L.; Hardie, S.M.; Rodway, P. Pause before you respond: handedness influences response style on the Tower of Hanoi task. *Laterality* **2004**, *9*, 133–147. [CrossRef] [PubMed]
60. Branson, N.J.; Rogers, L.J. Relationship between paw preference strength and noise phobia in *Canis. familiaris*. *J. Comp. Psychol.* **2006**, *120*, 176–183. [CrossRef] [PubMed]
61. Batt, L.S.; Batt, M.S.; Baguley, J.A.; McGreevy, P.D. Lateralization and salivary cortisol. *J. Vet. Behav.* **2009**, *4*, 216–222. [CrossRef]
62. Schneider, L.A.; Delfabbro, P.H.; Burns, N.R. Temperament and lateralization in the domestic dog (*Canis. familiaris*). *J. Vet. Behav.* **2013**, *8*, 124–134. [CrossRef]
63. Marshall-Pescini, S.; Barnard, S.; Branson, N.J.; Valsecchi, P. The effect of preferential paw usage on dogs' (*Canis. familiaris*) performance in a manipulative problem-solving task. *Behav. Process.* **2013**, *100*, 40–43. [CrossRef] [PubMed]
64. Siniscalchi, M.; Quaranta, A.; Rogers, L.J. Hemispheric specialization in dogs for processing different acoustic stimuli. *PLoS ONE* **2008**, *3*, e3349. [CrossRef] [PubMed]
65. Found, R.; St. Clair, C.C. Ambidextrous ungulates have more flexible behavior, bolder personalities and migrate less. *R. Soc. Open Sci.* **2017**, *4*, 160958. [CrossRef] [PubMed]
66. Rogers, L.J. Development and function of lateralization in the avian brain. *Brain Res. Bull.* **2008**, *76*, 235–244. [CrossRef] [PubMed]
67. Alonso, Y. Lateralization of visually guided behavior during feeding in zebra finches (*Taeniapygia. guttata*). *Behav. Process.* **1988**, *43*, 257–263. [CrossRef]
68. Magat, M.; Brown, C. Laterality enhances cognition in Australian parrots. *Proc. R. Soc. B* **2009**, *276*, 4155–4162. [CrossRef] [PubMed]
69. Nottebohm, F.; Stokes, T.M.; Leonard, C.M. Central control of song in the canary, *Serinus. canarius*. *J. Comp. Neurol.* **1976**, *165*, 457–486. [CrossRef] [PubMed]
70. Rogers, L.J.; Anson, J.M. Lateralisation of function in the chicken fore-brain. *Pharmacol. Biochem. Behav.* **1979**, *10*, 679–686. [CrossRef]
71. Güntürkün, O.; Diekamp, B.; Manns, M.; Nottlemann, F.; Prior, H.; Schwartz, A.; Skiba, M. Asymmetry pays: Visual lateralization improves discrimination success in pigeons. *Curr. Biol.* **2000**, *10*, 1079–1081. [CrossRef]
72. Güntürkün, O.; Kesch, S. Visual lateralization during feeding in pigeons. *Behav. Neurosci.* **1987**, *101*, 433–435. [CrossRef] [PubMed]
73. Rogers, L.J.; Bolden, S. Light-dependent development and asymmetry of visual projections. *Neurosci. Lett.* **1991**, *121*, 63–67. [CrossRef]
74. Rogers, L.J.; Zucca, P.; Vallortigara, G. Advantage of having a lateralized brain. *Proc. R. Soc. Lond. B* **2004**, *271*, S420–S422. [CrossRef] [PubMed]
75. Rogers, L.J. Early experiential effects on laterality: Research on chicks has relevance to other species. *Laterality* **1997**, *2*, 199–219. [PubMed]
76. Rogers, L.J. Evolution of hemispheric specialisation: Advantages and disadvantages. *Brain Lang.* **2000**, *73*, 236–253. [CrossRef] [PubMed]
77. Dharmaretnam, M.; Rogers, L.J. Hemispheric specialization and dual processing in strongly versus weakly lateralized chicks. *Behav. Brain Res.* **2005**, *162*, 62–70. [CrossRef] [PubMed]
78. Archer, G.S.; Mench, J.A. Exposing avian embryos to light affects post-hatch anti-predator fear responses. *Appl. Anim. Behav. Sci.* **2017**, *186*, 80–84. [CrossRef]
79. Chiandetti, C.; Regolin, L.; Rogers, L.J.; Vallortigara, G. Effects of light stimulation of embryos on the use of position-specific and object-specific cues in binocular and monocular domestic chicks (*Gallus gallus*). *Behav. Brain Res.* **2005**, *163*, 10–17. [CrossRef] [PubMed]
80. Tommasi, L.; Vallortigara, G. Encoding of geometric and landmark information in the left and right hemispheres of the avian brain. *Behav. Neurosci.* **2001**, *115*, 602–613. [CrossRef] [PubMed]
81. Tommasi, L.; Gagliardo, A.; Andrew, R.J.; Vallortigara, G. Separate processing mechanisms for encoding geometric and landmark information in the avian hippocampus. *Eur. J. Neurosci.* **2003**, *17*, 1695–1702. [CrossRef] [PubMed]

82. Chiandetti, C.; Vallortigara, G. Effects of embryonic light stimulation on the ability to discriminate left from right in the domestic chick. *Behav. Brain Res.* **2009**, *198*, 240–246. [CrossRef] [PubMed]
83. Brown, C.; Magat, M. Cerebral lateralization determines hand preferences in Australian parrots. *Biol. Lett.* **2011**, *7*, 496–498. [CrossRef] [PubMed]
84. Sovrano, V.A.; Andrew, R.J. Eye use during viewing a reflection: behavioural lateralization in zebrafish larvae. *Behav. Brain Res.* **2006**, *167*, 226–231. [CrossRef] [PubMed]
85. Brown, C.; Bibost, A.-L. Laterality is linked to personality in the black-lined rainbowfish, *Melanotaenia. nigrans*. *Behav. Ecol. Sociobiol.* **2014**, *68*, 999–1005. [CrossRef]
86. Dadda, M.; Koolhaas, W.H.; Domenici, P. Behavioural asymmetry affects escape performance in a teleost fish. *Biol. Lett.* **2010**, *6*, 414–417. [CrossRef] [PubMed]
87. Chivers, D.P.; McCormick, M.I.; Bridie, J.M.A.; Mitchell, M.D.; Gonçalves, E.J.; Bryshun, R.; Ferrari, M.C.O. At odds with the group: changes in lateralization and escape performance reveal conformity and conflict in fish schools. *Proc. R. Soc. Lond. B* **2016**, *283*, 20161127. [CrossRef] [PubMed]
88. Dadda, M.; Bisazza, A. Does brain asymmetry allow efficient performance of simultaneous tasks? *Anim. Behav.* **2006**, *72*, 523–529. [CrossRef]
89. Kurvers, R.H.J.; Krause, S.; Viblanc, P.E.; Herbert-Read, J.E.; Zaslansky, P.; Domenici, P.; Marras, S.; Steffensen, J.F.; Svendsen, M.B.S.; Wilson, A.D.M.; et al. The evolution of lateralization in group hunting sailfish. *Curr. Biol.* **2017**, *27*, 521–526. [CrossRef] [PubMed]
90. Sovrano, V.A.; Dadda, M.; Bisazza, A. Lateralized fish perform better than nonlateralized fish in spatial orientation tasks. *Behav. Brain Res.* **2005**, *163*, 122–127. [CrossRef] [PubMed]
91. Lucon-Xiccato, T.; Chivers, D.P.; Mitchell, M.D.; Ferrari, M.C.O. Prenatal exposure to predation affects predator recognition learning via lateralization plasticity. *Behav. Ecol.* **2017**, *28*, 253–259. [CrossRef]
92. Dadda, M.; Zandona, E.; Agrillo, C.; Bisazza, A. The costs of hemispheric specialization in a fish. *Proc. R. Soc. Lond. B* **2009**, *276*, 4399–4407. [CrossRef] [PubMed]
93. Rogers, L.J.; Deng, C. Light experience and lateralization of the two visual pathways in the chick. *Behav. Brain Res.* **1999**, *98*, 277–287. [CrossRef]
94. Güntürkün, O. Ontogeny of visual asymmetry in pigeons. In *Comparative Vertebrate Lateralization*; Rogers, L.J., Andrew, R.J., Eds.; Cambridge University Press: Cambridge, UK, 2002; pp. 247–273.
95. Rogers, L.J.; Sink, H.S. Transient asymmetry in the projections of the rostral thalamus to the visual hyperstriatum of the chicken, and reversal of its direction by light exposure. *Exp. Brain Res.* **1988**, *70*, 378–384. [CrossRef] [PubMed]
96. Rogers, L.J.; Robinson, T.; Ehrlich, D. Role of the supraoptic decussation in the development of asymmetry of brain function in the chicken. *Dev. Brain Res.* **1986**, *28*, 33–39. [CrossRef]
97. Rogers, L.J. Eye and ear Preferences. In *Lateralized Brain Functions: Methods in Human and Non-Human Species*; Rogers, L.J., Vallortigara, G., Eds.; Springer NeuroMethods Series; Humana Press: New York, NY, USA, 2017; Volume 122, pp. 79–102.
98. Parsons, C.H.; Rogers, L.J. Role of the tectal and posterior commissures in lateralization in the avian brain. *Behav. Brain Res.* **1993**, *54*, 153–164. [CrossRef]
99. Manns, M.; Römling, J. The impact of asymmetrical light input on cerebral hemisphere specialization and interhemispheric cooperation. *Nat. Commun.* **2012**, *3*, 696. [CrossRef] [PubMed]
100. Rogers, L.J.; Andrew, R.J.; Burne, T.H.J. Light exposure of the embryo and development of behavioural lateralization in chicks: I. Olfactory responses. *Behav. Brain Res.* **1998**, *97*, 195–200. [CrossRef]
101. Andrew, R.J.; Johnston, A.N.B.; Robins, A.; Rogers, L.J. Light exposure of the embryo and development of behavioural lateralization in chicks: II. Choice of a familiar versus unfamiliar model social partner. *Behav. Brain Res.* **2004**, *155*, 67–76. [CrossRef] [PubMed]
102. Barth, K.A.; Miklosi, A.; Watkins, J.; Bianco, I.H.; Wilson, S.W.; Andrew, R.J. fsi Zebrafish show concordant reversal of laterality of viscera, neuroanatomy, and a subset of al responses. *Curr. Biol.* **2005**, *15*, 844–850. [CrossRef] [PubMed]
103. Heyers, D.; Manns, M.; Luksch, H.; Güntürkün, O.; Mouritsen, H. A visual pathway links brain structures active during magnetic compass orientation in migratory birds. *PLoS ONE* **2007**, *2*, e937. [CrossRef] [PubMed]

104. Chiandetti, C. Manipulation of strength of cerebra lateralization via embryonic light stimulation in birds. In *Lateralized Brain Functions: Methods in Human and Non-Human Species*; Rogers, L.J., Vallortigara, G., Eds.; Neuromethods; Springer Protocols; Humana Press: New York, NY, USA, 2017; Volume 122, pp. 611–631.
105. Schwarz, I.M.; Rogers, L.J. Testosterone: A role in the development of brain asymmetry in the chick. *Neurosci. Lett.* **1992**, *146*, 167–170. [CrossRef]
106. Rogers, L.J.; Rajendra, S. Modulation of the development of light-initiated asymmetry in chick thalamofugal visual projections by oestradiol. *Exp. Brain Res.* **1993**, *93*, 89–94. [CrossRef] [PubMed]
107. Becking, T.; Geuze, R.H.; Groothuis, T.G.G. Investigating effects of steroid hormones on lateralization of brain and behavior. In *Lateralized Brain Functions: Methods in Human and Non-Human Species*; Rogers, L.J., Vallortigara, G., Eds.; Neuromethods; Springer Protocols; Humana Press: New York, NY, USA, 2017; Volume 122, pp. 633–666.
108. Hausmann, M. Why sex hormones matter for neuroscience: A very short review on sex, sex hormones, and functional brain asymmetries. *J. Neurosci. Rev.* **2017**, *95*, 40–49. [CrossRef] [PubMed]

15

Lateralized Functions in the Dog Brain

Marcello Siniscalchi *, Serenella d'Ingeo and Angelo Quaranta

Department of Veterinary Medicine, Section of Behavioral Sciences and Animal Bioethics, University of Bari "Aldo Moro", 70121 Bari, Italy; serenella.dingeo@uniba.it (S.I.); angelo.quaranta@uniba.it (A.Q.)

* Correspondence: marcello.siniscalchi@uniba.it

Academic Editor: Lesley J. Rogers

Abstract: Understanding the complementary specialisation of the canine brain has been the subject of increasing scientific study over the last 10 years, chiefly due to the impact of cerebral lateralization on dog behaviour. In particular, behavioural asymmetries, which directly reflect different activation of the two sides of the dog brain, have been reported at different functional levels, including motor and sensory. The goal of this review is not only to provide a clear scenario of the experiments carried out over the last decade but also to highlight the relationships between dogs' lateralization, cognitive style and behavioural reactivity, which represent crucial aspect relevant for canine welfare.

Keywords: dog; lateralization; emotion; behaviour; physiology

---

1. Introduction

Brain hemispheres specialise to process and analyse information in an asymmetrical way: this is a phenomenon widely reported in the animal kingdom [1,2] and, as shown by the increasing scientific study over the last decade, it is now well manifested also in canine species. Based on findings derived from experiments carried on different animal models, clear evidence exists that basic lateralized neural mechanisms are very similar across vertebrate brains with a specialisation of the left hemisphere in the control of routine behaviours, responding to features that are invariant and repeated, and with the specialisation of the right hemisphere in detecting novelty (unexpected stimuli) and in the expression of intense emotions, such as aggression and fear [3,4].

In this review, our first aim is to provide a comprehensive overview of the experiments carried out in dogs providing extensive evidence of hemispheric asymmetries in function, structure and behaviour. Our second aim in this paper is to analyse lateralized patterns specifically involved in emotional processing by the dog brain and how the study of emotional lateralization could represent a valid and interesting tool to contribute to the improvement of canine welfare and management.

In dogs, deepening the knowledge of cerebral lateralization with particular regard to emotional processing is particularly interesting since behavioural asymmetries which indirectly reflect lateralized cognitive processing of emotions can be easily detected (e.g., paw preference, nostril use, and tail wagging) and can give insight into the different valences of an emotion felt by the animal. The latter is crucial not only for a better understanding of canine cognition but also for the improvement of dogs' training and handling during several activities within the human community (e.g., animal-assisted therapy, police and rescue work, and guides for vision impaired people).

2. Sensory Lateralization

The complementary specialisation of dogs' brain hemispheres is clearly apparent at different sensory levels, including vision [5], hearing [6–10] and what is considered to be the most relevant sensory domain for canine species, namely olfaction [11,12].

Asymmetries of dogs' visual sensory channels have been observed by studying their asymmetrical head-turning response to bidimensional visual stimuli presented during feeding behaviour [5]. The experimental set-up consisted of the presentation of black silhouette drawings of different animal models (a dog, a cat and a snake) to the dog's right and left visual hemifields using two retro-illuminated panels. When stimuli were presented at the same time in the two visual hemifields, dogs preferentially turned the head with their left eye leading in response to alarming stimuli (the snake silhouette that is considered to be an alarming stimulus for most mammals [13] or the cat silhouette displaying a defensive threat posture). Given that, in dogs, neural structures located in the right hemisphere are mainly fed by inputs from the left visual hemifield and vice versa (crossing of fibres at the optic nerve level is 75% [14]), left head turns in response to threatening stimuli are consistent with the specialisation of the right side of the brain for expressing intense emotion including fear (snake) and aggression (cat with an arched lateral displayed body and erected tail). The latter specialisation of the right hemisphere has been reported in several animal models (reviewed in [1,2]).

It is interesting to note that left head turns (right hemisphere activation) lead to shorter latencies to react and longer latencies to resume feeding (i.e., higher emotional response). Moreover, during monocular presentation, higher responsiveness to stimuli presented in the left visual hemifield was observed, and this was irrespective of the type of stimulus. Overall, these results support the hypothesis that in canine species, as well as in other mammals, the neural sympathetic mechanisms controlling the "fight or flight" behavioural response are mainly under the activation of the right hemisphere [15]. In dogs, it is interesting to note that both in vivo [16] (Computed Tomography (CT) brain scanning) and post mortem techniques [17] have revealed a right-biased hemispheric asymmetry with the right hemisphere greater than the left; the latter could reflect the right hemisphere specialisation for intense emotional activities like fight or flight reactions, which are related to aggressive and defensive-escape behaviours.

As in dogs, a number of animals exhibit aggressive and defensive behaviours when the right hemisphere is active. Chicks, for example, respond strongly to a potential predator (silhouette of a predatory bird) seen in their left visual field (right hemisphere) [18,19]); very similar results were reported in toads, which showed stronger avoidance responses when a model snake was presented on their left side than when it was on their right side [20]. In domestic animals, horses approached by a potential threatening stimulus (a human opening an umbrella) reacted more (i.e., moving further away) when the approach was from their left side than when it was from their right side [21].

There is now evidence that the auditory sensory system in the dog brain also works in an asymmetrical way depending on the type of acoustic stimulus [6,8,9]. Specifically, during feeding behaviour, dogs' head orienting responses to different sounds played at the same time from two speakers placed symmetrically with respect to the subjects' head were recorded [6] (see Figure 1A). When thunderstorm playbacks were presented, dogs consistently turned the head with their left ear leading and, given that the direction of the head turn is an unconditioned response indicating a contralateral hemispheric advantage in attention to the auditory stimulus [22], this result supported the right hemisphere specialization in processing alarming stimuli. In a way similar to that previously reported about vision, in this experimental condition, left-head orienting turns also led to longer latencies to resume feeding from the bowl. On the other hand, dogs consistently turned the head with their right ear leading in response to playbacks of canine vocalizations ("disturbance" and "isolation" calls) supporting the role of the left hemisphere in the analysis of familiar conspecific calls, as reported in other species (non-human primates [23], horses [24], cats [25] and sea lions [26]). Nevertheless, in dogs, conspecific vocalizations are not always processed by the left hemisphere, since the right hemisphere is used for processing vocalizations when they elicit intense emotion [6,7].

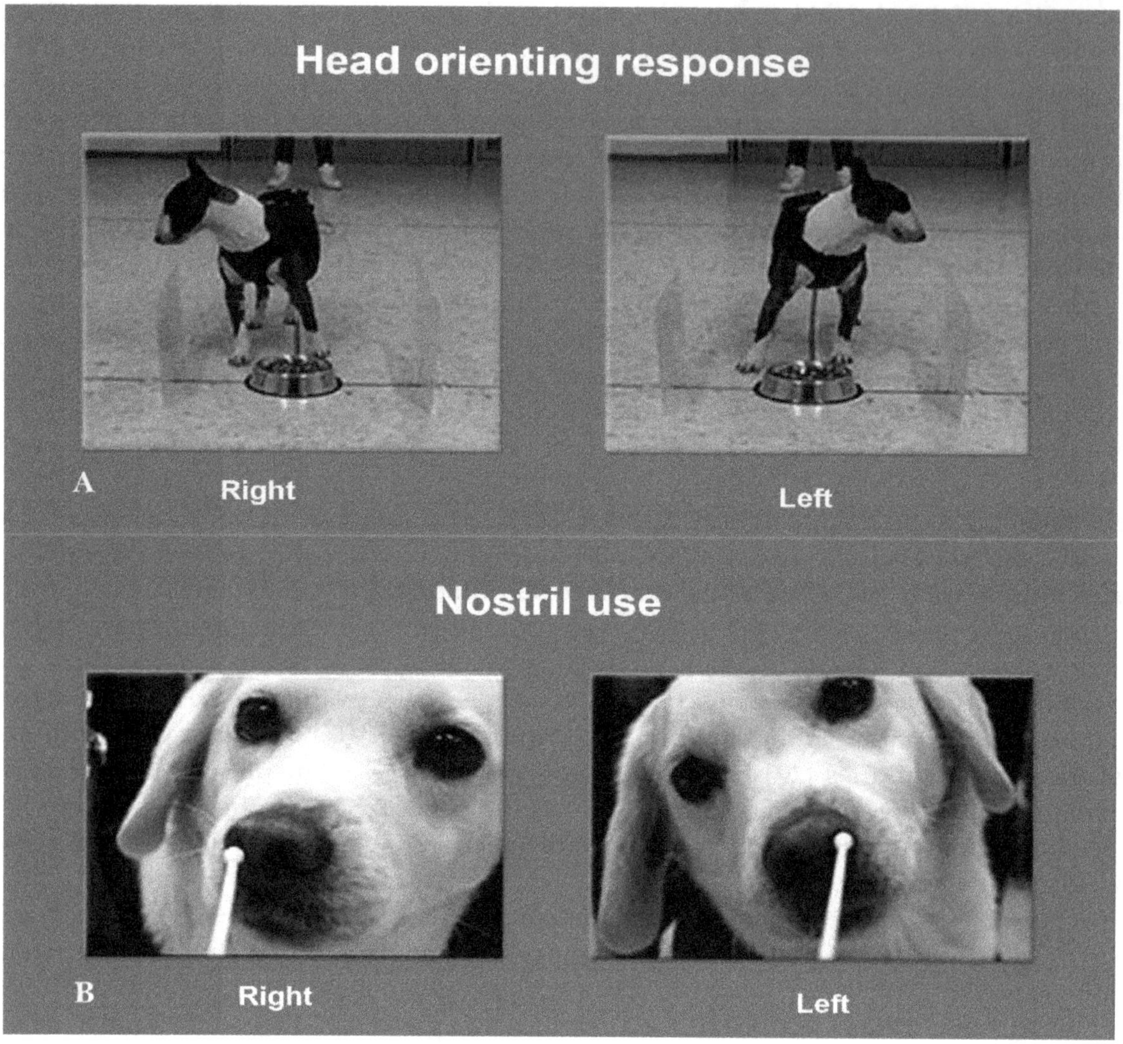

Figure 1. Behavioural techniques used to study functional lateralization in dogs: (**A**) head-orienting response used to study auditory lateralization; and (**B**) left and right nostril use during sniffing of different olfactory stimuli.

In dogs, the left hemisphere advantage in processing vocalizations of familiar conspecifics seems dependent on the calls' temporal features, since the presentation of the reversed version of the same canine call caused the loss of the right bias in the head turning response [27].

Head orienting response methods have been used in dogs to study possible lateralized neural mechanisms in processing human speech [8]. Results revealed that dogs consistently turned their head to the right during presentation of human spoken commands with artificially increased segmental cues (i.e., higher salience of meaningful phonemic components); moreover, a significant left-turning bias was observed in response to manipulated commands with increased supra-segmental vocal cues (i.e., higher salience of intonation component). These results have been confirmed by recent neuroimaging studies and overall suggest a convergent lateralized brain specialisation between canine and human species for processing speech [9].

Regarding olfaction, asymmetries in nostril use have been observed during free sniffing behaviour of odorants that differ in terms of emotional valence [11,28]. Briefly, cotton swabs installed on a digital video camera were used to present odorants to dogs (see Figure 1B). The camera was installed on a tripod in the centre of a large silent room. A frame-by-frame analysis of nostril use video footages revealed a clear right nostril bias during sniffing of clearly arousing odours for dogs (e.g., adrenaline and veterinary sweat). Given that, in dogs, the olfactory nervous fibres, which drive odour information from peripheral receptors to the olfactory cortex, are uncrossed, right nostril use indicates a prevalent right hemisphere activation [29]. The latter was consistent with the previously reported right hemisphere involvement in analysing alarming/threatening stimuli and had direct implication for dogs' welfare and training since, for example, the constant use of the right nostril during olfactory inspection of a human being could reveal an increased arousal state of the animal, even in the absence of clear behavioural signs (this could be useful in those activities like animal-assisted therapy in which dogs must possess advanced behavioural control skills in order to help them handle high arousal situations and consequently it is not always easy to detect stress increase directly from behavioural signs).

When non-aversive stimuli were presented (e.g., food, lemon, and canine vaginal secretions), right nostril use was observed only during the first presentations indicating the initial involvement of the right hemisphere in the analysis of novelty (this bias was not evident for initial sniffing of food probably because of its reduced valence as a novel stimulus). Furthermore, a shift from the right to the left nostril use was observed with repeated stimulus presentations, indicating the prevalent control of sniffing behaviour by the left hemisphere when routine responses to odour stimuli emerge as a result of familiarization [1,2,30,31]. Left hemisphere specialisation in routine tasks has been observed in pigeons [32], wild stilts [33], toads [34] and chickens [35]. In the latter case, during a routine task of finding food, chicks using the right eye (left hemisphere) and not the left eye learn to find food grains scattered on a back-ground of distracting pebbles (similar to the grains).

There is now evidence that dogs' olfaction works in an asymmetrical way for processing both conspecific and heterospecific odours collected during different emotional events [12]. In particular, during sniffing of canine odours collected in a stressful situation (i.e., an "isolation" situation in which dogs were isolated from their owners in an unfamiliar environment), a consistent use of the right nostril was observed (right hemisphere activity). Moreover, when human odorants were presented to dogs, a significant left-nostril bias (left hemisphere activation) was found for sniffing olfactory stimuli collected from humans during a fearful situation (emotion-eliciting movies) and physical stress. The observed opposite nostril use pattern in response to conspecific and heterospecific odorants suggests that dog's olfaction uses different sensory pathways to extract emotional cues from canine and human chemosignals. Furthermore, an interesting hypothesis about the left nostril use during sniffing at human sweat collected during a fear situation and physical stress is that these heterospecific chemosignals (probably produced during the escape behavioural response to a predator) could elicit dogs' prey drive (i.e., approaching behavioural tendencies) to the stimuli through the selective activation of the left hemisphere. The evidence that, in dogs [36], as in other animal models (e.g., toads [34] and birds [33]), neural structures on the left side of the brain are involved in the control of predatory behaviour supports this hypothesis.

3. Paw Preferences

Asymmetries of motor functions have been widely reported in various vertebrate and invertebrate species, including the dog [1,2]. There is now a growing body of literature on motor lateralization in dogs, focused mainly on behavioural lateralization in the form of forelimb preferential use. In recent studies, paw preference has been assessed using several tasks: removal of a adhesive plaster from the eye [17,37] or of a piece of tape from the nose [38–42], removal of a blanket from the head [43], retrieval of food [44,45] from a toy object (namely the "Kong", see Figure 2) [46–50] or a metal can [43 paw-shaking [43], first foot placed forward to depart from a standing or sitting position [49,51] or during a run [52] and stabilization of a ball [39] and hindlimb raising behaviour during urination [53

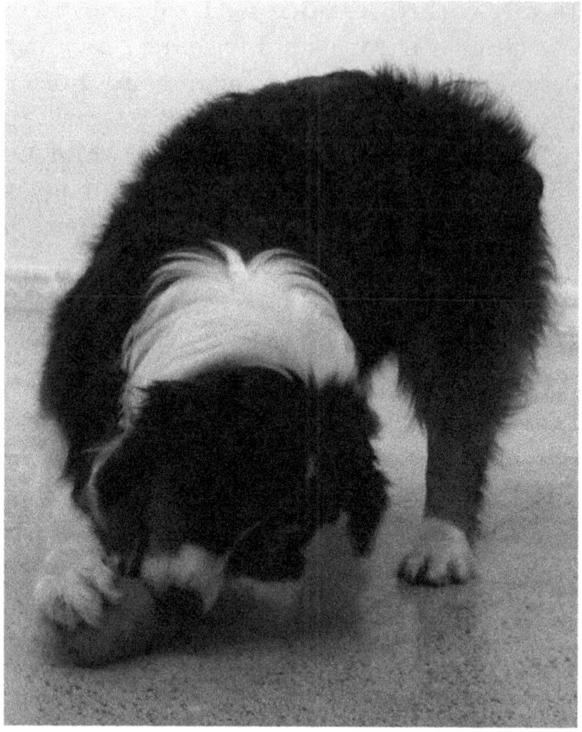

Figure 2. Motor lateralization: right paw use during stabilization of a food object (namely the "Kong").

The existence of motor asymmetries at a population level is currently a subject of wide debate. It has been reported in several species, including humans [54], non-human primates [55,56], rats [57], humpback whales [58] and common European toads [59] but studies on other animals, as for example marmosets [60], sheep [61,62], cats [63] and horses [64,65], has shown a motor bias only at the individual-level. However, the same species may also display a limb preference at the level of population or at the individual level depending on the task, as found in monkeys [66,67], cats [68] and sheep [69].

Motor lateralization in dogs is stable between breeds and over time [41,46] but variable between sexes. Although a few studies have reported an association between paw preference and sex at a population level but in opposite directions, with males showing a left-paw and females a right-paw preference [29,43,47], this seems to be inconsistent with other findings, which describe no population bias [17,39,41,46,51]. These conflicting results suggest that sex hormone status could be influential on the development of individual motor laterality but further investigations are necessary to accurately determine if this is the case.

There have been several recent studies that revealed an interesting association between emotional functioning and limb preference in animals, including dogs. It is well established that in primates motor bias is associated with differences in the behaviour of individuals and their emotional states. In particular, left-handed/pawed animals displayed more fear responses, higher stress levels and levels of reactivity than right-handed/pawed animals [4,70,71]. The latter, instead, were more likely to approach new objects and showed more social behaviours to capture a prey (chimpanzees: [72], marmosets: [73,74]). These behavioural differences match the known specialization of the hemisphere involved in the control of motor functions (contralateral to the preferred limb). Therefore, the limb preferential use could be indicative of the subject's personality type and its likelihood of expressing a positive or negative emotional functioning. Recent studies have reported indeed that left-handed marmosets have a negative cognitive bias compared to right-handed marmosets, which display a positive cognitive bias [75]. Concerning dogs, Branson and Rogers [46] showed that dogs with weaker motor lateralization were more reactive when exposed to potentially threatening stimuli (thunderstorm and fireworks sounds) since they displayed more stressed behaviours than lateralized subjects. Dogs with stronger paw preference are otherwise more confident and relaxed in an unfamiliar environment and when presented with novel stimuli [76]; on the contrary, they are less able in a problem-solving task, to manipulate and explore a new object to obtain food than ambilateral subjects [76].

Given these findings, preferential limb use could be employed as a measure to assess vulnerability to stress and welfare risk in animals [4] and also in dogs. Consequently, it is essential to correctly categorize subjects as left- or right-pawed, choosing a motor test that provides reliable information about dogs' dominant paw, in order to make inference about dogs' dominant hemisphere and their ability to cope with stress. Wells et al. [48] recently investigated whether dogs use their dominant paw in the most common motor test employed in this species, namely the Kong test. They found that dogs use their non-dominant paw to stabilize the Kong to obtain food and their dominant paw for postural support. These findings need to be considered for correct implications on animals' welfare and emotional vulnerability.

Therefore, the evaluation of paw preferential use could provide notable information regarding a dog's predisposition to solve future behavioural problems or about its suitability for work. It has been demonstrated, indeed, that the direction of laterality is predictive of success in a Guide Dog Training Programme; in particular, right-pawed dogs were more successful in completing the training than left-pawed and ambilateral subjects [77].

Considering that behavioural differences in dogs' response to different situations are linked with motor lateralization and that dogs' temperament plays an important role in the selection of dogs (for working or adoptions), Schneider and colleagues [50] examined the relationship between paw preference and temperament. They found no differences between lateralized and non-lateralized dogs in the score obtained by a questionnaire completed by owners, aside from stranger-directed aggression scale, where lateralized subjects registered higher scores than the ambilateral ones. This may suggest the existence of a lateralized component in that particular type of aggressive response but further investigations are required. Moreover, recent findings show that behavioural signs of fear and distress displayed in a given situation and motor laterality are not associated with cortisol concentration in saliva samples [42].

However, it would be interesting in the near future to deepen our understanding of the relationship between motor laterality and emotional functioning since knowing the direction of paw preference of a dog we could correctly assess the strategy to be employed to preserve and improve its welfare.

Motor laterality is also associated with the analysis of visuospatial information, as we recently found in our research. Specifically, agility trained dogs with weaker paw preference were less attentive in performing agility exercises and displayed greater latency in the wave poles task (i.e., dogs' ability to work around pole obstacles that are secured in a straight line to a metal base) when the owner was positioned in its left visual field [78]. These results clearly show that stimuli with high emotional valence (the owner) could influence specific cognitive abilities, particularly when the right hemisphere processes them. In a more recent study, we reported that visuospatial attention is strictly related to motor lateralization since left-pawed dogs exhibited left visuospatial bias, right-pawed dogs a reversed rightward bias, while ambilateral dogs displayed no bias [79]. The existence of such a relationship has significant implications for animal welfare since it establishes a basis on which to develop new therapies for the rehabilitation of visual attention during pathological conditions (namely, unilateral spatial neglect); it could also help humans to improve canine training techniques, choosing the correct side to handle dogs and how to capture their attention easily.

The importance of paw preference assessment as a useful tool to preserve animal welfare derives also from the evidence of a direct relationship between dogs' motor laterality and immune response via an asymmetrical modulation exerted by the autonomic nervous system [38,80–82]. Right-pawed and left-pawed dogs exhibit different patterns of immune response, in particular the former displayed higher granulocytes percentage, number of γ-globulins [38], anti-rabies antibody titres and interferon gamma (IFN-γ) serum level [80] while the latter showed higher lymphocytes number [38] and higher expression of specific interleukin genes (IL-2 and IL-6) after immune challenge [81]. Furthermore, ambidextrous dogs exhibit a significantly higher increase of catecholamine levels after immunization with rabies vaccine than lateralized subjects [82].

The direction of dogs paw preference is also related to anatomical asymmetries of the brain. Aydınlıoğlu et al. [45] found a variation in callosal size, particularly in its posterior segment (namely the isthmus) that was larger in right-preferent dogs than left-pawed subjects. Post mortem analyses also showed morphological asymmetries in canine hippocampi, which were associated with both sex (males larger than females) and paw preference. Female left-pawed dogs showed indeed larger hippocampi than the right ones [44]. In light of this evidence, motor lateralization may be considered as a direct consequence of brain structural asymmetries that could be, more broadly, the likely cause of cerebral specialization of functions.

4. Tail-Wagging as a Tool to Study the Asymmetrical Representation of Emotional Processing in the Dog Brain

Tail wagging represents an interesting model to study competition or cooperation between brain hemispheres in the control of behavioural response to emotional stimuli mainly for two reasons:

(1) Dogs move their tails in an asymmetrical way in response to different emotional stimuli [83].
(2) Studies on behavioural asymmetries associated with lateralized brain functions have usually focused on asymmetric use of paired organs (e.g., forelimbs) but not of a medial organ (i.e., the tail). In order to test asymmetries in tail wagging behaviour, family pet dogs of mixed breeds were placed in a large rectangular wooden box with an opening at the centre of one of its shorter sides to allow subjects to view the different stimuli (see Figure 3). Different emotional stimuli were presented as follows: the dog's owner; an unknown person; an unfamiliar dog with agonistic approach behaviour; and a cat. Tail wagging was analysed frame by frame from video footages recorded through a video camera placed on the ceiling of the box (see Figure 3).

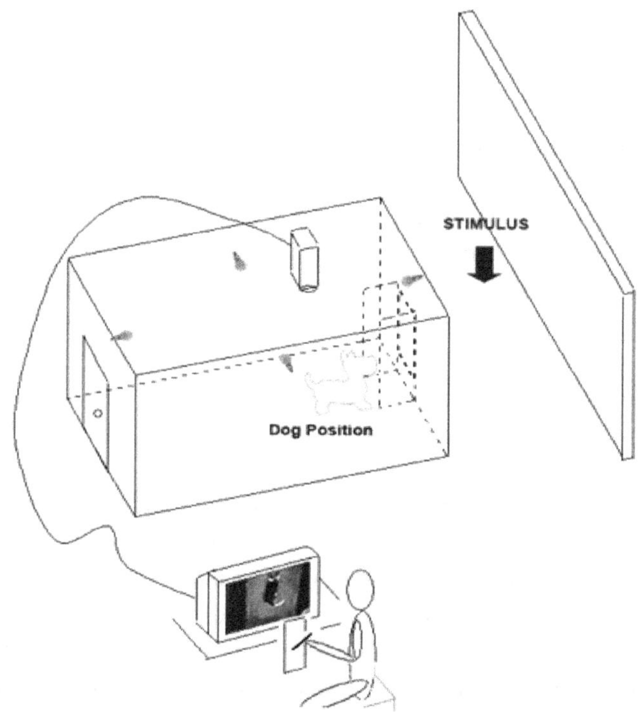

Figure 3. Schematic representation of the testing apparatus used to study asymmetric tail-wagging behaviour.

Results revealed that both direction and amplitude of tail wagging movements were related to the emotional valence of the stimulus. Specifically, when dogs looked at stimuli with a positive emotional valence (e.g., their owner), there was a higher amplitude of tail wagging to the right. On the other hand, during presentation of negative emotional stimuli (an unfamiliar dog with a clear agonistic behaviour), a left bias in tail wagging appeared. Given that the movement of the tail depends on the contralateral side of the brain [84], results are consistent with Davidson's laterality-valence hypothesis about the specialization of the left hemisphere for the control of approaching behavioural responses (right-wag → positive stimulus) and the dominant role of the right hemisphere for the control of withdrawal responses (left-wag → negative stimulus) [85]. In dogs, similar results were reported in the work of Racca et al. [86] in which subjects presented with pictures of expressive dog faces exhibited a left gaze bias (right hemisphere activation) while looking at negative conspecific facial expressions and a right gaze bias (left hemisphere activation) when looking at positive ones. The amplitude of tail-wagging movements is also a determinant cue for estimating "quantitatively" the level of arousal elicited by different emotional stimuli: during presentations of an unfamiliar human being, dogs significantly wagged their tails to the right side of their bodies but with less amplitude than towards the owner, whereas the sight of a cat once again elicited right side tail-wagging movements with less amplitude than towards the unfamiliar human being. The right side tail-wagging bias observed during cat presentations would probably reflect the tendency of dogs to approach the stimulus under the left hemisphere control of prey-drive behaviour.

In order to test whether or not dogs detect this asymmetry, in a more recent experiment, 43 dogs of various breeds were shown movies of other dogs or black silhouettes manipulated in order to display prevalent right or left sided tail-wagging or no wagging at all [87]. In addition, dogs' emotional response to movies were evaluated by measuring the subjects' behaviour and cardiac activity. Results revealed that when dogs saw movies of a conspecific exhibiting prevalent left-sided tail wagging, they had an increased cardiac activity and higher stress behaviours. Moreover, when observing movies of conspecific with right-sided tail wagging movements, dogs exhibited more relaxed behaviours with a normal cardiac activity (i.e., heart rate values similar to those of the dogs during resting) suggesting that the canine species is sensitive to the asymmetric tail movement of conspecifics, which has direct implication for understanding dog social behaviour. Different results were reported in a previous study in which the approach behaviour of free-ranging dogs to the asymmetric tail wagging of a life-size robotic dog replica was recorded [88]. Results revealed a preference to approach the robotic model (i.e., without stopping) when its tail was wagging to the left side. Authors reported that a possible explanation for the stop response during the approach to the model moving its tail with a clear bias to the right may originate when tested dogs are presented with a signal that would otherwise be positive (right wag) yet is not accompanied by additional reciprocal visual or acoustical responses by the robotic model. Another possible explanation for the different results between the two experiments is that, in the first experiment, tail movements were taken by real dogs (i.e., biological movements) while in the second they were artificially reproduced by a robotic model (even in the presence of a good dog-replica robotic movements are not properly biological).

5. Conclusions

Overall, there is clear evidence that functional lateralization has profound connections with cognition in dogs. A greater understanding of this association may certainly contribute to improve dog welfare and the relationship between dogs and humans. Non-invasive techniques of measuring lateralization (e.g., paw preference or tail wagging) could constitute a reliable, simple and direct tool of evaluating dogs' cognitive style and emotional affective states, providing elements that could enhance every-day management practice and improve both dogs' welfare and behavioural medicine.

Acknowledgments: There were no funding sponsors that had any role in the writing of this manuscript or in any other capacity in preparing and publishing this manuscript.

Author Contributions: The authors contributed equally to this manuscript.

References

1. Rogers, L.J.; Andrew, R.J. *Comparative Vertebrate Lateralization*; Cambridge University Press: New York, NY, USA, 2002; p. 660. ISBN: 0521781612.
2. Rogers, L.J.; Vallortigara, G.; Andrew, R.J. *Divided Brains. The Biology and Behaviour of Brain Asymmetries*; Cambridge University Press: New York, NY, USA, 2013; p. 229. ISBN: 0521604850.
3. MacNeilage, P.F.; Rogers, L.J.; Vallortigara, G. Origins of the left and right brain. *Sci. Am.* **2009**, *301*, 60–67. [CrossRef] [PubMed]
4. Rogers, L.J. Relevance of brain and behavioural lateralization to animal welfare. *Appl. Anim. Behav. Sci.* **2010**, *127*, 1–11. [CrossRef]
5. Siniscalchi, M.; Sasso, R.; Pepe, A.M.; Vallortigara, G.; Quaranta, A. Dogs turn left to emotional stimuli. *Behav. Brain Res.* **2010**, *208*, 516–521. [CrossRef] [PubMed]
6. Siniscalchi, M.; Quaranta, A.; Rogers, L.J. Hemispheric specialization in dogs for processing different acoustic stimuli. *PLoS ONE* **2008**, *3*, e3349. [CrossRef] [PubMed]
7. Reinholz-Trojan, A.; Włodarczyk, E.; Trojan, M.; Kulczyński, A.; Stefańska, J. Hemispheric specialization in domestic dogs (*Canis familiaris*) for processing different types of acoustic stimuli. *Behav. Process.* **2012**, *91*, 202–205. [CrossRef] [PubMed]
8. Ratcliffe, V.F.; Reby, D. Orienting asymmetries in dogs' responses to different communicatory components of human speech. *Curr. Biol.* **2014**, *24*, 2908–2912. [CrossRef] [PubMed]
9. Andics, A.; Gácsi, M.; Faragó, T.; Kis, A.; Miklósi, A. Voice-sensitive regions in the dog and human brain are revealed by comparative fMRI. *Curr. Biol.* **2014**, *24*, 574–578. [CrossRef] [PubMed]
10. Andics, A.; Gábor, A.; Gácsi, M.; Faragó, T.; Szabó, D.; Miklósi, A. Neural mechanisms for lexical processing in dogs. *Science* **2016**, *353*, 1030–1032. [CrossRef] [PubMed]
11. Siniscalchi, M.; Sasso, R.; Pepe, A.M.; Dimatteo, S.; Vallortigara, G.; Quaranta, A. Sniffing with right nostril: Lateralization of response to odour stimuli by dogs. *Anim. Behav.* **2011**, *82*, 399–404. [CrossRef]
12. Siniscalchi, M.; d'Ingeo, S.; Quaranta, A. The dog nose "KNOWS" fear: Asymmetric nostril use during sniffing at canine and human emotional stimuli. *Behav. Brain Res.* **2016**, *304*, 34–41. [CrossRef] [PubMed]
13. LoBue, V.; DeLoache, J.S. Detecting the snake in the grass: Attention to fear relevant stimuli by adults and young children. *Psychol. Sci.* **2008**, *19*, 284–289. [CrossRef] [PubMed]
14. Fogle, B. The Dog's Mind. Pelham Editions: London, UK, 1992; p. 203. ISBN: 072071964X.
15. Wittling, W. Brain asymmetry in the control of autonomic-physiologic activity. In *Brain Asymmetry*; Davidson, R.J., Hugdahl, K, Eds.; MIT Press: Cambridge, UK, 1995; pp. 305–357. ISBN: 9780262041447.
16. Siniscalchi, M.; Franchini, D.; Pepe, A.M.; Sasso, R.; Dimatteo, S.; Vallortigara, G.; Quaranta, A. Volumetric assessment of cerebral asymmetries in dogs. *Laterality* **2011**, *16*, 528–536. [CrossRef] [PubMed]
17. Tan, U.; Caliskan, S. Allometry and asymmetry in the dog brain: The right-hemisphere is heavier regardless of paw preferences. *Int. J. Neurosci.* **1987**, *35*, 189–194. [CrossRef] [PubMed]
18. Rogers, L.J. Evolution of hemispheric specialisation: Advantages and disadvantages. *Brain Lang.* **2000**, *73*, 236–253. [CrossRef] [PubMed]
19. Dharmaretnam, M.; Rogers, L.J. Hemispheric specialization and dual processing in strongly versus weakly lateralized chicks. *Behav. Brain Res.* **2005**, *162*, 62–70. [CrossRef] [PubMed]
20. Lippolis, G.; Bisazza, A.; Rogers, L.J.; Vallortigara, G. Lateralization of predator avoidance responses in three species of toads. *Laterality* **2002**, *7*, 163–183. [CrossRef] [PubMed]
21. Austin, N.P.; Rogers, L.J. Asymmetry of flight and escape turning responses in horses. *Laterality* **2007**, *12*, 464–474. [CrossRef] [PubMed]
22. Scheumann, M.; Zimmermann, E. Sex-specific asymmetries in communication sound perception are not related to hand preference in an early primate. *BMC Biol.* **2008**, *6*, 3. [CrossRef] [PubMed]
23. Poremba, A.; Malloy, M.; Saunders, R.C.; Carson, R.E.; Herscovitch, P.; Mishkin, M. Species-specific calls evoke asymmetric activity in the monkey's temporal lobes. *Nature* **2004**, *427*, 448–451. [CrossRef] [PubMed]
24. Basile, M.; Boivin, S.; Boutin, A.; Blois-Heulin, C.; Hausberger, M.; Lemasson, A. Socially dependent auditory laterality in domestic horses (*Equus caballus*). *Anim. Cogn.* **2009**, *12*, 611–619. [CrossRef] [PubMed]

25. Siniscalchi, M.; Laddago, S.; Quaranta, A. Auditory lateralization of conspecific and heterospecific vocalizations in cats. *Laterality* **2016**, *21*, 215–227. [CrossRef] [PubMed]
26. Böye, M.; Güntürkün, O.; Vauclair, J. Right ear advantage for conspecific calls in adults and subadults, but not infants, California sea lions (*Zalophus californianus*): Hemispheric specialization for communication? *Eur. J. Neurosci.* **2005**, *21*, 1727–1732. [CrossRef] [PubMed]
27. Siniscalchi, M.; Lusito, R.; Sasso, R.; Quaranta, A. Are temporal features crucial acoustic cues in dog vocal recognition? *Anim. Cogn.* **2012**, *15*, 815–821. [CrossRef] [PubMed]
28. Siniscalchi, M. Olfactory lateralization. In *Lateralized Brain Functions*; Rogers, L.J., Vallortigara, G., Eds.; Humana press: New York, NY, USA, 2017; pp. 103–120. ISBN: 9781493967230.
29. Siniscalchi, M. Olfaction and the Canine Brain. In *Canine Olfaction Science and Law*; Jezierski, T., Ensminger, J., Papet, L.E., Eds.; CRC Press: Boca Raton, FL, USA, 2016; pp. 31–37. ISBN: 1482260239.
30. Vallortigara, G.; Chiandetti, C.; Sovrano, V.A. Brain asymmetry (animal). *WIREs Cogn. Sci.* **2011**, *2*, 146–157. [CrossRef] [PubMed]
31. Vallortigara, G. Comparative neuropsychology of the dual brain: A stroll through left and right animals' perceptual worlds. *Brain Lang.* **2000**, *73*, 189–219. [CrossRef] [PubMed]
32. Güntürkün, O.; Kesh, S. Visual lateralization during feeding in pigeons. *Behav. Neurosci.* **1987**, *101*, 433–435. [CrossRef] [PubMed]
33. Ventolini, N.; Ferrero, E.A.; Sponza, S.; Chiesa, A.D.; Zucca, P.; Vallortigara, G. Laterality in the wild: Preferential hemifield use during predatory and sexual behaviour in the black-winged stilt. *Anim. Behav.* **2005**, *69*, 1077–1084. [CrossRef]
34. Robins, A.; Rogers, L.J. Lateralised prey catching responses in the toad (*Bufo marinus*): Analysis of complex visual stimuli. *Anim. Behav.* **2004**, *68*, 567–575. [CrossRef]
35. Rogers, L.J. Early experiential effects on laterality: Research on chicks has relevance to other species. *Laterality* **1997**, *2*, 199–219. [CrossRef] [PubMed]
36. Siniscalchi, M.; Pergola, G.; Quaranta, A. Detour behaviour in attack-trained dogs: Left-turners perform better than right-turners. *Laterality* **2013**, *18*, 282–293. [CrossRef] [PubMed]
37. Tan, U. Paw preferences in dogs. *Int. J. Neurosci.* **1987**, *32*, 825–829. [CrossRef] [PubMed]
38. Quaranta, A.; Siniscalchi, M.; Frate, A.; Vallortigara, G. Paw preference in dogs: Relations between lateralised behaviour and immunity. *Behav. Brain Res.* **2004**, *153*, 521–525. [CrossRef] [PubMed]
39. Poyser, F.; Caldwell, C.; Cobba, M. Dog paw preference shows liability and sex differences. *Behav. Process.* **2006**, *73*, 216–221. [CrossRef] [PubMed]
40. Batt, L.S.; Batt, M.S.; McGreevy, P.D. Two tests for motor laterality in dogs. *J. Vet. Behav.* **2007**, *2*, 47–51. [CrossRef]
41. Batt, L.S.; Batt, M.S.; Baguley, J.A.; McGreevy, P.D. Stability of motor lateralisation in maturing dogs. *Laterality* **2008**, *13*, 468–479. [CrossRef] [PubMed]
42. Batt, L.S.; Batt, M.S.; Baguley, J.A.; McGreevy, P.D. The relationships between motor lateralization, salivary cortisol concentrations and behavior in dogs. *J. Vet. Behav.* **2009**, *4*, 216–222. [CrossRef]
43. Wells, D.L. Lateralised behaviour in the domestic dog, *Canis familiaris*. *Behav. Process.* **2003**, *61*, 27–35. [CrossRef]
44. Aydınlıoğlu, A.; Arslan, K.; Cengiz, N.; Ragbetli, M.; Erdoğan, E. The relationships of dog hippocampus to sex and paw preference. *Int. J. Neurosci.* **2006**, *116*, 77–88. [CrossRef] [PubMed]
45. Aydınlıoğlu, A.; Arslan, K.; Rıza Erdoğan, A.; Cetin Rağbetli, M.; Keleş, P.; Diyarbakırlı, S. The relationship of callosal anatomy to paw preference in dogs. *Eur. J. Morphol.* **2000**, *38*, 128–133. [CrossRef]
46. Branson, N.J.; Rogers, L.J. Relationship between paw preference strength and noise phobia in *Canis familiaris*. *J. Comp. Psychol.* **2006**, *120*, 176–183. [CrossRef] [PubMed]
47. McGreevy, P.D.; Brueckner, A.; Branson, N.J. Motor laterality in four breeds of dog. *J. Vet. Behav.* **2010**, *5*, 318–323. [CrossRef]
48. Wells, D.L.; Hepper, P.G.; Milligan, A.D.; Barnard, S. Comparing lateral bias in dogs and humans using the Kong™ ball test. *Appl. Anim. Behav. Sci.* **2016**, *176*, 70–76. [CrossRef]
49. Tomkins, L.M.; Thomson, P.C.; McGreevy, P.D. First-stepping Test as a measure of motor laterality in dogs (*Canis familiaris*). *J. Vet. Behav.* **2010**, *5*, 247–255. [CrossRef]
50. Schneider, L.A.; Delfabbro, P.H.; Burns, N.R. Temperament and lateralization in the domestic dog (*Canis familiaris*). *J. Vet. Behav.* **2013**, *8*, 124–134. [CrossRef]

51. Van Alphen, A.; Bosse, T.; Frank, I.; Jonker, C.M.; Koeman, F. Paw preference correlates to task performance in dogs. In *27th Annual Conference of the Cognitive Science Society*; Cognitive Science Society: Stresa, Italy, 2005; pp. 2248–2253.
52. Hackert, R.; Maes, L.D.; Herbin, M.; Libourel, P.A.; Abourachid, A. Limb preference in the gallop of dogs and the halfbound of pikas on flat ground. *Laterality* **2008**, *13*, 310–319. [CrossRef] [PubMed]
53. Gough, W.; McGuire, B. Urinary posture and motor laterality in dogs (*Canis lupus familiaris*) at two shelters. *Appl. Anim. Behav. Sci.* **2015**, *168*, 61–70. [CrossRef]
54. McManus, I.C. *Right Hand, Left Hand: The Origins of Asymmetry in Brains, Bodies, Atoms, and Cultures*; Weidenfeld & Nicolson: London, UK, 2002; ISBN: 9780674016132.
55. Diamond, A.C.; McGrew, W.C. True handedness in the cotton-top tamarin (*Saguinus oedipus*)? *Primates* **1994**, *35*, 69–77. [CrossRef]
56. Laska, M. Manual laterality in spider monkeys (*Ateles geoffroyi*) solving visually and tactually guided food-reaching tasks. *Cortex* **1996**, *32*, 717–726. [CrossRef]
57. Güven, M.; Elalmis, D.D.; Binokay, S.; Tan, U. Population-level right-paw preference in rats assessed by a new computerized food-reaching test. *Int. J. Neurosci.* **2003**, *113*, 1675–1689. [CrossRef] [PubMed]
58. Clapham, P.J.; Leimkuhler, E.; Gray, B.K.; Mattila, D.K. Do humpback whales exhibit lateralized behaviour? *Anim. Behav.* **1995**, *50*, 73–82. [CrossRef]
59. Bisazza, A.; Cantalupo, C.; Robins, A.; Rogers, L.J.; Vallortigara, G. Right-pawedness in toads. *Nature* **1996**, *379*, 408. [CrossRef]
60. Hook, M.A.; Rogers, L.J. Development of hand preferences in marmosets (*Callithrix jacchus*) and effects of ageing. *J. Comp. Psychol.* **2000**, *114*, 263–271. [CrossRef] [PubMed]
61. Anderson, D.M.; Murray, L.W. Sheep laterality. *Laterality* **2013**, *18*, 179–193. [CrossRef] [PubMed]
62. Morgante, M.; Gianesella, M.; Versace, E.; Contalbrigo, L.; Casella, S.; Cannizzo, C.; Piccione, G.; Stelletta, C. Preliminary study on metabolic profile of pregnant and non pregnant ewes with high or low degree of behavioral lateralization. *Anim. Sci. J.* **2010**, *81*, 722–730. [CrossRef] [PubMed]
63. Pike, A.V.L.; Maitland, D.P. Paw preferences in cats (*Felis silvestris catus*) living in a household environment. *Behav. Process.* **1997**, *39*, 241–247. [CrossRef]
64. Austin, N.P.; Rogers, L.J. Limb preferences and lateralization of aggression, reactivity and vigilance in feral horses, *Equus caballus*. *Anim. Behav.* **2012**, *83*, 239–247. [CrossRef]
65. Austin, N.P.; Rogers, L.J. Lateralization of agonistic and vigilance responses in Przewalski horses (*Equus przewalskii*). *Appl. Anim. Behav. Sci.* **2014**, *151*, 43–50. [CrossRef]
66. Hook, M.A.; Rogers, L.J. Visuospatial reaching preferences of common marmosets (*Callithrix jacchus*): An assessment of individual biases across a variety of tasks. *J. Comp. Psychol.* **2008**, *122*, 41–51. [CrossRef] [PubMed]
67. Fagot, J.; Vauclair, J. Manual laterality in nonhuman primates: A distinction between handedness and manual specialization. *Psychol. Bull.* **1991**, *109*, 76–89. [CrossRef] [PubMed]
68. Wells, D.L.; Millsopp, S. Lateralized behaviour in the domestic cat, *Felis silvestris catus*. *Anim. Behav.* **2009**, *78*, 537–541. [CrossRef]
69. Versace, E.; Morgante, M.; Pulina, G.; Vallortigara, G. Behavioural lateralization in sheep (*Ovis aries*). *Behav. Brain Res.* **2007**, *184*, 72–80. [CrossRef] [PubMed]
70. Braccini, S.N.; Caine, N.G. Hand preference predicts reactions to novel foods and predators in marmosets (*Callithrix geoffroyi*). *J. Comp. Psychol.* **2009**, *123*, 18. [CrossRef] [PubMed]
71. Rogers, L.J. Hand and paw preferences in relation to the lateralized brain. *Philos. Trans. R. Soc. B* **2009**, *364*, 943–954. [CrossRef] [PubMed]
72. Hopkins, W.D.; Bennett, A.J. Handedness and approach-avoidance behaviour in chimpanzees (*Pan troglodytes*). *J. Exp. Psychol.* **1994**, *20*, 413–418. [CrossRef]
73. Cameron, R.; Rogers, L.J. Hand preference of the common marmoset, problem solving and responses in a novel setting. *J. Comp. Psychol.* **1999**, *113*, 149–157. [CrossRef]
74. Gordon, D.J.; Rogers, L.J. Differences in social and vocal behavior between left- and right-handed common marmosets. *J. Comp. Psychol.* **2010**, *124*, 402–411. [CrossRef] [PubMed]
75. Gordon, D.J.; Rogers, L.J. Cognitive bias, hand preference and welfare of common marmosets. *Behav. Brain Res.* **2015**, *287*, 100–108. [CrossRef] [PubMed]

76. Marshall-Pescini, S.; Barnard, S.; Branson, N.J.; Valsecchi, P. The effect of preferential paw usage on dogs' (*Canis familiaris*) performance in a manipulative problem-solving task. *Behav. Process.* **2013**, *100*, 40–43. [CrossRef] [PubMed]
77. Tomkins, L.M.; Thomson, P.C.; McGreevy, P.D. Associations between motor, sensory and structural lateralisation and guide dog success. *Vet. J.* **2012**, *192*, 359–367. [CrossRef] [PubMed]
78. Siniscalchi, M.; Bertino, D.; Quaranta, A. Laterality and performance of agility-trained dogs. *Laterality* **2014**, *19*, 219–234. [CrossRef] [PubMed]
79. Siniscalchi, M.; d'Ingeo, S.; Fornelli, S.; Quaranta, A. Relationship between visuospatial attention and paw preference in dogs. *Sci. Rep.* **2016**, *6*, 31682. [CrossRef] [PubMed]
80. Quaranta, A.; Siniscalchi, M.; Frate, A.; Iacoviello, R.; Buonavoglia, C.; Vallortigara, G. Lateralised behaviour and immune response in dogs: relations between paw preference and interferon-gamma, interleukin-10 and IgG antibodies production. *Behav. Brain Res.* **2006**, *166*, 236–240. [CrossRef] [PubMed]
81. Quaranta, A.; Siniscalchi, M.; Albrizio, M.; Volpe, S.; Buonavoglia, C.; Vallortigara, G. Influence of behavioural lateralization on interleukin-2 and interleukin-6 gene expression in dogs before and after immunization with rabies vaccine. *Behav. Brain Res.* **2008**, *186*, 256–260. [CrossRef] [PubMed]
82. Siniscalchi, M.; Sasso, R.; Pepe, A.M.; Dimatteo, S.; Vallortigara, G.; Quaranta, A. Catecholamine plasma levels following immune stimulation with rabies vaccine in dogs selected for their paw preferences. *Neurosci. Lett.* **2010**, *476*, 142–145. [CrossRef] [PubMed]
83. Quaranta, A.; Siniscalchi, M.; Vallortigara, G. Asymmetric tail-wagging responses by dogs to different emotive stimuli. *Curr. Biol.* **2007**, *17*, R199–R201. [CrossRef] [PubMed]
84. Buxton, D.F.; Goodman, D.C. Motor function and the corticospinal tracts in the dog and raccoon. *J. Comp. Neurol.* **1967**, *129*, 341–360. [CrossRef] [PubMed]
85. Davidson, R.J. Well-being and affective style: Neural substrates and biobehavioural correlates. *Phil. Trans. R. Soc. B* **2004**, *359*, 1395–1411. [CrossRef] [PubMed]
86. Racca, A.; Guo, K.; Meints, K.; Mills, D.S. Reading faces: differential lateral gaze bias in processing canine and human facial expressions in dogs and 4-year-old children. *PLoS ONE* **2012**, *7*, e36076. [CrossRef] [PubMed]
87. Siniscalchi, M.; Lusito, R.; Vallortigara, G.; Quaranta, A. Seeing left- or right-asymmetric tail wagging produces different emotional responses in dogs. *Curr. Biol.* **2013**, *23*, 2279–2282. [CrossRef] [PubMed]
88. Artelle, K.A.; Dumoulin, L.K.; Reimchen, T.E. Behavioral responses of dogs to asymmetrical tail wagging of a robotic dog replica. *Laterality* **2011**, *16*, 129–135. [CrossRef] [PubMed]

The Genetics of Asymmetry: Whole Exome Sequencing in a Consanguineous Turkish Family with an Overrepresentation of Left-Handedness

Sebastian Ocklenburg [1,*,†], Ceren Barutçuoğlu [1,†], Adile Öniz Özgören [2], Murat Özgören [2], Esra Erdal [3], Dirk Moser [4], Judith Schmitz [1], Robert Kumsta [4] and Onur Güntürkün [1]

1 Institute of Cognitive Neuroscience, Biopsychology, Ruhr-University, 44780 Bochum, Germany; crn.barutcuoglu@gmail.com (C.B.); judith.schmitz@rub.de (J.S.); onur.guentuerkuen@rub.de (O.G.)
2 Department of Biophysics, Faculty of Medicine, Dokuz Eylül University, 35340 Izmir, Turkey; adile.oniz@gmail.com (A.Ö.Ö.); murat.ozgoren@deu.edu.tr (M.Ö.)
3 Department of Medical Biology, Faculty of Medicine, Dokuz Eylül University, 35340 Izmir, Turkey; esra.erdal@deu.edu.tr
4 Genetic Psychology, Faculty of Psychology, Ruhr-University, 44780 Bochum, Germany; Dirk.Moser@rub.de (D.M.); robert.kumsta@rub.de (R.K.)
* Correspondence: sebastian.ocklenburg@rub.de
† These authors contributed equally.

Academic Editor: Lesley Rogers

Abstract: Handedness is the most pronounced behavioral asymmetry in humans. Genome-wide association studies have largely failed to identify genetic loci associated with phenotypic variance in handedness, supporting the idea that the trait is determined by a multitude of small, possibly interacting genetic and non-genetic influences. However, these studies typically are not capable of detecting influences of rare mutations on handedness. Here, we used whole exome sequencing in a Turkish family with history of consanguinity and overrepresentation of left-handedness and performed quantitative trait analysis with handedness lateralization quotient as a phenotype. While rare variants on different loci showed significant association with the phenotype, none was functionally relevant for handedness. This finding was further confirmed by gene ontology group analysis. Taken together, our results add further evidence to the suggestion that there is no major gene or mutation that causes left-handedness.

Keywords: handedness; hemispheric asymmetries; genetics; ontogenesis; consanguineous marriage

1. Introduction

Handedness is a heritable trait [1] and, historically, it was thought that left-handedness was determined by a major gene effect [2]. This idea was based on the statistical distribution of the phenotype, but has since been refuted by molecular studies. In particular, the fact that genome-wide associations studies (GWAS) consistently failed to identify a gene that explains enough phenotypic variance to qualify as a single-gene explanation has disproven single gene theories [3,4]. Thus, most authors today agree that handedness is likely to be a multifactorial trait that is determined by several different genetic and non-genetic factors (e.g., [5–8]). A number of contributing loci have been identified by GWAS and candidate gene studies using handedness questionnaires or hand skill tests like the pegboard test as phenotypes, e.g., *LRRTM1*, *PCSK6* and *AR* [9–15]. However, the general understanding is that there is likely a large number of yet unidentified genetic contributions to handedness [5]. Besides replication of published loci, identification of new candidate genes therefore is one of the major aims of current research on handedness genetics. Since GWAS in healthy cohorts are unlikely to identify rare genetic variants relevant for handedness, other methods to identify candidate genes should also be considered.

One possible way to increase statistical power to detect relevant candidate genes for handedness without the need for overly large cohorts is testing population isolates with reduced genetic heterogeneity and overrepresentation of left-handedness. For example, Somers et al. [16] performed a genome-wide genetic linkage study of left-handedness and language lateralization in a sample of 368 subjects from a population isolate in the Netherlands. Due to the geographical isolation of the town that the subjects were recruited from, as well as a genetic bottleneck event in the early 17th century, founders in the sample of Somers et al. [16] showed lower genetic heterogeneity than random samples from the Dutch population. The sample was deliberately enriched for left-handedness, as the authors only selected families that had left-handed subjects in at least two generations, with at least two left-handed family members per generation. This resulted in a sample in which 24% of participants were left-handed, roughly 2.5 as many as in the general population. While Somers et al. [16] did not observe any genome-wide evidence for linkage in handedness, there was at least suggestive evidence for linkage for left-handedness in the 22q13 region. Somers et al. [16] argued that the absence of any significant linkage indicates that there is no major gene coding for handedness and it is likely to be a polygenic complex trait.

In addition to testing populations that show lower genetic heterogeneity than the general population due to a genetic bottleneck in the past and a more or less isolated way of living, another methodological option to detect genetic variants that influence handedness is to test families with a history of consanguineous marriage and an overrepresentation of left-handedness. This method has for example been used by Kavaklioglu et al. [17]. These authors used whole exome sequencing in 17 members of an extended family from Pakistan that practiced consanguineous marriage and had an overrepresentation of non-right-handed members (about 40%). Neither multipoint linkage analysis across all autosomes nor single-point analysis of exomic variation resulted in any clear candidate genes or mutations, leading Kavaklioglu et al. [17] to conclude, similar to Somers et al. [16], that handedness is a polygenic complex trait and not driven by a major gene or single mutation.

Although neither of these studies observed any significant effects, this does not necessarily imply that rare mutations could not affect handedness in other samples. Thus, more research in similar samples in other regions is needed. Also, previous studies in bottleneck populations analyzed handedness as a dichotomous variable (e.g., right-handedness/non-right-handedness). However, it is commonly measured as a continuous variable using a lateralization quotient (LQ) [18], ranging from −100 (consistent left-handedness) to +100 (consistent right-handedness). Interestingly, findings from a recent PCSK6 candidate gene study on handedness showed that the direction and degree of handedness might underlie differential genetic influences [9]. Thus, using the LQ as a phenotype instead of differentiating between left- and right-handers could potentially yield interesting insights into the genetics of handedness. To this end, we performed whole exome sequencing in nine members of an extended Eastern Turkish family that practices consanguineous marriage and has an overrepresentation of left-handedness. We then conducted a quantitative trait analysis with handedness LQ as a trait. Our hypothesis was that if there was indeed a major gene effect of a rare variant in this cohort, this variant should be significantly related to handedness LQ. If no such association was found, this would further confirm the idea that handedness is not driven by a major gene effect.

2. Materials and Methods

2.1. Participants

All participants were from Turkey, specifically from the vicinity of Şanlı Urfa, a city in the east of Turkey. This area was chosen as it has a higher prevalence of kin marriage compared to other regions of Turkey. The study was approved by the ethics committee of Dokuz Eylül University, Faculty of Medicine, İzmir, Turkey. All participants were treated in accordance with the declaration of Helsinki.

All participants gave written informed consent, and in case of participants younger than 18 years, the parents also gave written informed consent. Subjects were compensated for participating in the experiment with a gift of high quality Turkish sweets, as they refused to take money as reimbursement. Nine members of the family, two female and seven male, with a mean age of 29.33 (SD = 13.07; range: 11–46 years) agreed to participate in the study (Figure 1). Verbal interviews confirmed at least four consanguineous marriages between living family members and a family history of previous consanguineous marriages. None of the participants had a history of any psychiatric diseases or neurological diseases.

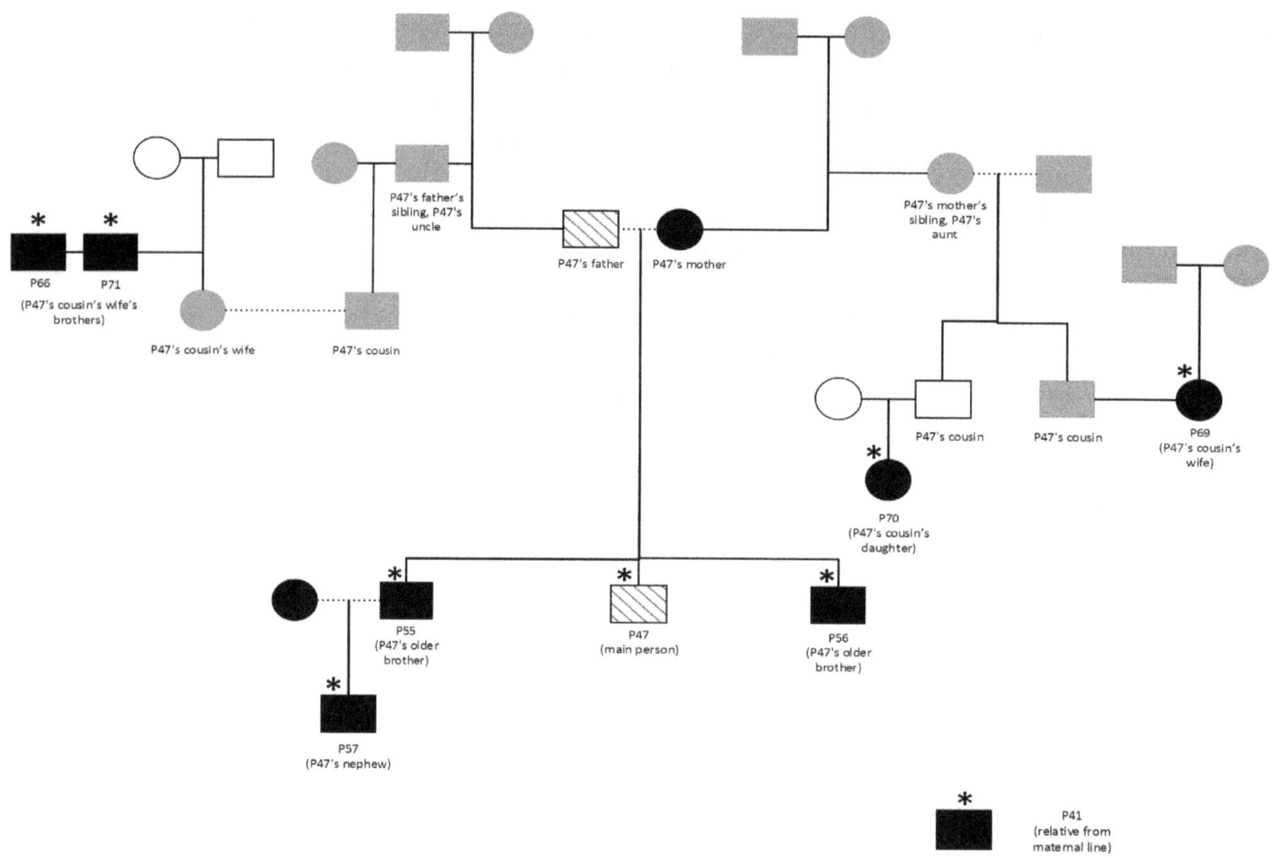

Figure 1. Family tree for the investigated cohort. Squares indicate male family members, circles indicate female family members. Asterisks indicate family members that participated in the present study. For these family members, handedness was determined using the Edinburgh Handedness Inventory (EHI). For other family members shown in the figure, handedness was assessed by verbal report. Black indicates left-handedness, white right-handedness and white with black shading ambidexterity. For family members with grey symbols, no information about handedness could be obtained. Consanguineous marriages are indicated by dotted lines. Consanguineous marriages were also performed by several family members of earlier generations not shown in this figure, as confirmed by verbal report.

2.2. *Phenotyping*

2.2.1. Edinburgh Handedness Inventory

Handedness was assessed with a Turkish translation of the EHI [18]. In this questionnaire, participants have to indicate whether they prefer to use left or right hand for ten different activities which are hand preference in writing, drawing, throwing a ball, using scissors, a toothbrush, a knife (without fork), a spoon, and a broom (upper hand), striking a match, and opening a box. An individual LQ can be calculated using the Formula $LQ = [(R - L)/(R + L)] \times 100$ (R = the number of right-hand preferences; L = the number of left-hand preferences) as based on participants' answers. The LQ has a range between +100 and −100. Positive values indicate right-handedness and negative values indicate left-handedness. At the same time, higher absolute values indicate more consistent handedness and lower absolute values indicate more inconsistent handedness or ambidexterity.

2.2.2. Pegboard Test

In addition to questionnaires like the EHI that assess hand preference, hand skill can be assessed with motor tasks such as placing dots in squares or circles on a sheet of paper as quickly as possible [19,20], or picking up matches placed on a table as quickly as possible [19]. The most commonly used measure is the so-called "pegboard task" (e.g., [15,21,22]) that was also utilized to determine participants manual hand skills in the present study. The test consists of measuring the time taken by the subjects to move, with each hand separately, a row of 10 pegs on a board from one location to another. The test is repeated three times for each hand. The measure of relative hand skill (PegQ) is calculated as the difference between the average times for the left hand (L) and the right hand (R), (L − R), divided by the average time for both hands combined, (L + R)/2 [15]. A positive PegQ demonstrates superior relative right-hand skill, and a negative PegQ demonstrates superior relative left-hand skill.

2.2.3. Dichotic Listening Task

The Dichotic Listening Task is a noninvasive behavioral test to determine language lateralization. During a dichotic listening test, two different consonant-vowel (CV) syllables are presented to participants simultaneously using headphones, one to the right ear and one to the left ear. The syllables used in the present study were "BA, DA, GA, KA, PA, TA" [23]. Participants are instructed to indicate the syllable which they heard best by pressing a button [23]. Overall, 72 stimulus pairs were presented with Sony stereo headphones type MDR-ZX100 using Presentation software (https://www.neurobs.com/). The stimuli consisted of two times presenting all possible 36 combinations of the six syllables, including homonyms (e.g., BA-BA). Syllables were spoken by a native Turkish speaker and were provided by Dokuz Eylül University, Faculty of Medicine, Biophysics Department. Voice-onset times were controlled for.

2.3. Collection of DNA Samples

For the non-invasive collection of high quality DNA, saliva samples were collected using Oragene-DNA OG-500 saliva self-collection kits. These kits were used since they ensure DNA sample stability at room temperature for a prolonged time, which was essential since data collection took place in a field study without permanent access to refrigeration. From each participant, 2 mL of saliva were collected.

2.4. Whole Exome Sequencing

DNA was extracted from saliva samples and purified according to the kit protocol. All samples passed initial quality control with OD260/OD280 ratios between 1.6 and 2.0, and were then shipped to GATC Biotech AG (Konstanz, Germany), a service provider for DNA sequencing and bioinformatics (www.gatc-biotech.com). In addition to the nine samples from the family, we also included one sample of an unrelated right-hander from Turkey, to differentiate possible regional exome variation from true rare variants specific for the family, in addition to comparison against other reference genomes (see below). All samples passed a second DNA quality control performed by GATC. "INVIEW HUMAN EXOME" (http://www.gatc-biotech.com/de/produkte/inview-applikationen/inview-human-exome.html) was chosen as the whole exome sequencing platform. The array used was an Agilent Genomics SureSelectXT All Exon V5 (Agilent Technologies, Santa Clara, CA, USA). Mapping to the UCSC Genome Browser *Homo Sapiens* reference genome (hg19) was performed using BWA (Burrows-Wheeler Aligner; http://bio-bwa.sourceforge.net/ [24], with default parameters.

On average, 99.13% of high quality reads were mapped to the reference genome (see Table S1 for mapped read metrics for all samples). Removal of polymerase chain reaction (PCR) duplicates was conducted using Picard (http://broadinstitute.github.io/picard/) and local realignment using GATK (Genome Analysis Toolkit; https://software.broadinstitute.org/gatk/) [25]. On average, 93.99% of the exome was covered with a sequence depth read of at least 10× (see Table S2 for the depth of coverage summary). single-nucleotide polymorphism (SNP) and InDel calling was performed using GATK's UnifiedGenotyper (https://software.broadinstitute.org/gatk/documentation/tooldocs/current/org_broadinstitute_gatk_tools_walkers_genotyper_UnifiedGenotyper.php) [25], with a Bayesian genotype likelihood model. Subsequently, variant annotations were performed using snpEff (http://snpeff.sourceforge.net/) [26]. Further analysis of exome data and quantitative trait analysis was performed using "QIAGEN Ingenuity Variant Analysis" (http://www.ingenuity.com/products/variant-analysis) (see results for analysis pathway). The quantitative trait test that was used represents a continuous version of the Sequence Kernel Association Test (SKAT) where each sample is associated with a continuous quantity (in our case handedness LQ) instead of a case and control label. The underlying test is a variance component score test, based on a linear mixed effects model where the impact of rare variants is taken into account as random effects and co-variants are included as fixed affects. The quantitative trait test determines asymptotic p-values that are calculated approximately using Kuonens saddlepoint method. Furthermore, Gene ontology (GO) analysis was performed using the webtool WebGestalt (http://bioinfo.vanderbilt.edu/webgestalt/). This was done in order to identify whether associated gene variants were involved in GO groups with functional significance for handedness development (e.g., left-right axis differentiation or nervous system development). The minimum number of genes included in each GO group was set to five, and analyses were corrected for hypergeometric testing ($p < 0.001$) using false discovery rate (FDR) correction [27].

3. Results

3.1. Phenotyping

All nine family members investigated were left-handed according to EHI results (mean LQ: −84.44, standard deviation: 26.51; range: −100 to −20). The person from whom the control sample was obtained was right-handed (LQ: 100). Analysis of pegboard data showed that seven family members showed superior left hand skill and two family members slightly superior right hand skills (mean PegQ: −0.17, standard deviation: 0.15; range: −0.45 to 0.04). The control person showed superior right hand skills (PegQ: 0.19). For the dichotic listening data, three family members showed a left ear advantage (33.33%) and six showed the typical right ear advantage (66.66%). Dichotic listening data were analyzed non-parametrically due to the small sample size. In absolute number, family members on average reported more syllables presented to the right ear (35.67, standard deviation: 9.72) than to the left ear (29.56, standard deviation: 6.50), but this difference failed to reach significance (Z: −1.31, $p = 0.19$). To determine whether this nonsignificant result was indicating a real absence of an effect or rather was an artefact due to the small sample size, we also analyzed the data with a bootstrapped t-test for dependent comparisons with 5000 iterations. As this comparison also failed to reach significance ($p = 0.26$) it is likely that family members indeed did not show the typical right ear advantage found in the population.

3.2. Sequencing Results

Overall, the analysis detected 299,431 variants on 19,576 genes in family members that were non-identical to the reference genome. As a first step, variants with a call quality less than 20 and all variants in highly variable exonic regions were excluded, narrowing down the number of variants to 235,339 on 19,075 genes. We then excluded all variants that were present in less than at least seven of the nine family members (77.78%), resulting in 9714 variants on 4376 genes. This was done in order to include only variants that were consistently typical for the sample. Furthermore, all variants with a frequency higher than 3% in the 1000Genomes project (http://www.1000genomes.org/) were excluded, as we focused on detecting rare variants. This step resulted in 810 variants on 411 genes left in the analysis. Afterwards, only variants likely to cause loss of function of a gene were included using the "Predicted deleterious" filter, resulting in 116 variants on 69 genes. This was done to only include causal genetic variants that affect protein function. As a last step, quantitative trait analysis was performed to include only variants that showed significant relations with handedness LQ with p-values of at least $p < 0.01$. This analysis revealed 49 variants on 26 genes that were significantly associated with the phenotype (see Table 1). Most of these genes were involved in general cellular processes and only very few were associated with the brain or neuronal processes specifically.

Table 1. Rare gene variants statistically associated with the phenotype. IDs from the Single Nucleotide Polymorphism Database (dbSNP) are given when available. Likely gene functions were determined using PubMed (http://www.ncbi.nlm.nih.gov/gene). (Chr. = chromosome).

Chr.	Gene	dbSNP ID	Likely Function
2	*ANKRD36C*	202102082	Ion channel inhibitor activity
3	*MUC20*	2688539 3828408	Cellular protein metabolism
4	*ZNF595*	-	Regulation of DNA transcription
4	*FRG1*	199978807 201142987	Associated with facioscapulohumeral muscular dystrophy
7	*MUC3A*	71540917 775174499 747768677 759956700 796070497 796719496 796627084 796799995 796422604 796558082 796345426 796976589 62483696	Cellular protein metabolism
10	*FRG2*	200347477	Protein coding in the nucleus
11	*MUC6*	770290437 34490696 200644196 796934918 111641154 112301388 78265558	Cellular protein metabolism/ production of gastric mucin
11	*MUC5AC*	74390930 749291344	Cellular protein metabolism
11	*TRIM49*	74584169	Protein-protein interactions, preferentially expressed in testis
14	*HOMEZ*	148005528	Regulation of DNA transcription
15	*GOLGA6L2*	76062343	Protein binding
16	*CBFA2T3*	71395351 71395352	Transcription corepressor activity

Table 1. *Cont.*

Chr.	Gene	dbSNP ID	Likely Function
17	*CCDC144NL*	73298040	Affects blood copper, selenium and zinc
17	*KCNJ12*	77987694 80335301	Encodes an inwardly rectifying K+ channel in neurons, heart and muscle cells.
17	*RECQL5*	142406301	DNA helicase activity
18	*CNDP1*	10663835	Encodes a member of the M20 metalloprotease family that is specifically expressed in the brain
19	*MUC16*	4992693	Cellular protein metabolism
19	*ZNF443*	62114866	Regulation of DNA transcription
19	*SIGLEC11*	9676436 78673790	Anti-inflammatory and immunosuppressive signaling
21	*BAGE2*	9808647	Melanoma antigen
21	*BAGE5*	113315187	Melanoma antigen
X	*RBMX*	76876438 74463481 74667874 35899675 77794331	RNA binding

Gene ontology (GO) analysis showed that the identified genes were significantly enriched within nine GO groups. The majority of these GO groups were related to protein glycosylation (see Table 2). The remaining GO group was "Golgi lumen".

Table 2. Results of the GO group analysis. *p*-values are Benjamini-Hochberg corrected.

GO Group	Genes	Adjusted *p*-Value
O-glycan processing	5	0.0000002
Protein O-linked glycosylation	5	0.0000005
Post-translational protein modification	5	0.00005
Protein glycosylation	5	0.0001
Macromolecule glycosylation	5	0.0001
Glycosylation	5	0.0001
Glycoprotein biosynthetic process	5	0.0002
Glycoprotein metabolic process	5	0.0005
Golgi lumen	5	0.0000007

4. Discussion

Handedness is a trait that has been related to both cognitive ability [28] and psychopathology [29], making the identification of genetic factors underlying its ontogenesis highly interesting for cognitive neuroscientists and clinical psychologists alike. Here, we performed whole exome sequencing in nine members of an extended Eastern Turkish family with a long history of consanguineous marriage and an overrepresentation of left-handedness. For the first time, we used quantitative trait analysis in such a cohort in order to identify rare genetic variants that were associated with handedness.

The results from the EHI clearly revealed that all nine tested family members were left-handers and, for most family members, these findings were also supported by the results of the pegboard test. Family members showed reduced language lateralization. While in the general population about 95% of individuals show left hemispheric language dominance, in our sample only 66.66% of individuals showed a right-ear advantage during dichotic listening and there was no significant right-ear advantage. This number is however only slightly lower than the 70–80% observed in left-handed samples [30]. Given the small sample size of the present study, we would assume that our data are within the normal range for left-handed populations.

The quantitative trait analysis revealed rare variants on 49 loci on 26 genes that were significantly associated with the EHI LQ. However, the biological significance of these genes for handedness remains unclear. As handedness represents a functional asymmetry between the left and right motor cortices in controlling for fine motor skills [6], one would expect genes involved in shaping this phenotype to be specifically expressed in the brain or spinal cord. Moreover, they should have functional relevance for left-right axis development or nervous system development or function in the broadest sense. Almost all of the genes that were associated with handedness LQ in the present study did not meet these criteria, as they were involved in general cellular or regulatory processes not specific for nervous tissue. Furthermore, some genes clearly were relevant for function in body parts other than the brain, making an involvement in handedness development highly unlikely. Only two out of 26 genes showed a functional relevance for neuronal functioning in the broadest sense. The first of these genes, *KCNJ12* (potassium voltage-gated channel subfamily J member 12), encodes a functional inward rectifier potassium channel [31]. Functionally, most studies have linked it to the heart (e.g., [32]) or muscle [33] function, but also tumerogenesis [34]. While a recent study suggested that protein-protein interactions between a G protein-gated inwardly rectifying potassium channel (Kir3), G proteins and G protein-coupled neurotransmitter receptors might be functionally relevant for GABA-B receptors [35], direct evidence linking *KCNJ12* to a specific function in the central nervous system is sparse. While Stonehouse et al. [36] could show that the inwardly rectifying potassium ion channel encoded by *KCNJ12* in humans can be localized in sections of rat hindbrain and dorsal root ganglia tissue, there is no evidence for a functional link to handedness development so far. The second gene, *CNDP1* (carnosine dipeptidase 1), encodes a member of the M20 metalloprotease family which acts as carnosinase. While it is expressed in the brain, most studies have linked it to susceptibility for diabetic nephropathy in human diabetic patients (e.g., [37]), with no evidence for a direct functional link to handedness. Thus, the analysis of functionally relevant rare variants did not result in any evidence for a major gene or mutation determining handedness in our cohort.

This interpretation was further supported by the result of the GO analysis. Out of nine GO groups that reached significance, seven were linked to glycosylation, an enzymatic process that attaches glycans to other molecules. Glycosylation represents an important post-translational modification of proteins in a vast number of different tissues. While congenital disorders of glycosylation have been shown to affect central nervous function [38], glycosylation has also been related to the development and progression of several different types of cancer and other diseases unrelated to the brain [39]. Interestingly, it has been shown that inbreeding in human populations strongly affects the glycosylation of human plasma proteins, potentially leading to the increased prevalence of tumors that has been reported in certain isolated populations as well as other phenotypic changes [40]. Thus, it is likely that the significant effects for glycosylation-related GO groups were an effect of inbreeding and only by happenstance were associated with the handedness phenotype. The other three significant GO groups also were unlikely to affect handedness, as they either represented processes unrelated to the brain or were too general ("Golgi lumen" "post-translational protein modification") to specifically be involved in the formation of the functional motor cortex asymmetry underlying handedness.

The present study contains several methodological aspects that have the potential to be optimized in future studies. Clearly, testing a larger group of family members with a consanguineous background would be ideal. Unfortunately, we were only able to recruit left-handed family members in the present study, but for future studies including both left-and right-handers from the same family would by optimal. Also, for quantitative trait analyses, larger cohorts would be favorable, if recruitment is possible. This would be particularly important as the GATK protocol used for variant calling in the present study gives optimal results with sample sizes of 30 or larger. Moreover, in our cohort there was the possibility that some of the individuals (e.g., P69, see Figure 1) married in with potentially their own forms of left-handedness, and do not necessarily share a genetic basis with the other members of the family. This could have confounded the analysis and should be controlled for when recruiting cohorts for future studies. Moreover, the test used to determine quantitative trait association did not account for different degrees of relatedness, but for a weakly heritable trait this is unlikely to bias the results. As rare variants might be highly cohort-specific, more studies in cohorts with diverse ethnic backgrounds are needed to completely exclude a possible influence of major rare variants on handedness. Another possible criticism of our data could be that it is unclear to what extent an overrepresentation of left-handedness is a specific characteristic of the sample that was investigated in our study or the general population it comes from. While there is no specific published data on handedness in the vicinity of Şanlı Urfa, studies in Turkish samples indicate that the frequency of left-handedness in Turkey is between 6% and 11% [41–43], which is in line with what has been found in other populations worldwide (around 10%). Tan reports the incidence of familial left-handedness in Turkey to be around 28.4% [43], which is lower than the 39.3% that has been reported in a large American sample [44]. Thus, the over-representation of left-handedness observed in our sample is typical for this family, not the general population in Turkey.

5. Conclusions

Taken together, both the analysis of single rare variants and the analysis of GO groups revealed no indication for a rare variant that could realistically determine handedness. Thus, our analysis in a Turkish cohort with lower genetic heterogeneity than the general population independently replicates previous findings from similar studies in Dutch [16] and Pakistani [17] cohorts. Thus, our study supports the conclusions of these studies that handedness is likely to be determined by complex polygenic and/or epigenetic factors [45].

Acknowledgments: This work was supported by the Deutsche Forschungsgemeinschaft through Gu 227/16-1 to O.G. The authors also acknowledge support by the DFG Open Access Publication Funds of the Ruhr-Universität Bochum. We would like to thank Ahmet Çini, Macide Barutçuoğlu and Monika Güntürkün for their help with data collection.

Author Contributions: Onur Güntürkün and Sebastian Ocklenburg conceived and designed the experiments; Ceren Barutçuoğlu and Onur Güntürkün performed the experiments; Ceren Barutçuoğlu, Judith Schmitz and Sebastian Ocklenburg analyzed the data; Adile Öniz Özgören, Murat Özgören, Esra Erdal, Robert Kumsta and Dirk Moser contributed reagents/materials/analysis tools; Sebastian Ocklenburg wrote the paper.

References

1. Lien, Y.J.; Chen, W.J.; Hsiao, P.C.; Tsuang, H.C. Estimation of heritability for varied indexes of handedness. *Laterality* **2015**, *20*, 469–482. [CrossRef] [PubMed]
2. Annett, M. Tests of the right shift genetic model for two new samples of family handedness and for the data of McKeever (2000). *Laterality* **2008**, *13*, 105–123. [CrossRef] [PubMed]
3. Armour, J.A.; Davison, A.; McManus, I.C. Genome-wide association study of handedness excludes simple genetic models. *Heredity* **2014**, *112*, 221–225. [CrossRef] [PubMed]
4. Eriksson, N.; Macpherson, J.M.; Tung, J.Y.; Hon, L.S.; Naughton, B.; Saxonov, S.; Avey, L.; Wojcicki, A.; Pe'er, I.; Mountain, J. Web-based, participant-driven studies yield novel genetic associations for common traits. *PLoS Genet.* **2010**, *6*, e1000993. [CrossRef] [PubMed]
5. McManus, I.C.; Davison, A.; Armour, J.A. Multilocus genetic models of handedness closely resemble single-locus models in explaining family data and are compatible with genome-wide association studies. *Ann. NY Acad. Sci.* **2013**, *1288*, 48–58. [CrossRef] [PubMed]

6. Ocklenburg, S.; Beste, C.; Güntürkün, O. Handedness: A neurogenetic shift of perspective. *Neurosci. Biobehav. Rev.* **2013**, *37*, 2788–2793. [CrossRef] [PubMed]
7. Ocklenburg, S.; Beste, C.; Arning, L.; Peterburs, J.; Güntürkün, O. The ontogenesis of language lateralization and its relation to handedness. *Neurosci. Biobehav. Rev.* **2014**, *43*, 191–198. [CrossRef] [PubMed]
8. Rentería, M.E. Cerebral asymmetry: A quantitative, multifactorial, and plastic brain phenotype. *Twin Res. Hum. Genet.* **2012**, *15*, 401–413. [CrossRef] [PubMed]
9. Arning, L.; Ocklenburg, S.; Schulz, S.; Ness, V.; Gerding, W.M.; Hengstler, J.G.; Falkenstein, M.; Epplen, J.T.; Güntürkün, O.; Beste, C. PCSK6 VNTR Polymorphism Is Associated with Degree of Handedness but Not Direction of Handedness. *PLoS ONE* **2013**, *8*, e67251. [CrossRef] [PubMed]
10. Arning, L.; Ocklenburg, S.; Schulz, S.; Ness, V.; Gerding, W.M.; Hengstler, J.G.; Falkenstein, M.; Epplen, J.T.; Güntürkün, O.; Beste, C. Handedness and the X chromosome: The role of androgen receptor CAG-repeat length. *Sci. Rep.* **2015**, *5*. [CrossRef] [PubMed]
11. Brandler, W.M.; Morris, A.P.; Evans, D.M.; Scerri, T.S.; Kemp, J.P.; Timpson, N.J.; St. Pourcain, B.; Smith, G.D.; Ring, S.M.; Stein, J.; et al. Common variants in left/right asymmetry genes and pathways are associated with relative hand skill. *PLoS Genet.* **2013**, *9*, e1003751. [CrossRef] [PubMed]
12. Francks, C.; Maegawa, S.; Laurén, J.; Abrahams, B.S.; Velayos-Baeza, A.; Medland, S.E.; Colella, S.; Groszer, M.; McAuley, E.Z.; Caffrey, T.M.; et al. LRRTM1 on chromosome 2p12 is a maternally suppressed gene that is associated paternally with handedness and schizophrenia. *Mol. Psychiatr.* **2007**, *12*, 1129–1139. [CrossRef] [PubMed]
13. Leach, E.L.; Prefontaine, G.; Hurd, P.L.; Crespi, B.J. The imprinted gene LRRTM1 mediates schizotypy and handedness in a nonclinical population. *J. Hum. Genet.* **2014**, *59*, 332–336. [CrossRef] [PubMed]
14. Robinson, K.J.; Hurd, P.L.; Read, S.; Crespi, B.J. The PCSK6 gene is associated with handedness, the autism spectrum, and magical ideation in a non-clinical population. *Neuropsychologia* **2016**, *84*, 205–212. [CrossRef] [PubMed]
15. Scerri, T.S.; Brandler, W.M.; Paracchini, S.; Morris, A.P.; Ring, S.M.; Richardson, A.J.; Talcott, J.B.; Stein, J.; Monaco, A.P. PCSK6 is associated with handedness in individuals with dyslexia. *Hum. Mol. Genet.* **2011**, *20*, 608–614. [CrossRef] [PubMed]
16. Somers, M.; Ophoff, R.A.; Aukes, M.F.; Cantor, R.M.; Boks, M.P.; Dauwan, M.; de Visser, K.L.; Kahn, R.S.; Sommer, I.E. Linkage analysis in a Dutch population isolate shows no major gene for left-handedness or atypical language lateralization. *J. Neurosci.* **2015**, *35*, 8730–8736. [CrossRef] [PubMed]
17. Kavaklioglu, T.; Ajmal, M.; Hameed, A.; Francks, C. Whole exome sequencing for handedness in a large and highly consanguineous family. *Neuropsychologia* **2015**, *93*, 342–349. [CrossRef] [PubMed]
18. Oldfield, R.C. The assessment and analysis of handedness: The Edinburgh inventory. *Neuropsychologia* **1971**, *9*, 97–113. [CrossRef]
19. McManus, I.C. Right- and left- hand skill: Failure of the right shift model. *Br. J. Psychol.* **1985**, *76*, 1–34. [CrossRef] [PubMed]
20. Bryden, M.P.; Tapley, S.M. A group test for the assessment of performance between the hands. *Neuropsychologia* **1985**, *23*, 215–221.
21. Annett, M. *Left, Right, Hand and Brain: The Right Shift Theory*; Lawrence Erlbaum Associates: Mahwah, NJ, USA, 1985.
22. Annett, M. *Handedness and Brain Asymmetry: The Right Shift Theory*; Psychology Press: Abingdon, UK, 2002.
23. Hugdahl, K.; Eichele, T.; Rimol, L.M. The effect of voice-onset-time on dichotic listening with consonant–vowel syllables. *Neuropsychologia* **2006**, *44*, 191–196.
24. Li, H.; Durbin, R. Fast and accurate short read alignment with Burrows-Wheeler transform. *Bioinformatics* **2009**, *25*, 1754–1760. [CrossRef] [PubMed]
25. DePristo, M.A.; Banks, E.; Poplin, R.; Garimella, K.V.; Maguire, J.R.; Hartl, C.; Philippakis, A.A.; del Angel, G.; Rivas, M.A.; Hanna, M.; et al. A framework for variation discovery and genotyping using next-generation DNA sequencing data. *Nat. Genet.* **2011**, *43*, 491–498. [CrossRef] [PubMed]
26. Cingolani, P.; Platts, A.; Wang, L.L.; Coon, M.; Nguyen, T.; Wang, L.; Land, S.J.; Lu, X.; Ruden, D.M. A program for annotating and predicting the effects of single nucleotide polymorphisms, SnpEff: SNPs in the genome of Drosophila melanogaster strain w1118; iso-2; iso-3. *Fly* **2012**, *6*, 80–92. [CrossRef] [PubMed]
27. Benjamini, Y.; Hochberg, Y. Controlling the False Discovery Rate: A Practical and Powerful Approach to Multiple Testing. *J. R. Stat. Soc. B* **1995**, *57*, 289–300.

28. Somers, M.; Shields, L.S.; Boks, M.P.; Kahn, R.S.; Sommer, I.E. Cognitive benefits of right-handedness: A meta-analysis. *Neurosci. Biobehav. Rev.* **2015**, *51*, 48–63. [CrossRef] [PubMed]
29. Hirnstein, M.; Hugdahl, K. Excess of non-right-handedness in schizophrenia: Meta-analysis of gender effects and potential biases in handedness assessment. *Br. J. Psychiatr.* **2014**, *205*, 260–267. [CrossRef] [PubMed]
30. Foundas, A.L.; Corey, D.M.; Hurley, M.M.; Heilman, K.M. Verbal dichotic listening in right and left-handed adults: laterality effects of directed attention. *Cortex* **2006**, *42*, 79–86. [CrossRef]
31. Kaibara, M.; Ishihara, K.; Doi, Y.; Hayashi, H.; Ehara, T.; Taniyama, K. Identification of human Kir2.2 (KCNJ12) gene encoding functional inward rectifier potassium channel in both mammalian cells and Xenopus oocytes. *FEBS Lett.* **2002**, *531*, 250–254. [CrossRef]
32. Kiesecker, C.; Zitron, E.; Scherer, D.; Lueck, S.; Bloehs, R.; Scholz, E.P.; Pirot, M.; Kathöfer, S.; Thomas, D.; Kreye, V.A.; et al. Regulation of cardiac inwardly rectifying potassium current IK1 and Kir2.x channels by endothelin-1. *J. Mol. Med.* **2006**, *84*, 46–56. [CrossRef] [PubMed]
33. Karkanis, T.; Li, S.; Pickering, J.G.; Sims, S.M. Plasticity of KIR channels in human smooth muscle cells from internal thoracic artery. *Am. J. Physiol. Heart. Circ. Physiol.* **2003**, *284*, H2325–H2334. [CrossRef] [PubMed]
34. Lee, I.; Park, C.; Kang, W.K. Knockdown of inwardly rectifying potassium channel Kir2.2 suppresses tumorigenesis by inducing reactive oxygen species-mediated cellular senescence. *Mol. Cancer Ther.* **2010**, *9*, 2951–2959. [CrossRef] [PubMed]
35. Fowler, C.E.; Aryal, P.; Suen, K.F.; Slesinger, P.A. Evidence for association of GABA(B) receptors with Kir3 channels and regulators of G protein signalling (RGS4) proteins. *J. Physiol.* **2007**, *580*, 51–65. [CrossRef] [PubMed]
36. Stonehouse, A.H.; Grubb, B.D.; Pringle, J.H.; Norman, R.I.; Stanfield, P.R.; Brammar, W.J. Nuclear immunostaining in rat neuronal cells using two anti-Kir2.2 ion channel polyclonal antibodies. *J. Mol. Neurosci.* **2003**, *20*, 189–194. [CrossRef]
37. Sauerhöfer, S.; Yuan, G.; Braun, G.S.; Deinzer, M.; Neumaier, M.; Gretz, N.; Floege, J.; Kriz, W.; van der Woude, F.; Moeller, M.J. L-carnosine, a substrate of carnosinase-1, influences glucose metabolism. *Diabetes* **2007**, *56*, 2425–2432. [CrossRef] [PubMed]
38. Barone, R.; Fiumara, A.; Jaeken, J. Congenital disorders of glycosylation with emphasis on cerebellar involvement. *Semin. Neurol.* **2014**, *34*, 357–366. [CrossRef] [PubMed]
39. Drake, R.R. Glycosylation and cancer: moving glycomics to the forefront. *Adv. Cancer Res.* **2015**, *126*, 1–10. [PubMed]
40. Polašek, O.; Leutenegger, A.L.; Gornik, O.; Zgaga, L.; Kolcic, I.; McQuillan, R.; Wilson, J.F.; Hayward, C.; Wright, A.F.; Lauc, G.; et al. Does inbreeding affect N-glycosylation of human plasma proteins? *Mol. Genet. Genom.* **2011**, *285*, 427–432.
41. Ertas, U.; Canakçi, E. Prevalence and handedness correlates of recurrent aphthous stomatitis in the Turkish population. *J. Publ. Health Dent.* **2004**, *64*, 151–156.
42. Canakci, V.; Akgül, H.M.; Akgül, N.; Canakci, C.F. Prevalence and handedness correlates of traumatic injuries to the permanent incisors in 13–17-year-old adolescents in Erzurum, Turkey. *Dent. Traumatol.* **2003**, *19*, 248–254. [CrossRef] [PubMed]
43. Tan, U. The distribution of the Geschwind scores to familial left-handedness. *Int. J. Neurosci.* **1988**, *42*, 85–105. [CrossRef] [PubMed]
44. Spiegler, B.J.; Yeni-Komshian, G.H. Incidence of left-handed writing in a college population with reference to family patterns of hand preference. *Neuropsychologia* **1983**, *21*, 651–659. [CrossRef]
45. Ocklenburg, S.; Schmitz, J.; Moinfar, Z.; Moser, D.; Klose, R.; Lor, S.; Kunz, G.; Tegenthoff, M.; Faustmann, P.; Francks, C.; et al. Epigenetic regulation of lateralized fetal spinal gene expression underlies hemispheric asymmetries. *eLife* **2017**, *1*, e22784. [CrossRef] [PubMed]

Permissions

All chapters in this book were first published by MDPI; hereby published with permission under the Creative Commons Attribution License or equivalent. Every chapter published in this book has been scrutinized by our experts. Their significance has been extensively debated. The topics covered herein carry significant findings which will fuel the growth of the discipline. They may even be implemented as practical applications or may be referred to as a beginning point for another development.

The contributors of this book come from diverse backgrounds, making this book a truly international effort. This book will bring forth new frontiers with its revolutionizing research information and detailed analysis of the nascent developments around the world.

We would like to thank all the contributing authors for lending their expertise to make the book truly unique. They have played a crucial role in the development of this book. Without their invaluable contributions this book wouldn't have been possible. They have made vital efforts to compile up to date information on the varied aspects of this subject to make this book a valuable addition to the collection of many professionals and students.

This book was conceptualized with the vision of imparting up-to-date information and advanced data in this field. To ensure the same, a matchless editorial board was set up. Every individual on the board went through rigorous rounds of assessment to prove their worth. After which they invested a large part of their time researching and compiling the most relevant data for our readers.

The editorial board has been involved in producing this book since its inception. They have spent rigorous hours researching and exploring the diverse topics which have resulted in the successful publishing of this book. They have passed on their knowledge of decades through this book. To expedite this challenging task, the publisher supported the team at every step. A small team of assistant editors was also appointed to further simplify the editing procedure and attain best results for the readers.

Apart from the editorial board, the designing team has also invested a significant amount of their time in understanding the subject and creating the most relevant covers. They scrutinized every image to scout for the most suitable representation of the subject and create an appropriate cover for the book.

The publishing team has been an ardent support to the editorial, designing and production team. Their endless efforts to recruit the best for this project, has resulted in the accomplishment of this book. They are a veteran in the field of academics and their pool of knowledge is as vast as their experience in printing. Their expertise and guidance has proved useful at every step. Their uncompromising quality standards have made this book an exceptional effort. Their encouragement from time to time has been an inspiration for everyone.

The publisher and the editorial board hope that this book will prove to be a valuable piece of knowledge for researchers, students, practitioners and scholars across the globe.

List of Contributors

Arianna Felisatti and Martin H. Fischer
Department of Psychology, University of Potsdam, Karl-Liebknecht-Strasse 24-25 House 14, D-14476 Potsdam OT Golm, Germany

David Aagten-Murphy
Department of Psychology, University of Potsdam, Karl-Liebknecht-Strasse 24-25 House 14, D-14476 Potsdam OT Golm, Germany
Neuraltrain GmbH, Friedrichstr. 68, 10117 Berlin, Germany

Jochen Laubrock
Department of Psychology, University of Potsdam, Karl-Liebknecht-Strasse 24-25 House 14, D-14476 Potsdam OT Golm, Germany
Department of Psychology, Brandenburg Medical School Theodor Fontane Fehrbelliner Straße 38, 16816 Neuruppin, Germany

Samuel Shaki
Department of Behavioral Sciences and Psychology, Ariel University, Ariel 40700, Israel

Almira Kustubayeva and Altyngul Kamzanova
Center for Cognitive Neuroscience, Department of Biophysics, Biomedicine, and Neuroscience, Al-Farabi Kazakh National University, Almaty 050040, Kazakhstan
Center for Cognitive Neuroscience, Department of Psychology, Al-Farabi Kazakh National University, Almaty 050040, Kazakhstan

Sandugash Kudaibergenova and Veronika Pivkina
Center for Cognitive Neuroscience, Department of Psychology, Al-Farabi Kazakh National University, Almaty 050040, Kazakhstan

Gerald Matthews
Institute for Simulation and Training, University of Central Florida, Orlando, FL 32826, USA

Kazuhiko Sawada and Shiori Kamiya
Department of Nutrition, Faculty of Medical and Health Sciences, Tsukuba International University, Tsuchiura, Ibaraki 300-0051, Japan

Ichio Aoki
Department of Molecular Imaging and Theranostics, National Institute of Radiological Sciences, National Institutes for Quantum and Radiological Science and Technology (QST), Chiba 263-8555, Japan
Institute for Quantum Life Science (iQLS), QST, Chiba 263-8555, Japan

Beatrice Bonati
Department of Chemistry, Life Sciences and Environmental Sustainability, University of Parma, Parco Area delle Scienze 11/A, 43124 Parma, Italy

Caterina Quaresmini
Department of Psychology and Cognitive Sciences, University of Trento, 38068 Rovereto (Trento), Italy

Gionata Stancher
Rovereto Civic Museum Foundation, 38068 Rovereto (Trento), Italy
Center for Mind/Brain Sciences, University of Trento, 38068 Rovereto (Trento), Italy

Valeria Anna Sovrano
Department of Psychology and Cognitive Sciences, University of Trento, 38068 Rovereto (Trento), Italy
Center for Mind/Brain Sciences, University of Trento, 38068 Rovereto (Trento), Italy

Giulia Prete and Luca Tommasi
Department of Psychology, Health and Territory, G. d'Annunzio University of Chieti-Pescara, Chieti 66013, Italy

Mara Fabri
Department of Clinical and Experimental Medicine, Neuroscience and Cell Biology Section, Polytechnic University of Marche, Ancona 60121, Italy

Nicoletta Foschi
Regional Epilepsy Centre, Neurological Clinic, Ospedali Riuniti, Ancona 60126, Italy

Dennis Gehring, Wolfgang Wiltschko and Roswitha Wiltschko
FB Biowissenschaften, Goethe-Universität Frankfurt am Main, Max-von-Laue-Str. 13, D-60438 Frankfurt am Main, Germany

Onur Güntürkün
Abteilung Biopsychologie, Fakultät für Psychologie, Ruhr-Universität Bochum, D-44780 Bochum, Germany
Stellenbosch Institute for Advanced Study (STIAS), Wallenberg Research Centre at Stellenbosch University, Stellenbosch 7600, South Africa
Institute of Cognitive Neuroscience, Biopsychology, Ruhr-University, 44780 Bochum, Germany
Institute of Cognitive Neuroscience, Biopsychology, Department of Psychology, Ruhr-University Bochum, 44801 Bochum, Germany

Gisela Kaplan
School of Science and Technology, University of New England, Armidale, NSW 2351, Australia

Cinzia Chiandetti
Department of Life Sciences, University of Trieste, I-34127 Trieste, Italy

Bastien S. Lemaire
Institute of applied biology (IBFA), University of Caen, 14000 Caen, France
Center for Mind/Brain Sciences, University of Trento, I-38068 Rovereto, Italy

Elisabetta Versace
Center for Mind/Brain Sciences, University of Trento, I-38068 Rovereto, Italy

Giorgio Vallortigara
Center for Mind/Brain Sciences, University of Trento, Piazza della Manifattura 1, I-38068 Rovereto, Italy
Center for Mind/Brain Sciences, University of Trento, I-38068 Rovereto, Italy

Maria Elena Miletto Petrazzini
Department of Biomedical Sciences, University of Padova, Via Bassi 58-b, 35131 Padova, Italy

Alessandra Pecunioso and Marco Dadda
Department of General Psychology, University of Padova, Via Venezia 8, 35131 Padova, Italy

Christian Agrillo
Department of General Psychology, University of Padova, Via Venezia 8, 35131 Padova, Italy
Padua Neuroscience Center, University of Padova, Via 8 Febbraio 2, 35122 Padova, Italy

Natalie Uomini
Department of Linguistic and Cultural Evolution, Max Planck Institute for the Science of Human History, Kahlaische Strasse 10, 07745 Jena, Germany

Rebecca Lawson
School of Psychology, University of Liverpool, Eleanor Rathbone Building, Bedford Street South, Liverpool L69 7ZA, UK

Elisa Frasnelli
Center for Mind/Brain Sciences, University of Trento, Piazza della Manifattura 1, I-38068 Rovereto, Italy

Janet Mertzen
Institute of Cognitive Neuroscience, Biopsychology, Department of Psychology, Ruhr-University Bochum, 44801 Bochum, Germany

Sebastian Ocklenburg
Institute of Cognitive Neuroscience, Biopsychology, Department of Psychology, Ruhr-University Bochum, 44801 Bochum, Germany
Institute of Cognitive Neuroscience, Biopsychology, Ruhr-University, 44780 Bochum, Germany

Jutta Peterburs
Institute of Medical Psychology and Systems Neuroscience, University of Münster, 48149 Münster, Germany

Gina M. Grimshaw
Cognitive and Affective Neuroscience Lab, School of Psychology, Victoria University of Wellington, 6140Wellington, New Zealand

Lesley J. Rogers
School of Science and Technology, University of New England, Armidale, NSW 2351, Australia

Marcello Siniscalchi, Serenella d'Ingeo and Angelo Quaranta
Department of Veterinary Medicine, Section of Behavioral Sciences and Animal Bioethics, University of Bari "Aldo Moro", 70121 Bari, Italy

Ceren Barutçuoğlu
Institute of Cognitive Neuroscience, Biopsychology, Ruhr-University, 44780 Bochum, Germany

Judith Schmitz
Institute of Cognitive Neuroscience, Biopsychology, Ruhr-University, 44780 Bochum, Germany
Institute of Cognitive Neuroscience, Biopsychology, Department of Psychology, Ruhr-University Bochum, 44801 Bochum, Germany

Adile Öniz Özgören and Murat Özgören
Department of Biophysics, Faculty of Medicine, Dokuz Eylül University, 35340 Izmir, Turkey

Esra Erdal
Department of Medical Biology, Faculty of Medicine, Dokuz Eylül University, 35340 Izmir, Turkey

Dirk Moser and Robert Kumsta
Genetic Psychology, Faculty of Psychology, Ruhr-University, 44780 Bochum, Germany

Mark A. Eckert, Kenneth I. Vaden Jr. and Brittany T. Glaze
Hearing Research Program, Department of Otolaryngology-Head and Neck Surgery, Medical University of South Carolina, Charleston, SC 29425, USA

Federico Iuricich
Visual Computing Division, School of Computing, Clemson University, Clemson, SC 29634, USA

Index